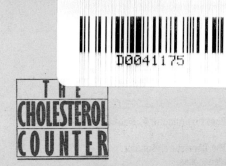

# THE CHOLESTEROL COUNTER

ANNETTE B. NATOW, Ph.D., R.D., and JO-ANN HESLIN, M.A., R.D., are the authors of seven books on nutrition, including *The Pocket Encyclopedia of Nutrition, No-Nonsense Nutrition for Kids* and *Megadoses: Vitamins as Drugs* (all available from Pocket Books). They are faculty members of Adelphi University and previously taught at Downstate Medical Center and New York University. They have held editorial positions at the *Journal of Nutrition for the Elderly, American Baby* and *Prevention* magazines, and are regular contributors to health magazines and journals.

---

LOOK FOR
ANNETTE B. NATOW
AND JO-ANN HESLIN'S

*The Fat Counter*
and
*The Calcium Counter*

COMING SOON
FROM
POCKET BOOKS

**Books by Annette B. Natow and Jo-Ann Heslin**

The Cholesterol Counter
Megadoses
No-Nonsense Nutrition for Kids
The Pocket Encyclopedia of Nutrition

Published by POCKET BOOKS

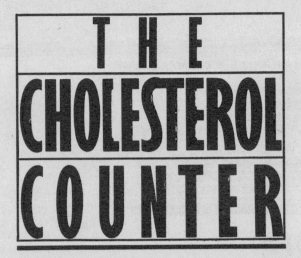

# THE CHOLESTEROL COUNTER

## Expanded and Updated

Annette Natow, Ph.D., R.D.,
and Jo-Ann Heslin, M.A., R.D.

**POCKET BOOKS**

New York   London   Toronto   Sydney   Tokyo

An *Original* Publication of POCKET BOOKS

POCKET BOOKS, a division of Simon & Schuster Inc.
1230 Avenue of the Americas, New York, NY 10020

ISBN: 0-671-67890-6

First Pocket Books revised printing March 1989

10  9  8  7  6  5  4  3  2  1

POCKET and colophon are trademarks of
Simon & Schuster Inc.

Printed in the U.S.A.

To our families, who support us through every project:
Harry, Allen, Irene, Sarah, Laura, Marty, George, Emily,
Steven, Joseph, Kristen and Karen

# ACKNOWLEDGMENTS

Without the tireless cooperation of Steven and Laura, *Cholesterol Counter* would never have been completed. A special thanks to Abe and Lillie Lefkowitz, who were there when we really needed them.

Our thanks also go to all the food manufacturers who graciously shared their data.

# AUTHORS' NOTE

Sources of Data

Values in this counter have been obtained from the Composition of Foods, United States Department of Agriculture: Dairy and Egg Products, Agricultural Handbook No. 8-1; Spices and Herbs, Agricultural Handbook No. 8-2; Fats and Oils, Agricultural Handbook No. 8-4; Poultry, Agricultural Handbook No. 8-5; Soups, Sauces and Gravies, Agricultural Handbook No. 8-6; Sausages and Luncheon Meats, Agricultural Handbook No. 8-7; Fruit and Fruit Juices, Agricultural Handbook No. 8-9; Pork Products, Agricultural Handbook No. 8-10; Vegetables and Vegetable Products, Agricultural Handbook No. 8-11; Nut and Seed Products, Agricultural Handbook No. 8-12; Beef Products, Agricultural Handbook No. 8-13; Beverages, Agricultural Handbook No. 8-14; Finfish and Shellfish Products, Agricultural Handbook No. 8-15; Legumes and Legume Products, Agricultural Handbook No. 8-16.

Nutritive values of foods, United States Department of Agriculture, Home and Garden Bulletin No. 72.

Bowes & Church's Food Values of Portions Commonly Used (Philadelphia, PA: J.B. Lippincott Co., 1985).

Nutrients in Foods (Cambridge, MA: Nutrition Guild, 1983).

Information from food labels, manufacturers and processors. The values are based on research conducted prior to October 1988. Manufacturer's ingredients are subject to change, so current values may vary from those listed in the book.

"If only half a dozen foods were available the matter would be quickly settled."

MARY SWARTZ ROSE, PH.D.
*Feeding the Family*
The MacMillan Company
1919

# CONTENTS

## PART I
## Brand Name and Generic Foods

## xxvi    CONTENTS

## PART II
## Restaurant, Take-Out and Fast-Food Chains

## APPENDIX
# Baby Foods

# WHAT IS CHOLESTEROL?

High Cholesterol is a major risk factor for heart disease.
High Cholesterol is a major risk factor for stroke.
High Cholesterol increases your risk of colon and rectal cancer.
High Cholesterol plus high blood pressure may cause hearing loss.
High Cholesterol, fat-rich diets may cause gallstones.

Did you know that every year more than half a million Americans die from coronary heart disease—heart attack and stroke? That's more than the number of people who die from all forms of cancer! Heart attack and stroke disable even more people than they kill. Coronary heart disease is a disease not only of the old. One out of five men has a heart attack before he is fifty. Often, the heart attack or stroke that causes death or disability is the first sign you get that something is wrong.

Research shows that high cholesterol levels are one of the most important risk factors for heart disease. Lowering your cholesterol lowers your risk.

### What is cholesterol?

Cholesterol is a white, waxy, fatlike substance that is part of every cell in your body. Cholesterol is important to body function. Hormones, nerve coverings, vitamin D, bile (used for digestion), and the fat that keeps your skin soft (sebum) are all made from cholesterol. Cholesterol makes up a major part of your brain. Cholesterol is needed by the body, but when the blood level of cholesterol in your blood gets too high, it's not healthy. Some of that extra cholesterol can be deposited on the artery wall, narrowing it and interfering with normal blood flow.

### Where does cholesterol come from?

We get some cholesterol every time we eat any animal foods. Meat, poultry, fish, eggs, milk, yogurt, cheese and butter are all animal foods and contain cholesterol. Egg yolk is a major source of cholesterol. An average yolk contains about 270 milligrams. The egg white does not have any cholesterol. Caviar and organ meats like liver, heart and brains are very high in cholesterol.

There is no cholesterol in any food that grows in the ground. Vegetable oils, peanut butter, vegetables, fruits, cereals and grains contain no cholesterol.

Cholesterol is also made in the body. In fact most people make three times as much cholesterol as they get in the food they eat.

### How do I know if my blood cholesterol is too high?

It is estimated that only ten percent of all American adults know their cholesterol level. The National Cholesterol Education Program recommends that all adults over age twenty find out their total cholesterol level. A blood test can tell you. Below are average blood cholesterol levels of Americans, but they are not the most healthy levels.

## AVERAGE BLOOD CHOLESTEROL LEVELS*

| AGE | MALES | FEMALES |
|-----|-------|---------|
| 20–29 | 175 | 165 |
| 30–39 | 195 | 180 |
| 40–49 | 210 | 200 |
| 50–59 | 215 | 225 |
| 60–69 | 215 | 230 |
| 70 + | 205 | 230 |

*Adapted from "American Heart Association Special Report: Recommendation for the Treatment of Hyperlipidemia: A Joint Statement of the Nutrition Committee and the Council on Arteriosclerosis of the American Heart Association," *Circulation*, 69(1984):433a.

For adults, a cholesterol level over 200 milligrams is considered too high. If your cholesterol is above 200 milligrams your risk for heart disease and other problems is increased.

## CHOLESTEROL VALUES THAT PLACE YOU AT RISK*

| AGE | MODERATE RISK | HIGH RISK |
|-----|---------------|-----------|
| 20–29 | 200–220 | Over 220 |
| 30–39 | 220–240 | Over 240 |
| 40 | 240–260 | Over 260 |

**Lowering Blood Cholesterol to Prevent Heart Disease: Consensus Conference," *Journal of the American Medical Association*, 253(1985):2080.

### *If my cholesterol is higher than 200, what should I do?*

In late 1987 the federal government, along with over twenty health organizations, issued guidelines to help identify and treat people whose blood cholesterol levels were too high. This will affect one in four Americans.

People with desirable cholesterol levels of under 200 milligrams were advised only to recheck the level every five years.

People with levels above 200 milligrams were advised to go on a cholesterol-lowering diet that is low in cholesterol, fats and saturated fats.

Many foods are high in all three—cholesterol, fats and saturated fats. By lowering your intake of high cholesterol foods, you reduce your intake of other fats as well and lower your risk for heart disease.

For each one percent decrease in blood cholesterol level, you reduce your risk of heart disease by two percent. Even the smallest change is to your benefit.

In the government guidelines for lowering cholesterol, the Step I diet for those whose cholesterol levels are 200 to 239 milligrams recommends eating less than 300 milligrams of cholesterol a day. Those people whose cholesterol levels are 240 milligrams and over are advised to restrict their cholesterol intake to less than 200 milligrams per day.

## GUIDELINES FOR CHOLESTEROL INTAKE*

| CHOLESTEROL LEVEL IN THE BLOOD | MG OF CHOLESTEROL YOU CAN EAT EACH DAY |
| --- | --- |
| 200–239 mg | less than 300 mg a day |
| 240 mg and over | less than 200 mg a day |

*Adapted from material provided by National Cholesterol Education Program, National Heart, Lung and Blood Institute, National Institutes of Health, 1987

### What about taking drugs to lower my cholesterol?

Some people who have a high cholesterol level may not be able to lower it enough by diet changes alone. They may need to use a drug in addition to making changes in the way they eat. Drugs used most often are cholestyramine, colestipol and niacin.

Cholestyramine (Questran) and colestipol (Colestid) are resins that increase the excretion of cholesterol from the body. Major side effects are constipation, bloating and gas. They are unpleasant to take.

Niacin (nicotinic acid, a B vitamin) causes intense flushing and itching of the skin right after you take it. Major side effects are rashes and upset stomach. It can worsen diabetes and gout.

Lovastatin (Mevacor), a new drug approved by the FDA in late 1987, is recommended to be used with caution because there has not yet been time to evaluate its long-term effects. It is recommended for use when other drugs do not work.

Probucol (Lorelco) and Gemfibrozil (Lopid) are reserved for use when diet and other medications are not effective.

# COUNT UP
# YOUR CHOLESTEROL

Most of us eat too much cholesterol each day.

We eat on the run and pick foods high in fat. By the end of the day we've eaten too much cholesterol.

You know that you shouldn't be eating a lot of cholesterol. You want to cut back. But it's not easy since you are not really sure which foods are high in cholesterol and which foods are not. With the *Cholesterol Counter* it's simple to find out which foods have cholesterol and to reduce the amount you are eating.

Let's look at a typical day. Are the food choices familiar? Let's see just how much cholesterol this sample day contains and how we can reduce the amount with better food choices.

## CHOLESTEROL COUNTING:
## A SAMPLE DAY OF POOR FOOD CHOICES

|  | CHOLESTEROL (MG) |
|---|---|
| **Breakfast** | |
| Orange juice (½ cup) | 0 |
| Scrambled eggs | 427 |
| Bacon (2 slices) | 10 |
| Toast (1 slice) | 0 |
| Butter (1 tsp) | 10 |
| Coffee & Cream (1 Tbsp) | 6 |
| **Lunch** | |
| Cheeseburger | |
|   Hamburger (3 oz) | 80 |
|   American cheese (1 slice) | 25 |
|   Roll | 0 |
|   Catsup | 0 |
| French fries | 0 |
| Vanilla shake | 29 |
| **Snack** | |
| Pound cake (1 slice) | 46 |
| Coffee & | 0 |
|   Cream (1 Tbsp) | 6 |
| **Dinner** | |
| Batter-dipped fried chicken (½ breast) | 119 |
| Baked potato & | 0 |
|   Sour cream (2 Tbsp) | 14 |
| Tossed salad & | 0 |
|   Thousand Island dressing (¼ cup) | 20 |
| Apple pie (1 slice) | 10 |
| Tea & | 0 |
|   Sugar | 0 |
| **TV Snack** | |
| Rich vanilla ice cream (1 cup) | 88 |
| **Total Cholesterol:** | **890** |

This is too much cholesterol for one day—almost 3 times the recommended level of 300 milligrams a day. Now you can see how easy it is to take in more cholesterol than you need.

## CHOLESTEROL COUNTING:
## A SAMPLE DAY OF WISE FOOD CHOICES

| | CHOLESTEROL (MG) |
|---|---|
| **Breakfast** | |
| Orange juice (4 oz) | 0 |
| Cheerios & | |
| Lowfat milk (½ cup) | 5 |
| Toast (1 slice) & | 0 |
| Jelly | 0 |
| Coffee & | 0 |
| Lowfat milk (2 Tbsp) | 1 |
| **Lunch** | |
| Hamburger (3 oz) | 80 |
| Roll | 0 |
| Catsup | 0 |
| French fries | 0 |
| Cola | 0 |
| **Snack** | |
| Pear | 0 |
| **Dinner** | |
| Roasted chicken breast, no skin (½ breast) | 73 |
| Baked potato & | 0 |
| Plain yogurt (2 Tbsp or 1 oz) | 2 |
| Tossed salad & | 0 |
| Oil & vinegar dressing (2 Tbsp) | 0 |
| Fruit cocktail (½ cup) | 0 |
| Tea & | 0 |
| Sugar | 0 |
| **TV Snack** | |
| Vanilla ice milk (1 cup) | 18 |
| **Total Cholesterol:** | **179** |

Wise food choices! A much healthier intake of cholesterol for the day.

Now it's your turn to count your cholesterol. Note everything you eat today, then look up the cholesterol in each food you have eaten and see how much cholesterol you ate today. While you're at it, jot down the calories, too!

## CHOLESTEROL COUNTING:
## A SAMPLE WORKSHEET

| FOOD | AMOUNT | CHOLESTEROL (MG) | CALORIES |
|------|--------|------------------|----------|
| **Breakfast** | | | |
| **Snack** | | | |
| **Lunch** | | | |
| **Snack** | | | |
| **Dinner** | | | |
| **Snack** | | | |

### TOTAL CHOLESTEROL:        CALORIES:

Did your cholesterol total more than 300 milligrams for the day? If it did, you need to start counting cholesterol and making wiser food choices.

## CHOLESTEROL COUNTING:
## A SAMPLE WORKSHEET

| FOOD | AMOUNT | CHOLESTEROL (MG) | CALORIES |
|------|--------|------------------|----------|

**Breakfast**

**Snack**

**Lunch**

**Snack**

**Dinner**

**Snack**

## TOTAL CHOLESTEROL:        CALORIES:

Did your cholesterol total more than 300 milligrams for the day? If it did, you need to start counting cholesterol and making wiser food choices.

# EIGHT STEPS
# TO LOWER CHOLESTEROL

1. Use liquid vegetable oils. Choose olive, canola, corn, soybean, sunflower, safflower and cottonseed oils.

2. Limit amount of meat eaten. Do not use liver, brains or other organ meats. Poultry, shellfish and other fish also should be eaten in small portions.

3. Use lean cuts of meat; trim off all visible fat. Cook without added fat. Bake, broil or roast to further reduce fat. Remove skin from poultry and fish.

4. Use more beans, grains, pasta, rice and vegetables to make up for the smaller portions of meat, fish and poultry.

5. Avoid coffee whiteners (nondairy creamers) and whipped toppings.

6. Limit eggs to three a week, including those used in cooking and desserts. Two egg whites can be substituted for one egg.

7. Use skim milk, skim milk cheese, ice milk and lowfat yogurt. Avoid butter, cream, ice cream, sour cream and whole milk.

8. When using margarine, salad dressing or gravy, use a teaspoon or tablespoon to measure out a portion.

# USING YOUR
# CHOLESTEROL COUNTER

This book lists the cholesterol and calorie content of over 8000 foods. For the first time, information about cholesterol values is at your fingertips. Now you will find it easy to follow a low-cholesterol diet.

Before *Cholesterol Counter* it was impossible to tell how much cholesterol there was in prepared foods since most do not list cholesterol information on the label. Fresh foods like meat, chicken, fish and cheese do not even have a label. The same goes for take-out items like potato salad, coleslaw, quiche, or foods bought at the bakery. How can you tell how much cholesterol there is in a burger or taco that you enjoy at the local fast-food restaurant? *Cholesterol Counter* lists them all!

The second edition is divided into two main sections. Part I, Brand Name and Generic Foods, lists foods alphabetically. For each group, you will find brand-name foods listed first in alphabetical order, followed by an alphabetical listing of generic foods.

If you want to know how much cholesterol is in the hamburger you are having for lunch, look under BEEF, where you will find a beef patty or a microwave hamburger sandwich listed. If you are making a homemade hamburger, look under ROLL, where you will find the hamburger roll listed alphabetically. For foods like FRENCH TOAST, PASTA or TUNA, simply look for the specific food alphabetically in the complete listing. For example, FRENCH TOAST is found on page 178, listed alphabetically between FRENCH BEANS and FROG LEG. Two slices have 224 milligrams of cholesterol.

Part II, Restaurant, Take-out and Fast-Food Chains, contains an alphabetical listing of 21 popular chains. Fast foods like BURGER KING, DOMINO'S PIZZA, TACO BELL and WENDY'S are listed alphabetically under the chain's name. For example McDONALD'S is listed on page 483 under M.

If you are eating at home, simply look up the individual foods you are eating and total the cholesterol for the meal. For example, your dinner may consist of:

|  | CHOLESTEROL (MG) |
|---|---|
| 2 rib lamb chops, broiled | 132 |
| Broccoli w/ Cheese Sauce (Birds Eye) | 6 |
| Long Grain & Wild Rice (Minute Rice) | 10 |
| Pecan Pie (Mrs. Smith's) | 30 |
| Glass of white wine | 0 |
| TOTAL CHOLESTEROL FOR THE MEAL | 178 |

We have tried to include all foods for which cholesterol values are known. There will be some foods, however, that are not listed in *Cholesterol Counter* because the cholesterol values are not available for that particular food.

When you can't locate your favorite brand, look at other similar foods. You will probably find a brand food, a generic product or a home recipe that is like your favorite food. For example: You find that your favorite brand of vanilla yogurt is not listed. Ask yourself, "Is my favorite brand made from whole milk or is it lowfat?" If it is lowfat vanilla yogurt, on pages 456–57 you will find a generic listing for lowfat vanilla yogurt as well as an entry for Friendship Lowfat vanilla yogurt and Yoplait 150 vanilla yogurt. From these three entries you can quickly determine that lowfat vanilla yogurt has 14 milligrams or less cholesterol in a serving. You can then assume that your favorite brand has a comparable amount.

With your *Cholesterol Counter* as your guide, you will never again wonder how much cholesterol is in food. You will always be able to tell if a food is high in cholesterol, moderate in cholesterol or low in cholesterol. Your goal is to pick low-cholesterol foods each time you eat.

### Finding Cholesterol in the Foods You Eat

When you know the ingredients in a food you can tell if that food contains cholesterol. Read the ingredients list on the label or, if you are using a home recipe, read through the recipe ingredients. To find cholesterol-containing ingredients you need only remember this simple rule:

If it grows in the ground, the food does not contain cholesterol.

If it has feet, fins, wings or claws and can walk, swim or fly, the food does contain cholesterol.

Try out the rule. Which of the following foods has cholesterol?

Is there cholesterol in:

|  | YES | NO |
|---|---|---|
| Hamburger | X | |
| Sardines | X | |
| Lobster | X | |
| Chicken leg | X | |
| Cheddar cheese | X | |
| Milk | X | |
| Egg | X | |
| Peanut butter | | X |
| Apple | | X |
| Olive oil | | X |

The first seven foods all contain cholesterol. Hamburger comes from a steer. Sardines and lobsters are seafood. Chicken leg comes from a chicken. All of these have either feet, fins, wings or claws. Therefore, they all contain cholesterol. Cheddar cheese, milk and egg have cholesterol because they all come from an animal that has feet.

Peanut butter, apples and olive oil are all from plants that grow in the ground. Therefore, they have no cholesterol.

Now you know why all of the ingredients on the following list have cholesterol. These are the ingredients to look for on a label or in a recipe.

### INGREDIENTS THAT CONTAIN CHOLESTEROL
whole eggs
egg yolks
whole milk
lowfat milk
cream
ice cream
sour cream
yogurt (unless labeled nonfat)
cheese (unless labeled nonfat)
bacon or bacon fat
butter
lard
chicken fat
beef suet or tallow
liver
kidney
brains
meat (any variety)
fish (any variety)
poultry (any variety)

Here are some sample labels with the cholesterol containing ingredients in *italics*.

---

**KEEBLER STONE CREEK HEARTY RYE CRACKERS**
Enriched wheat flour containing niacin, reduced iron, thiamine mononitrate (vitamin B1) and riboflavin (vitamin B2), *animal* or vegetable shortening (*lard* or partially hydrogenated soybean oil), sugar, stone ground rye flour, stone ground corn flour, salt, molasses, dehydrated onion, leavening, spices, artificial color (caramel) and lecithin.

---

These crackers have only one ingredient that contains cholesterol, but it is the second ingredient listed after flour. This means that the crackers contain more lard or soybean oil than any other ingredient except flour. Note that lard or soybean oil may be used. You have no way of knowing which was used. It is safer to assume it is the lard and that the crackers contain cholesterol.

---

**NOODLE RONI CHICKEN AND MUSHROOM FLAVOR**
*Egg noodles,* food starch modified, natural flavors, *chicken fat,* hydrolyzed vegetable protein with dry yeast and soy flour, dried mushrooms, *dried chicken,* monosodium glutamate, dried onion, dried red pepper, onion tumeric, tricalcium phosphate, sugar, dried parsley, spice, dried garlic, disodium inosinate, disodium guanylate, freshness preserved with BHA, propylgallate, citric acid.

---

This side dish contains three sources of cholesterol: egg noodles, chicken fat and dried chicken.

FRENCH'S IDAHO MASHED POTATOES
Idaho potato granules (with sodium bisulfite, citric acid and BHA added to protect color and flavor), monoglycerides.

Although these instant mashed potatoes contain no cholesterol, the package directions tell you to add butter and milk. Both are sources of cholesterol. Even though you buy a cholesterol-free product, you may be adding cholesterol in the preparation.

To cut down on the cholesterol in the instant mashed potatoes, you could use margarine and skim milk in place of butter and whole milk.

# DEFINITIONS

**as prep (as prepared):** refers to food that has been prepared according to package directions

**cooked:** refers to food cooked without the addition of fat (oil, butter, margarine, etc.); steaming, poaching, broiling and dry roasting are examples of this type of preparation

**generic:** describes a food without a brand name

**home recipe:** describes homemade dishes; those included can be used as a guide to the cholesterol and calorie values of similar products you may prepare or take-out food you buy ready-to-eat

**lean and fat:** describes meat with some fat on its edges that is not cut away before cooking or poultry prepared with skin and fat as purchased

**lean only:** lean portion, trimmed of all visible fat

**tr (trace):** value used when a food contains less than one calorie or less than one mg of cholesterol

## ABBREVIATIONS

| | | |
|---|---|---|
| avg | = | average |
| diam | = | diameter |
| fl oz | = | fluid ounce |
| frzn | = | frozen |
| g | = | gram |
| lb | = | pound |
| lg | = | large |
| med | = | medium |
| mg | = | milligram |
| oz | = | ounce |
| pkg | = | package |
| prep | = | prepared |
| pt | = | pint |
| reg | = | regular |
| sm | = | small |
| sq | = | square |
| Tbsp | = | tablespoon |
| tr | = | trace |
| tsp | = | teaspoon |
| w/ | = | with |
| w/o | = | without |
| " | = | inch |
| < | = | less than |

# EQUIVALENT MEASURES

| | | |
|---|---|---|
| 1 tablespoon | = | 3 teaspoons |
| 4 tablespoons | = | ¼ cup |
| 8 tablespoons | = | ½ cup |
| 12 tablespoons | = | ¾ cup |
| 16 tablespoons | = | 1 cup |
| | | |
| 1000 milligrams | = | 1 gram |
| 28 grams | = | 1 ounce |

## LIQUID MEASUREMENTS

| | | |
|---|---|---|
| 2 tablespoons | = | 1 ounce |
| ¼ cup | = | 2 ounces |
| ½ cup | = | 4 ounces |
| ¾ cup | = | 6 ounces |
| 1 cup | = | 8 ounces |
| 2 cups | = | 1 pint |
| 4 cups | = | 1 quart |

## DRY MEASUREMENTS

| | | |
|---|---|---|
| 16 ounces | = | 1 pound |
| 12 ounces | = | ¾ pound |
| 8 ounces | = | ½ pound |
| 4 ounces | = | ¼ pound |

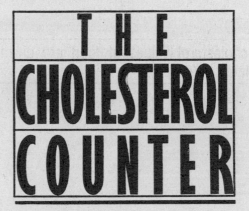

All cholesterol values of food are given in milligrams (mg).

# PART I

# Brand Name and Generic Foods

| FOOD | PORTION | CALORIES | CHOLESTEROL |
|------|---------|----------|-------------|

## ABALONE

**FRESH**

| | | | |
|------|---------|----------|-------------|
| fried | 3 oz | 161 | 80 |
| raw | 3 oz | 89 | 72 |

## ACEROLA

**FRESH**

| | | | |
|------|---------|----------|-------------|
| acerola | 1 fruit | 2 | 0 |

**JUICE**

| | | | |
|------|---------|----------|-------------|
| acerola | 1 oz | 6 | 0 |

## ADZUKI BEANS

**CANNED**

| | | | |
|------|---------|----------|-------------|
| sweetened | ½ cup | 351 | 0 |

**DRIED**

| | | | |
|------|---------|----------|-------------|
| cooked | 1 cup | 294 | 0 |
| raw | 1 cup | 649 | 0 |

**READY-TO-USE**

| | | | |
|------|---------|----------|-------------|
| yokan; sliced | ¼" slice | 36 | 0 |

## ALE

(*see* BEER AND ALE)

## ALFALFA

**SPROUTS**

| | | | |
|------|---------|----------|-------------|
| alfalfa sprouts | 1 cup | 40 | 0 |
| alfalfa sprouts | 1 Tbsp | 1 | 0 |

| FOOD | PORTION | CALORIES | CHOLESTEROL |
|------|---------|----------|-------------|

## ALMONDS

| FOOD | PORTION | CALORIES | CHOLESTEROL |
|------|---------|----------|-------------|
| Almond Butter (Erewhon) | 1 Tbsp | 90 | 0 |
| Blanched, Slivered, Whole or Sliced (Planters) | 1 oz | 170 | 0 |
| Dry Roasted (Planters) | 1 oz | 170 | 0 |
| Honey Roasted (Planters) | 1 oz | 170 | 0 |
| Shelled Almonds (Dole) | 1 oz | 170 | 0 |
| almond butter | 1 Tbsp | 101 | 0 |
| almond butter, honey and cinnamon | 1 Tbsp | 96 | 0 |
| almond meal, partially defatted | 1 oz | 116 | 0 |
| almond paste | 1 oz | 127 | 0 |
| dried, unblanched | 1 oz | 167 | 0 |
| dried, unblanched | 1 cup | 837 | 0 |
| dried, blanched | 1 oz | 166 | 0 |
| dry roasted, unblanched | 1 oz | 167 | 0 |
| oil roasted, blanched | 1 oz | 174 | 0 |
| oil roasted, unblanched | 1 oz | 176 | 0 |
| toasted, unblanched | 1 oz | 167 | 0 |
| whole, dried, blanched | 1 cup | 850 | 0 |

## AMARANTH

| FOOD | PORTION | CALORIES | CHOLESTEROL |
|------|---------|----------|-------------|
| Amaranth Flakes (Health Valley) | 1 oz | 110 | 0 |

| FOOD | PORTION | CALORIES | CHOLESTEROL |
| --- | --- | --- | --- |
| Amaranth w/ Banana (Health Valley) | 1 oz | 100 | 0 |
| Amaranth Crunch w/ Raisins (Health Valley) | 1 oz | 110 | 0 |
| Amaranth Pilaf (Health Valley) | 7.5 oz | 178 | 0 |
| amaranth; cooked | ½ cup | 59 | 0 |

## APPLE

| | | | |
| --- | --- | --- | --- |
| Spiced Apple Rings (White House) | 3.5 oz | 180 | 0 |
| applesauce, sweetened | ½ cup | 97 | 0 |
| applesauce, unsweetened | ½ cup | 53 | 0 |
| sliced, sweetened | ½ cup | 68 | 0 |
| **DRIED** Apples (Mariani) | ¼ cup | 150 | 0 |
| cooked w/ sugar | ½ cup | 116 | 0 |
| cooked w/o sugar | ½ cup | 172 | 0 |
| rings | 10 | 155 | 0 |
| **FRESH** apple | 1 | 81 | 0 |
| w/o skin; cooked | 1 cup | 91 | 0 |
| w/o skin; microwaved | 1 cup | 96 | 0 |
| w/o skin; sliced | 1 cup | 62 | 0 |
| **FROZEN** Apples, Glazed in Raspberry Sauce (Budget Gourmet) | 5 oz | 110 | 10 |
| sliced | ½ cup | 41 | 0 |

| FOOD | PORTION | CALORIES | CHOLESTEROL |
|---|---|---|---|
| **JUICE** | | | |
| Apple (Mott's) | 6 oz | 88 | 0 |
| Apple (Mott's) | 8.5 oz | 124 | 0 |
| Apple (Mott's) | 9.5 oz | 141 | 0 |
| Apple (Mott's) | 10 oz | 148 | 0 |
| Apple (Seneca) | 6 oz | 90 | 0 |
| Apple (Tree Top) | 6 oz | 90 | 0 |
| Apple frzn; as prep (Seneca) | 6 oz | 90 | 0 |
| Apple frzn; as prep (Tree Top) | 6 oz | 90 | 0 |
| Apple 100% Unsweetened (S&W) | 6 oz | 85 | 0 |
| Apple Cider (Tree Top) | 6 oz | 90 | 0 |
| Apple Cider frzn; as prep (Tree Top) | 6 oz | 90 | 0 |
| Apple Juice (Ocean Spray) | 6 oz | 90 | 0 |
| Apple Juice (White House) | 6 oz | 87 | 0 |
| Apple Juice 100% Pure (Kraft) | 6 oz | 80 | 0 |
| Apple Natural Style (Mott's) | 6 oz | 88 | 0 |

| FOOD | PORTION | CALORIES | CHOLESTEROL |
|---|---|---|---|
| Apple Unfiltered frzn; as prep (Tree Top) | 6 oz | 90 | 0 |
| Natural Apple frzn; as prep (Seneca) | 6 oz | 90 | 0 |
| apple | 1 cup | 116 | 0 |
| frzn; as prep | 1 cup | 111 | 0 |
| frzn; not prep | 6 oz | 349 | 0 |

## APRICOTS

| | | | |
|---|---|---|---|
| CANNED<br>Apricot Halves Unpeeled in Heavy Syrup (S&W) | ½ cup | 110 | 0 |
| Apricots Whole Peeled in Heavy Syrup (S&W) | ½ cup | 100 | 0 |
| apricots, heavy syrup w/ skin | 3 halves, 1¾ Tbsp liquid | 70 | 0 |
| apricots, juice pack w/ skin | 3 halves, 1¾ Tbsp liquid | 40 | 0 |
| apricots, light syrup w/ skin | 3 halves, 1¾ Tbsp liquid | 54 | 0 |
| apricots, water pack w/o skin | 2 fruits, 2 Tbsp liquid | 20 | 0 |
| apricots, water pack w/ skin | 3 halves | 22 | 0 |
| DRIED<br>Apricots (Mariani) | ¼ cup | 140 | 0 |

| FOOD | PORTION | CALORIES | CHOLESTEROL |
|---|---|---|---|
| halves | 10 | 83 | 0 |
| halves; cooked w/o sugar | ½ cup | 106 | 0 |
| FRESH apricots | 3 | 51 | 0 |
| FROZEN apricots | ½ cup | 119 | 0 |
| JUICE Nectar (S&W) | 6 oz | 100 | 0 |
| nectar | 1 cup | 141 | 0 |

## ARROWHEAD

| | | | |
|---|---|---|---|
| FRESH boiled | 1 med | 9 | 0 |
| raw | 1 med | 12 | 0 |

## ARTICHOKE

| | | | |
|---|---|---|---|
| CANNED Heart Marinated (S&W) | 3.5 oz | 225 | 0 |
| FRESH artichoke; cooked | 1 med | 53 | 0 |
| hearts; cooked | ½ cup | 37 | 0 |
| jerusalem, raw; sliced | ½ cup | 57 | 0 |
| raw | 1 med | 65 | 0 |
| FROZEN Artichoke Hearts (Birds Eye) | ½ cup | 32 | 0 |

| FOOD | PORTION | CALORIES | CHOLESTEROL |
|------|---------|----------|-------------|
| frzn; cooked | 9 oz pkg | 108 | 0 |
| frzn; not prep | 9 oz pkg | 96 | 0 |

## ASPARAGUS

| | | | |
|------|---------|----------|-------------|
| CANNED | | | |
| Cut Spears (Owatonna) | ½ cup | 20 | 0 |
| Spears Colossal Fancy (S&W) | ½ cup | 20 | 0 |
| Spears Fancy (S&W) | ½ cup | 18 | 0 |
| asparagus | ½ cup spears | 24 | 0 |
| FRESH | | | |
| asparagus, raw | ½ cup | 15 | 0 |
| asparagus; cooked | ½ cup | 22 | 0 |
| asparagus; cooked | 4 spears | 15 | 0 |
| FROZEN | | | |
| Cut (Birds Eye) | ½ cup | 23 | 0 |
| Spears (Birds Eye) | ½ cup | 24 | 0 |
| frzn; cooked | 4 spears | 17 | 0 |
| frzn; not prep | 10 oz | 69 | 0 |

## AVOCADO

| | | | |
|------|---------|----------|-------------|
| FRESH | | | |
| Avocado (California Avocados) | ½ | 153 | 0 |

| FOOD | PORTION | CALORIES | CHOLESTEROL |
|---|---|---|---|
| Avocado; mashed (California Avocados) | 1 cup | 407 | 0 |
| avocado | 1 | 324 | 0 |

## BACON
(*see also* BACON SUBSTITUTE)

| FOOD | PORTION | CALORIES | CHOLESTEROL |
|---|---|---|---|
| Armour Lower Salt; cooked | 1 strip | 38 | 6 |
| Armour Star; cooked | 1 strip | 38 | 6 |
| Oscar Mayer Center Cut; cooked | 1 strip (4.6 g) | 24 | 5 |
| Oscar Mayer Lower Salt; cooked | 1 strip (6.1 g) | 33 | 5 |
| Oscar Mayer; cooked | 1 strip (6 g) | 35 | 5 |
| bacon; cooked | 3 strips (19 g) | 109 | 16 |
| breakfast strips, beef; cooked | 3 strips (34 g) | 153 | 40 |
| breakfast strips, pork, raw | 3 strips (3 oz) | 264 | 47 |
| breakfast strips; cooked | 3 strips (34 g) | 156 | 36 |
| Canadian bacon; grilled | 2 slices (1.7 oz) | 86 | 27 |
| Canadian bacon; unheated | 1 pkg (6 oz) | 268 | 85 |
| pork | 3 slices (2 oz) | 378 | 46 |

## BACON SUBSTITUTE

| FOOD | PORTION | CALORIES | CHOLESTEROL |
|---|---|---|---|
| Bacon Bits (Oscar Mayer) | ¼ oz | 21 | 6 |

| FOOD | PORTION | CALORIES | CHOLESTEROL |
|------|---------|----------|-------------|
| Breakfast Strips Lean 'N Tasty Beef; cooked (Oscar Mayer) | 1 strip (12 g) | 46 | 13 |
| Breakfast Strips Lean 'N Tasty Pork; cooked (Oscar Mayer) | 1 strip (12 g) | 54 | 14 |
| Strips, frzn (Morningstar Farms) | 3.5 oz | 333 | 1 |
| bacon substitute | 1 strip | 25 | 0 |
| breakfast strips, beef, raw | 3 strips | 276 | 56 |

## BAGEL

| FOOD | PORTION | CALORIES | CHOLESTEROL |
|------|---------|----------|-------------|
| Big 'N Crusty (Lenders) | 1 | 230 | 0 |
| Blueberry (Lenders) | 1 | 190 | 0 |
| Cinnamon & Raisin (Sara Lee) | 1 | 240 | 0 |
| Egg (Sara Lee) | 1 | 250 | 20 |
| Onion (Sara Lee) | 1 | 230 | 0 |
| Plain (Lenders) | 1 | 150 | 0 |
| Plain (Sara Lee) | 1 | 230 | 0 |
| Poppy Seed (Sara Lee) | 1 | 230 | 0 |
| Sesame Seed (Sara Lee) | 1 | 260 | 0 |

## BAKING POWDER

| FOOD | PORTION | CALORIES | CHOLESTEROL |
|------|---------|----------|-------------|
| Calumet | 1 tsp | 3 | 0 |

| FOOD | PORTION | CALORIES | CHOLESTEROL |
|------|---------|----------|-------------|

## BAKING SODA

| Arm & Hammer (Church Dwight) | 1 tsp | 0 | 0 |

## BAMBOO SHOOTS

| CANNED | | | |
| bamboo shoots; sliced | 1 cup | 25 | 0 |
| FRESH | | | |
| cooked | ½ cup | 15 | 0 |
| raw | ½ cup | 21 | 0 |

## BANANA

| DRIED | | | |
| dehydrated powder | 1 Tbsp | 21 | 0 |
| FRESH | | | |
| Chiquita | 1 (3½ oz) | 110 | 0 |
| banana | 1 | 105 | 0 |

## BASS

| FRESH | | | |
| freshwater | 1 fillet (2.7 oz) | 903 | 54 |
| freshwater | 3 oz | 97 | 58 |
| sea, raw | 1 fillet (4.5 oz) | 125 | 53 |
| sea, raw | 3 oz | 82 | 35 |
| sea; cooked | 3 oz | 105 | 45 |
| sea; cooked | 1 fillet (3.5 oz) | 125 | 53 |

| FOOD | PORTION | CALORIES | CHOLESTEROL |
|---|---|---|---|
| striped, raw | 3 oz | 82 | 68 |
| striped, raw | 1 fillet (5.6 oz) | 154 | 127 |

## BEANS
*(see also individual names)*

| FOOD | PORTION | CALORIES | CHOLESTEROL |
|---|---|---|---|
| CANNED | | | |
| Boston Baked (Health Valley) | 4 oz | 110 | 0 |
| Cut Green Beans (Hanover) | ½ cup | 20 | 0 |
| Four Bean Salad (Hanover) | ½ cup | 80 | 0 |
| Maple Sugar Beans (S&W) | ½ cup | 150 | 0 |
| Mixed Bean Salad Marinated (S&W) | ½ cup | 90 | 0 |
| Pork 'N Beans (S&W) | ½ cup | 130 | 0 |
| Smokey Ranch Beans (S&W) | ½ cup | 130 | 0 |
| Vegetarian (Libby) | ½ cup | 130 | 0 |
| Vegetarian (Seneca) | ½ cup | 130 | 0 |
| Vegetarian w/ Miso (Health Valley) | 4 oz | 90 | 0 |
| baked beans, plain | ½ cup | 118 | 0 |
| baked beans, vegetarian | ½ cup | 118 | 0 |
| baked beans, w/ beef | ½ cup | 161 | 29 |
| baked beans, w/ franks | ½ cup | 182 | 8 |

| FOOD | PORTION | CALORIES | CHOLESTEROL |
|---|---|---|---|
| baked beans, w/ pork | ½ cup | 133 | 9 |
| baked beans, w/ pork & sweet sauce | ½ cup | 140 | 9 |
| baked beans, w/ pork & tomato sauce | ½ cup | 123 | 9 |
| **FROZEN** Romano Bean Medley (Hanover) | ½ cup | 25 | 0 |
| **HOME RECIPE** baked beans | ½ cup | 190 | 6 |
| refried beans | ½ cup | 43 | 2 |
| three bean salad | ¾ cup | 230 | 0 |
| **SPROUTS** bean sprouts, canned | ½ cup | 8 | 0 |

## BEECHNUTS

| | | | |
|---|---|---|---|
| dried | 1 oz | 164 | 0 |

## BEEF
(*see also* BEEF DISHES, VEAL)

Beef is graded according to its marbling, the little flecks of fat in the muscle. Beef graded "Prime" has the highest percentage of fat, followed by "Choice" with less fat and "Select" with the least fat.

| **CANNED** | | | |
|---|---|---|---|
| corned beef | 1 oz | 71 | 24 |
| corned beef | 1 slice (21 g) | 53 | 18 |
| stew w/vegetables | 1 cup | 186 | 33 |

| FOOD | PORTION | CALORIES | CHOLESTEROL |
|------|---------|----------|-------------|

**FRESH**
Note that the values for cooked beef may differ slightly from values
for raw beef. When meat is cooked some moisture and fat is lost,
changing the nutrition value slightly. As a rule of thumb it can be
assumed that a 4 oz raw portion will equal a 3 oz cooked portion
of meat.

| FOOD | PORTION | CALORIES | CHOLESTEROL |
|------|---------|----------|-------------|
| bottom round, lean & fat, Choice, raw | 4 oz | 256 | 72 |
| bottom round, lean & fat, Choice; braised | 3 oz | 224 | 81 |
| bottom round, lean & fat, Prime; braised | 3 oz | 253 | 81 |
| bottom round, lean & fat, Prime, raw | 4 oz | 256 | 72 |
| bottom round, lean & fat, Select, raw | 4 oz | 244 | 72 |
| bottom round, lean & fat, Select; braised | 3 oz | 215 | 81 |
| bottom round, lean only, Choice, raw | 4 oz | 172 | 68 |
| bottom round, lean only, Choice; braised | 3 oz | 191 | 81 |
| bottom round, lean only, Prime, raw | 4 oz | 180 | 68 |
| bottom round, lean only, Prime; braised | 3 oz | 212 | 81 |
| bottom round, lean only, Select, raw | 4 oz | 164 | 68 |
| bottom round, lean only, Select; braised | 3 oz | 182 | 81 |
| brisket, flat half, lean & fat; braised | 3 oz | 347 | 78 |

| FOOD | PORTION | CALORIES | CHOLESTEROL |
|---|---|---|---|
| brisket, flat half, lean only; braised | 3 oz | 223 | 77 |
| brisket, point half, lean & fat, raw | 4 oz | 336 | 80 |
| brisket, point half, lean only, raw | 4 oz | 152 | 68 |
| brisket, point half, lean only; braised | 3 oz | 181 | 81 |
| brisket, point half; braised | 3 oz | 311 | 81 |
| brisket, whole, lean & fat; braised | 3 oz | 332 | 79 |
| brisket, whole, lean only; braised | 3 oz | 205 | 79 |
| chuck arm pot roast, lean only, Choice; braised | 3 oz | 199 | 85 |
| chuck arm pot roast, lean only, Prime; braised | 3 oz | 222 | 85 |
| chuck arm pot roast, lean only, Select; braised | 3 oz | 189 | 85 |
| chuck arm pot roast, lean & fat, Choice; braised | 3 oz | 301 | 84 |
| chuck arm pot roast, lean & fat, Choice, raw | 4 oz | 296 | 80 |
| chuck arm pot roast, lean & fat, Prime, raw | 4 oz | 332 | 80 |
| chuck arm pot roast, lean & fat, Prime; braised | 3 oz | 332 | 84 |
| chuck arm pot roast, lean & fat, Select, raw | 4 oz | 268 | 76 |
| chuck arm pot roast, lean & fat, Select; braised | 3 oz | 287 | 84 |
| chuck arm pot roast, lean only, Choice, raw | 4 oz | 156 | 68 |

| FOOD | PORTION | CALORIES | CHOLESTEROL |
|---|---|---|---|
| chuck arm pot roast, lean only, Prime, raw | 4 oz | 176 | 68 |
| chuck arm pot roast, lean only, Select, raw | 4 oz | 148 | 68 |
| chuck blade roast, Select, raw | 4 oz | 296 | 80 |
| chuck blade roast, lean only, Choice; braised | 3 oz | 234 | 90 |
| chuck blade roast, lean only, Prime; braised | 3 oz | 270 | 90 |
| chuck blade roast, lean only, Select; braised | 3 oz | 218 | 90 |
| chuck blade roast, lean & fat, Choice, raw | 4 oz | 328 | 84 |
| chuck blade roast, lean & fat, Choice; braised | 3 oz | 330 | 87 |
| chuck blade roast, lean & fat, Prime, raw | 4 oz | 372 | 84 |
| chuck blade roast, lean & fat, Prime; braised | 3 oz | 354 | 87 |
| chuck blade roast, lean & fat, Select; braised | 3 oz | 311 | 88 |
| chuck blade roast, lean only, Choice, raw | 4 oz | 192 | 72 |
| chuck blade roast, lean only, Prime, raw | 4 oz | 232 | 72 |
| chuck blade roast, lean only, Select, raw | 4 oz | 172 | 72 |
| corned beef brisket, raw | 4 oz | 224 | 60 |
| corned beef brisket; cooked | 3 oz | 213 | 83 |
| eye of round, lean & fat, Choice, raw | 4 oz | 228 | 68 |

| FOOD | PORTION | CALORIES | CHOLESTEROL |
|---|---|---|---|
| eye of round, lean & fat, Choice; roasted | 3 oz | 207 | 62 |
| eye of round, lean & fat, Prime, raw | 4 oz | 252 | 68 |
| eye of round, lean & fat, Select, raw | 4 oz | 212 | 68 |
| eye of round, lean & fat, Select; roasted | 3 oz | 201 | 62 |
| eye of round, lean and fat, Prime; roasted | 3 oz | 213 | 61 |
| eye of round, lean only, Choice, raw | 4 oz | 152 | 60 |
| eye of round, lean only, Choice; roasted | 3 oz | 156 | 59 |
| eye of round, lean only, Prime; roasted | 3 oz | 168 | 59 |
| eye of round, lean only, Select, raw | 4 oz | 144 | 60 |
| eye of round, lean only, Select; roasted | 3 oz | 151 | 59 |
| eye of round, lean only, Prime, raw | 4 oz | 168 | 60 |
| flank, lean only, Choice; broiled | 3 oz | 207 | 60 |
| flank, lean only, Choice, raw | 3 oz | 192 | 56 |
| flank, lean only, Choice; braised | 3 oz | 208 | 60 |
| flank, lean & fat, Choice, raw | 4 oz | 220 | 60 |
| flank, lean & fat, Choice; braised | 3 oz | 218 | 61 |
| flank, lean & fat, Choice; broiled | 3 oz | 216 | 60 |

| FOOD | PORTION | CALORIES | CHOLESTEROL |
| --- | --- | --- | --- |
| ground, extra lean, raw | 4 oz | 265 | 78 |
| ground, extra lean; cooked medium | 3 oz | 213 | 70 |
| ground, extra lean; cooked well-done | 3 oz | 232 | 91 |
| ground, lean, raw | 4 oz | 298 | 85 |
| ground, lean; cooked medium | 3 oz | 227 | 66 |
| ground, lean; cooked well-done | 3 oz | 248 | 84 |
| ground, regular, raw | 4 oz | 351 | 96 |
| ground, regular; cooked medium | 3 oz | 244 | 74 |
| ground, regular; cooked well-done | 3 oz | 269 | 92 |
| lungs, raw | 4 oz | 104 | 274 |
| lungs; braised | 3 oz | 102 | 236 |
| porterhouse steak, lean only, Choice, raw | 4 oz | 180 | 68 |
| porterhouse steak, lean only, Choice; broiled | 3 oz | 185 | 68 |
| porterhouse steak, lean & fat, Choice, raw | 4 oz | 324 | 80 |
| porterhouse steak, lean & fat, Choice; broiled | 3 oz | 254 | 70 |
| rib eye small end, lean only, Choice, raw | 4 oz | 184 | 68 |
| rib eye small end, lean & fat, Choice, raw | 4 oz | 284 | 76 |
| rib eye small end, lean & fat, Choice; broiled | 3 oz | 250 | 70 |
| rib large end, lean & fat, Choice, raw | 4 oz | 404 | 84 |

| FOOD | PORTION | CALORIES | CHOLESTEROL |
|---|---|---|---|
| rib large end, lean & fat, Choice; broiled | 3 oz | 327 | 74 |
| rib large end, lean & fat, Choice; roasted | 3 oz | 316 | 72 |
| rib large end, lean & fat, Prime; broiled | 3 oz | 361 | 74 |
| rib large end, lean & fat, Prime, raw | 4 oz | 436 | 84 |
| rib large end, lean & fat, Prime; roasted | 3 oz | 346 | 72 |
| rib large end, lean & fat, Select, raw | 4 oz | 372 | 80 |
| rib large end, lean & fat, Select; broiled | 3 oz | 301 | 73 |
| rib large end, lean & fat, Select; roasted | 3 oz | 304 | 72 |
| rib large end, lean only, Choice, raw | 4 oz | 196 | 68 |
| rib large end, lean only, Choice; broiled | 3 oz | 203 | 70 |
| rib large end, lean only, Choice; roasted | 3 oz | 210 | 68 |
| rib large end, lean only, Prime; broiled | 3 oz | 250 | 70 |
| rib large end, lean only, Prime; roasted | 3 oz | 241 | 68 |
| rib large end, lean only, Select, raw | 4 oz | 180 | 68 |
| rib large end, lean only, Select; broiled | 3 oz | 183 | 70 |
| rib large end, lean only, Select; roasted | 3 oz | 197 | 68 |

| FOOD | PORTION | CALORIES | CHOLESTEROL |
|---|---|---|---|
| rib large end, lean only, Prime, raw | 4 oz | 240 | 68 |
| rib small end, lean & fat, Choice, raw | 4 oz | 356 | 80 |
| rib small end, lean & fat, Choice; broiled | 3 oz | 282 | 71 |
| rib small end, lean & fat, Choice; roasted | 3 oz | 312 | 72 |
| rib small end, lean & fat, Prime, raw | 4 oz | 396 | 80 |
| rib small end, lean & fat, Prime; broiled | 3 oz | 309 | 71 |
| rib small end, lean & fat, Prime; roasted | 3 oz | 357 | 72 |
| rib small end, lean & fat, Select, raw | 4 oz | 324 | 80 |
| rib small end, lean & fat, Select; broiled | 3 oz | 263 | 71 |
| rib small end, lean & fat, Select; roasted | 3 oz | 283 | 72 |
| rib small end, lean only, Choice, raw | 4 oz | 184 | 68 |
| rib small end, lean only, Choice; broiled | 3 oz | 191 | 68 |
| rib small end, lean only, Choice; broiled | 3 oz | 191 | 68 |
| rib small end, lean only, Choice; roasted | 3 oz | 206 | 68 |
| rib small end, lean only, Prime; broiled | 3 oz | 221 | 68 |
| rib small end, lean only, Prime; roasted | 3 oz | 259 | 68 |

| FOOD | PORTION | CALORIES | CHOLESTEROL |
| --- | --- | --- | --- |
| rib small end, lean only, Select, raw | 4 oz | 168 | 68 |
| rib small end, lean only, Select; broiled | 3 oz | 178 | 68 |
| rib small end, lean only, Select; roasted | 3 oz | 183 | 68 |
| rib small end, lean only, Prime, raw | 4 oz | 228 | 68 |
| rib whole, lean & fat, Choice, raw | 4 oz | 384 | 80 |
| rib whole, lean & fat, Choice; broiled | 3 oz | 313 | 73 |
| rib whole, lean & fat, Choice; roasted | 3 oz | 328 | 72 |
| rib whole, lean & fat, Prime, raw | 4 oz | 420 | 84 |
| rib whole, lean & fat, Prime; broiled | 3 oz | 347 | 73 |
| rib whole, lean & fat, Prime; roasted | 3 oz | 361 | 73 |
| rib whole, lean & fat, Select, raw | 4 oz | 352 | 80 |
| rib whole, lean & fat, Select; broiled | 3 oz | 289 | 72 |
| rib whole, lean & fat, Select; roasted | 3 oz | 306 | 72 |
| rib whole, lean only, Choice, raw | 4 oz | 192 | 68 |
| rib whole, lean only, Choice; broiled | 3 oz | 198 | 69 |
| rib whole, lean only, Choice; roasted | 3 oz | 209 | 68 |

| FOOD | PORTION | CALORIES | CHOLESTEROL |
|---|---|---|---|
| rib whole, lean only, Prime, raw | 4 oz | 232 | 68 |
| rib whole, lean only, Prime; broiled | 3 oz | 238 | 69 |
| rib whole, lean only, Prime; roasted | 3 oz | 248 | 68 |
| rib whole, lean only, Select, raw | 4 oz | 172 | 68 |
| rib whole, lean only, Select; broiled | 3 oz | 181 | 69 |
| rib whole, lean only, Select; roasted | 3 oz | 191 | 68 |
| round, lean only, Choice, raw | 4 oz | 156 | 64 |
| round, lean only, Choice; broiled | 3 oz | 165 | 70 |
| round, lean only, Select, raw | 4 oz | 152 | 64 |
| round, lean only, Select; broiled | 3 oz | 157 | 70 |
| round, lean & fat, Choice, raw | 4 oz | 272 | 76 |
| round, lean & fat, Choice; broiled | 3 oz | 233 | 71 |
| round, lean & fat, Select, raw | 4 oz | 260 | 76 |
| round, lean & fat, Select; broiled | 3 oz | 222 | 71 |
| shank crosscut, lean & fat, Choice, raw | 4 oz | 180 | 48 |
| shank crosscut, lean only, Choice, raw | 4 oz | 144 | 44 |
| shank, crosscut, lean & fat, Choice; simmered | 3 oz | 208 | 67 |

| FOOD | PORTION | CALORIES | CHOLESTEROL |
|------|---------|----------|-------------|
| shank, crosscut, lean only, Choice; simmered | 3 oz | 171 | 66 |
| short loin tenderloin, lean & fat, Choice, raw | 1 steak (6.6 oz) | 391 | 110 |
| short loin tenderloin, lean & fat, Prime, raw | 1 steak (5.5 oz) | 450 | 111 |
| short loin tenderloin, lean & fat, Prime; broiled | 1 steak (4 oz) | 362 | 99 |
| short loin tenderloin, lean & fat, Select, raw | 1 steak (5.5 oz) | 364 | 108 |
| short loin tenderloin, lean & fat, Select; broiled | 1 steak (4 oz) | 286 | 97 |
| short loin tenderloin, lean only, Choice, raw | 4 oz | 168 | 72 |
| short loin tenderloin, lean only, Prime, raw | 4 oz | 192 | 72 |
| short loin tenderloin, lean only, Select, raw | 4 oz | 160 | 72 |
| short loin top loin, lean & fat, Choice, raw | 1 steak (10.7 oz) | 886 | 212 |
| short loin top loin, lean & fat, Choice; broiled | 1 steak (8.2 oz) | 672 | 187 |
| short loin top loin, lean & fat, Prime, raw | 1 steak (10.7 oz) | 980 | 212 |
| short loin top loin, lean & fat, Prime; broiled | 1 steak (8 oz) | 774 | 183 |
| short loin top loin, lean & fat, Select, raw | 1 steak (10.7 oz) | 804 | 208 |
| short loin top loin, lean & fat, Select; broiled | 1 steak (8.1 oz) | 603 | 182 |
| short loin top loin, lean only, Choice, raw | 4 oz | 176 | 68 |

| FOOD | PORTION | CALORIES | CHOLESTEROL |
|---|---|---|---|
| short loin top loin, lean only, Prime, raw | 4 oz | 212 | 68 |
| short loin top loin, lean only, Select, raw | 4 oz | 156 | 68 |
| short loin, tenderloin, lean & fat, Choice; broiled | 3 oz | 230 | 73 |
| short loin, tenderloin, lean & fat, Choice; roasted | 3 oz | 262 | 74 |
| short loin, tenderloin, lean & fat, Choice; broiled | 1 steak (4.1 oz) | 314 | 100 |
| short loin, tenderloin, lean & fat, Prime; broiled | 3 oz | 270 | 73 |
| short loin, tenderloin, lean & fat, Prime; roasted | 3 oz | 305 | 75 |
| short loin, tenderloin, lean & fat, Select; broiled | 3 oz | 216 | 73 |
| short loin, tenderloin, lean & fat, Select; roasted | 3 oz | 245 | 74 |
| short loin, tenderloin, lean only, Choice; broiled | 3 oz | 176 | 72 |
| short loin, tenderloin, lean only, Choice; roasted | 3 oz | 189 | 73 |
| short loin, tenderloin, lean only, Prime; broiled | 3 oz | 197 | 72 |
| short loin, tenderloin, lean only, Prime; roasted | 3 oz | 217 | 73 |
| short loin, tenderloin, lean only, Select; broiled | 3 oz | 167 | 72 |
| short loin, tenderloin, lean only, Select; roasted | 3 oz | 177 | 73 |
| short loin, top loin, lean & fat, Choice; roasted | 3 oz | 243 | 68 |

| FOOD | PORTION | CALORIES | CHOLESTEROL |
|---|---|---|---|
| short loin, top loin, lean & fat, Prime; broiled | 3 oz | 288 | 68 |
| short loin, top loin, lean & fat, Select; broiled | 3 oz | 223 | 67 |
| short loin, top loin, lean only, Choice; broiled | 3 oz | 176 | 65 |
| short loin, top loin, lean only, Prime; broiled | 3 oz | 208 | 65 |
| short loin, top loin, lean only, Select; broiled | 3 oz | 162 | 65 |
| shortribs, lean & fat, Choice, raw | 4 oz | 440 | 88 |
| shortribs, lean & fat, Choice; braised | 3 oz | 400 | 80 |
| shortribs, lean only, Choice, raw | 4 oz | 196 | 68 |
| shortribs, lean only, Choice; braised | 3 oz | 251 | 79 |
| sirloin, wedge-bone, lean & fat, Choice; broiled | 3 oz | 240 | 77 |
| sirloin, wedge-bone, lean & fat, Choice; pan-fried | 3 oz | 288 | 84 |
| sirloin, wedge-bone, lean & fat, Prime; broiled | 3 oz | 271 | 77 |
| sirloin, wedge-bone, lean & fat, Select; broiled | 3 oz | 232 | 77 |
| sirloin, wedge-bone, lean only, Choice; broiled | 3 oz | 180 | 76 |
| sirloin, wedge-bone, lean only, Choice; pan-fried | 3 oz | 202 | 85 |
| sirloin, wedge-bone, lean only, Prime; broiled | 3 oz | 201 | 76 |

| FOOD | PORTION | CALORIES | CHOLESTEROL |
|---|---|---|---|
| sirloin, wedge-bone, lean only, Select; broiled | 3 oz | 170 | 76 |
| spleen, raw | 4 oz | 119 | 298 |
| spleen; braised | 3 oz | 123 | 295 |
| T-bone steak, lean & fat, Choice, raw | 4 oz | 348 | 80 |
| T-bone steak, lean only, Choice, raw | 4 oz | 180 | 68 |
| T-bone steak, lean & fat, Choice; broiled | 3 oz | 276 | 71 |
| T-bone steak, lean only, Choice; broiled | 3 oz | 182 | 68 |
| thymus, raw | 4 oz | 266 | 252 |
| thymus; braised | 3 oz | 271 | 250 |
| tip round, lean & fat, Choice, raw | 4 oz | 240 | 72 |
| tip round, lean & fat, Choice; roasted | 3 oz | 216 | 70 |
| tip round, lean & fat, Prime, raw | 4 oz | 256 | 76 |
| tip round, lean & fat, Prime; roasted | 3 oz | 242 | 71 |
| tip round, lean & fat, Select, raw | 4 oz | 220 | 72 |
| tip round, lean & fat, Select; roasted | 3 oz | 205 | 70 |
| tip round, lean only, Choice, raw | 4 oz | 152 | 68 |
| tip round, lean only, Choice; roasted | 3 oz | 164 | 69 |
| tip round, lean only, Prime, raw | 4 oz | 164 | 68 |

| FOOD | PORTION | CALORIES | CHOLESTEROL |
|---|---|---|---|
| tip round, lean only, Prime; roasted | 3 oz | 181 | 69 |
| tip round, lean only, Select, raw | 4 oz | 144 | 68 |
| tip round, lean only, Select; roasted | 3 oz | 156 | 69 |
| top round, lean & fat, Choice, raw | 4 oz | 196 | 68 |
| top round, lean & fat, Choice; pan-fried | 3 oz | 246 | 82 |
| top round, lean & fat, Choice; roasted | 3 oz | 181 | 72 |
| top round, lean & fat, Prime, raw | 4 oz | 212 | 68 |
| top round, lean & fat, Prime; broiled | 3 oz | 201 | 72 |
| top round, lean & fat, Select, raw | 4 oz | 188 | 68 |
| top round, lean & fat, Select; broiled | 3 oz | 176 | 72 |
| top round, lean only, Choice, raw | 4 oz | 152 | 64 |
| top round, lean only, Choice; broiled | 3 oz | 165 | 72 |
| top round, lean only, Choice; pan-fried | 3 oz | 193 | 83 |
| top round, lean only, Prime, raw | 4 oz | 176 | 64 |
| top round, lean only, Prime; broiled | 3 oz | 183 | 72 |
| top round, lean only, Select, raw | 4 oz | 144 | 64 |

| FOOD | PORTION | CALORIES | CHOLESTEROL |
|---|---|---|---|
| top round, lean only, Select; broiled | 3 oz | 156 | 72 |
| tripe, raw | 4 oz | 111 | 107 |
| wedge-bone sirloin, lean only, Choice, raw | 4 oz | 156 | 68 |
| wedge-bone sirloin, lean only, Prime, raw | 4 oz | 176 | 68 |
| wedge-bone sirloin, lean only, Select, raw | 4 oz | 148 | 68 |
| wedge-bone sirloin, lean & fat, Choice, raw | 4 oz | 300 | 80 |
| wedge-bone sirloin, lean & fat, Prime, raw | 4 oz | 328 | 80 |
| wedge-bone sirloin, lean & fat, Select, raw | 4 oz | 280 | 80 |

## BEEF DISHES

FROZEN

| FOOD | PORTION | CALORIES | CHOLESTEROL |
|---|---|---|---|
| Beef w/ Barbeque Sauce Sandwich (Microwave Chefwich) | 1 (5 oz) | 360 | 23 |
| Cheeseburger (Micro Magic) | 1 (4.75 oz) | 450 | 80 |
| Hamburger (Micro Magic) | 1 (4.75 oz) | 350 | 55 |
| ground patties, frzn, raw | 4 oz | 319 | 89 |
| patties; cooked medium | 3 oz | 240 | 80 |
| Hamburger Helper Beef Noodle; as prep (General Mills) | 6 oz | 326 | 61 |

| FOOD | PORTION | CALORIES | CHOLESTEROL |
|------|---------|----------|-------------|
| Hamburger Helper Cheeseburger Macaroni; as prep (General Mills) | 6 oz | 366 | 61 |
| Hamburger Helper Chili Tomato; as prep (General Mills) | 6 oz | 336 | 61 |
| Hamburger Helper Lasagne; as prep (General Mills) | 6 oz | 336 | 61 |
| HOME RECIPE | | | |
| sauerbraten | 3.5 oz | 190 | 75 |
| stew w/ vegetables | 1 cup | 209 | 61 |
| stroganoff | ¾ cup | 260 | 69 |
| swiss steak | 4.6 oz | 214 | 61 |

## BEER AND ALE

| FOOD | PORTION | CALORIES | CHOLESTEROL |
|------|---------|----------|-------------|
| Amstel Light | 12 oz | 95 | 0 |
| Anheuser Busch Natural Light | 12 oz | 110 | 0 |
| Bud Light | 12 oz | 108 | 0 |
| Coors Light | 12 oz | 105 | 0 |
| Guiness Kaliber (nonalcoholic) | 12 oz | 43 | 0 |
| Michelob Light | 12 oz | 134 | 0 |
| Miller Lite | 12 oz | 96 | 0 |
| Molson Light | 12 oz | 109 | 0 |
| Piels Light | 12 oz | 136 | 0 |
| Schlitz Light | 12 oz | 96 | 0 |
| Schaefer Light | 12 oz | 112 | 0 |
| Schmidts Light | 12 oz | 96 | 0 |

| FOOD | PORTION | CALORIES | CHOLESTEROL |
|------|---------|----------|-------------|
| ale | 12 oz | 155 | 0 |
| beer, light | 12 oz can | 100 | 0 |
| beer, regular | 12 oz can | 146 | 0 |
| light | 12 oz | 95 | 0 |
| malt beverage | 12 oz | 32 | 0 |
| regular | 12 oz | 150 | 0 |

## BEETS

| FOOD | PORTION | CALORIES | CHOLESTEROL |
|------|---------|----------|-------------|
| Cuts (Libby) | ½ cup | 35 | 0 |
| Cuts (Seneca) | ½ cup | 35 | 0 |
| Diced (Libby) | ½ cup | 35 | 0 |
| Diced (Seneca) | ½ cup | 35 | 0 |
| Diced Tender (S&W) | ½ cup | 40 | 0 |
| Harvard (Libby) | ½ cup | 80 | 0 |
| Harvard (Seneca) | ½ cup | 80 | 0 |
| Julienne French Style (S&W) | ½ cup | 40 | 0 |
| Pickled (Libby) | ½ cup | 35 | 0 |
| Pickled (Seneca) | ½ cup | 35 | 0 |
| Sliced (Libby) | ½ cup | 35 | 0 |

| FOOD | PORTION | CALORIES | CHOLESTEROL |
|---|---|---|---|
| Sliced (Seneca) | ½ cup | 35 | 0 |
| Sliced Pickled w/ Red Wine Vinegar (S&W) | ½ cup | 70 | 0 |
| CANNED Sliced Small Premium (S&W) | ½ cup | 40 | 0 |
| Whole (Libby) | ½ cup | 35 | 0 |
| Whole (Seneca) | ½ cup | 35 | 0 |
| Whole Extra Small Pickled (S&W) | ½ cup | 70 | 0 |
| Whole Small (S&W) | ½ cup | 40 | 0 |
| beets, harvard | ½ cup | 89 | 0 |
| beets, pickled | ½ cup | 75 | 0 |
| beets, sliced | ½ cup | 27 | 0 |
| FRESH beet greens, raw; chopped | ½ cup | 4 | 0 |
| beet greens; cooked | ½ cup | 20 | 0 |
| cooked | ½ cup | 26 | 0 |
| raw | 2 (5.7 oz) | 30 | 0 |

# BEVERAGES

(*see* BEER AND ALE, COFFEE, DRINK MIXER, FRUIT DRINKS, LIQUOR/
LIQUEUR, MINERAL WATER/BOTTLED WATER, SODA, TEA/HERBAL TEA,
WINE, WINE COOLERS)

| FOOD | PORTION | CALORIES | CHOLESTEROL |
|------|---------|----------|-------------|

## BISCUIT

| | | | |
|------|---------|----------|-------------|
| Buttermilk Biscuit Mix; not prep (Health Valley) | 1 oz | 100 | 0 |
| biscuit (home recipe) | 1.5 oz | 155 | 3 |

## BLACK BEANS

| | | | |
|------|---------|----------|-------------|
| cooked | 1 cup | 227 | 0 |
| raw | 1 cup | 661 | 0 |

## BLACKBERRIES

| | | | |
|------|---------|----------|-------------|
| CANNED in heavy syrup | ½ cup | 118 | 0 |
| FRESH blackberries | ½ cup | 37 | 0 |
| FROZEN blackberries | 1 cup | 97 | 0 |

## BLACKEYE PEAS

| | | | |
|------|---------|----------|-------------|
| DRIED Blackeye Peas (Hurst Brand) | 1 cup | 233 | 0 |

## BLINTZE

| | | | |
|------|---------|----------|-------------|
| cheese (home recipe) | 2 | 186 | 149 |

## BLUEBERRIES

| | | | |
|------|---------|----------|-------------|
| CANNED Blueberries in Heavy Syrup (S&W) | ½ cup | 111 | 0 |

| FOOD | PORTION | CALORIES | CHOLESTEROL |
|---|---|---|---|
| blueberries in heavy syrup | ½ cup | 112 | 0 |
| FRESH blueberries | 1 cup | 82 | 0 |
| FROZEN blueberries, unsweetened | 1 cup | 78 | 0 |
| sweetened | 1 cup | 187 | 0 |

## BLUEFISH

| | | | |
|---|---|---|---|
| FRESH raw | 3 oz | 105 | 50 |
| raw | 1 fillet (5.3 oz) | 186 | 88 |

## BORAGE

| | | | |
|---|---|---|---|
| FRESH cooked; chopped | 3½ oz | 25 | 0 |
| raw; chopped | ½ cup | 9 | 0 |

## BOYSENBERRIES

| | | | |
|---|---|---|---|
| CANNED in heavy syrup | ½ cup | 113 | 0 |
| FROZEN unsweetened | 1 cup | 66 | 0 |
| JUICE Boysenberry (Smucker's) | 8 oz | 120 | 0 |

## BRAINS

| | | | |
|---|---|---|---|
| FRESH beef, raw | 4 oz | 142 | 1890 |

| FOOD | PORTION | CALORIES | CHOLESTEROL |
|---|---|---|---|
| beef; pan-fried | 3 oz | 167 | 1696 |
| beef; simmered | 3 oz | 136 | 1746 |
| pork, raw | 3 oz | 108 | 1866 |
| pork; braised | 3 oz | 117 | 2169 |

## BRAN
(see CEREAL)

## BRAZIL NUTS
| dried, unblanched | 1 oz | 186 | 0 |

## BREAD
(see also BAGEL, BISCUIT, BREADSTICK, CROISSANT, ENGLISH MUFFIN, MUFFIN, ROLL, SCONE)

CANNED
| Brown Bread New England Recipe (S&W) | 2 slices | 76 | 0 |

FROZEN
| OH Boy! Garlic Bread | 2 oz | 202 | 0 |

HOME RECIPE
| banana | ½" slice | 116 | 25 |
| cornbread | 2"x2" piece (1.4 oz) | 107 | 28 |
| cornstick | 1 (1.3 oz) | 101 | 30 |
| date-nut | ½" slice | 92 | 15 |
| hush puppies | 1 (2 oz) | 147 | 45 |
| nut | 1 slice (1½ oz) | 127 | 13 |
| pita, whole wheat | 1 (6" diam) | 247 | 0 |

| FOOD | PORTION | CALORIES | CHOLESTEROL |
|---|---|---|---|
| pumpkin | 1 slice (1½ oz) | 127 | 28 |
| raisin | 1 slice (1½ oz) | 140 | 6 |
| whole wheat | 1 slice | 71 | 0 |
| **READY-TO-EAT** | | | |
| Bran'nola Country Oat | 1 slice | 90 | tr |
| Bran'nola Dark Wheat (Arnold) | 1 slice | 80 | tr |
| Bran'nola Hearty Wheat (Arnold) | 1 slice | 90 | tr |
| Bran'nola Nutty Grains (Arnold) | 1 slice | 90 | tr |
| Bran'nola Original (Arnold) | 1 slice | 70 | tr |
| Butter Crust (Freihofer's) | 1 slice | 70 | 0 |
| Canadian Oat (Freihofer's) | 1 slice | 80 | 0 |
| Cinnamon Oatmeal (Oatmeal Goodness) | 1 slice | 90 | 0 |
| Club Pullman (Freihofer's) | 1 slice | 70 | 0 |
| Cracked Wheat (Roman Meal) | 1 slice | 66 | 0 |
| Garlic Bread (Arnold) | 1 slice | 80 | 0 |
| Harvest Recipe 100% Whole Wheat (Roman Meal) | 1 slice | 66 | 0 |
| Hi-Fibre (Monks' Bread) | 1 slice | 50 | 0 |

| FOOD | PORTION | CALORIES | CHOLESTEROL |
|------|---------|----------|-------------|
| Honey Wheat Berry (Roman Meal) | 1 slice | 66 | 0 |
| Honey Wheat Berry Light (Roman Meal) | 1 slice | 40 | 0 |
| Honeybran Light (Roman Meal) | 1 slice | 40 | 0 |
| Italian, Francisco (Arnold) | 1 slice | 70 | 0 |
| Italian, Francisco, Thick Sliced (Arnold) | 1 slice | 70 | 0 |
| Italian, Light (Arnold) | 1 slice | 40 | tr |
| Italian, No Seeds (Freihofer's) | 1 slice | 70 | 0 |
| Italian, Seeded (Freihofer's) | 1 slice | 70 | 0 |
| Italian, Stick, unsliced (Arnold) | 1 oz | 90 | 0 |
| Lite Diet (Freihofer's) | 1 slice | 40 | 0 |
| Oat (Roman Meal) | 1 slice | 71 | 0 |
| Oat, Milk & Honey (Arnold) | 1 slice | 60 | tr |
| Oatmeal & Sunflower Seeds (Oatmeal Goodness) | 1 slice | 90 | 0 |
| Oatmeal & Bran (Oatmeal Goodness) | 1 slice | 90 | 0 |
| Oatmeal, Light (Arnold) | 1 slice | 40 | tr |
| Old Fashion (Freihofer's) | 1 slice | 70 | 0 |

| FOOD | PORTION | CALORIES | CHOLESTEROL |
|---|---|---|---|
| Pita, White, Regular Size (Sahara Bread) | 1 pocket (2 oz) | 160 | 0 |
| Pita, White, Mini Loaf (Sahara Bread) | 1 pocket (1 oz) | 80 | 0 |
| Pita, White, Large Size (Sahara Bread) | 1 pocket (3 oz) | 240 | 0 |
| Pita, Whole Wheat, Mini Loaf (Sahara Bread) | 1 pocket (1 oz) | 80 | 0 |
| Pita, Whole Wheat, Regular Size (Sahara Bread) | 1 pocket (2 oz) | 150 | 0 |
| Pumpernickel (Arnold) | 1 slice | 80 | 0 |
| Pumpernickel, Levy's (Arnold) | 1 slice | 80 | 0 |
| Raisin (Monks' Bread) | 1 slice | 70 | 0 |
| Raisin Tea Loaf (Arnold) | 1 slice | 70 | 2 |
| Raisin Orange (Arnold) | 1 slice | 70 | tr |
| Raisin, Sun Maid (Arnold) | 1 slice | 70 | 2 |
| Rite Diet (Freihofer's) | 2 slices | 90 | 0 |
| Rite Diet Wheat (Freihofer's) | 2 slices | 90 | 0 |
| Round Top (Roman Meal) | 1 slice | 67 | 0 |
| Rye, Dill, Seeded (Arnold) | 1 slice | 80 | 0 |
| Rye, Jewish, Seeded (Arnold) | 1 slice | 80 | 0 |

| FOOD | PORTION | CALORIES | CHOLESTEROL |
|---|---|---|---|
| Rye, Jewish, Unseeded (Arnold) | 1 slice | 80 | 0 |
| Rye, Levy's Real Jewish, Seeded (Arnold) | 1 slice | 80 | 0 |
| Rye, Levy's Real Jewish, Unseeded (Arnold) | 1 slice | 80 | 0 |
| Rye, Melba Thin (Arnold) | 1 slice | 40 | 0 |
| Rye, Stub Pullman (Freihofer's) | 1 slice | 70 | 0 |
| Sandwich Bread (Roman Meal) | 1 slice | 55 | 0 |
| Seven Grain (Roman Meal) | 1 slice | 68 | 0 |
| Seven Grain Light (Roman Meal) | 1 slice | 40 | 0 |
| Soft Rye Pumpernickel (Freihofer's) | 1 slice | 70 | 0 |
| Soft Rye, No Seeds (Freihofer's) | 1 slice | 70 | 0 |
| Soft Rye, Seeded (Freihofer's) | 1 slice | 70 | 0 |
| Soft Rye, Dill & Onion (Freihofer's) | 1 slice | 70 | 0 |
| Split Top Wheat (Freihofer's) | 1 slice | 70 | 0 |
| Split Top White (Freihofer's) | 1 slice | 70 | 0 |
| Sun Grain (Roman Meal) | 1 slice | 68 | 0 |

| FOOD | PORTION | CALORIES | CHOLESTEROL |
|------|---------|----------|-------------|
| Sunbeam King (Freihofer's) | 1 slice | 70 | 0 |
| Sunflower & Bran (Monks' Bread) | 1 slice | 70 | 0 |
| The Original (Freihofer's) | 1 slice | 70 | 0 |
| Wheat (Freihofer's) | 1½ slices | 70 | 0 |
| Wheat (Fresh Horizons) | 1 slice | 49 | 0 |
| Wheat Berry, Honey (Arnold) | 1 slice | 80 | tr |
| Wheat Cottage (America's Own) | 1 slice | 70 | 0 |
| Wheat Light (Roman Meal) | 1 slice | 40 | 0 |
| Wheat Oatmeal (Oatmeal Goodness) | 1 slice | 90 | 0 |
| Wheat, Brick Oven (Arnold) | 1 slice of 8 oz loaf | 60 | tr |
| Wheat, Brick Oven (Arnold) | 1 slice of 16 oz loaf | 60 | tr |
| Wheat, Brick Oven (Arnold) | 1 slice of 32 oz loaf | 90 | tr |
| Wheat, Golden Light (Arnold) | 1 slice | 40 | tr |
| Wheat, Less (Arnold) | 1 slice | 40 | 0 |
| Wheat, Small (Freihofer's) | 1½ slices | 70 | 0 |
| Wheat, Stone Ground 100% Whole (Arnold) | 1 slice | 50 | tr |

| FOOD | PORTION | CALORIES | CHOLESTEROL |
|------|---------|----------|-------------|
| Wheat, Stub Pullman (Freihofer's) | 1 slice | 70 | 0 |
| Wheat, Very Thin (Arnold) | 1 slice | 40 | tr |
| White (Freihofer's) | 1 slice | 70 | 0 |
| White (Fresh Horizons) | 1 slice | 50 | 0 |
| White (Monks' Bread) | 1 slice | 60 | 0 |
| White (Roman Meal) | 1 slice | 71 | 0 |
| White Cottage (America's Own) | 1 slice | 70 | 0 |
| White Light (Roman Meal) | 1 slice | 40 | 0 |
| White ½" Stub Pullman (Freihofer's) | 1 slice | 70 | 0 |
| White, 7/16" Stub Pullman (Freihofer's) | 1½ slices | 70 | 0 |
| White, Brick Oven (Arnold) | 1 slice of 8 oz loaf | 60 | tr |
| White, Brick Oven (Arnold) | 1 slice of 16 oz loaf | 60 | tr |
| White, Brick Oven (Arnold) | 1 slice of 32 oz loaf | 90 | tr |
| White, Country (Arnold) | 1 slice | 100 | tr |
| White, Less (Arnold) | 1 slice | 40 | 0 |
| White, Milk & Honey (Arnold) | 1 slice | 60 | tr |

| FOOD | PORTION | CALORIES | CHOLESTEROL |
|------|---------|----------|-------------|
| White, Very Thin (Arnold) | 1 slice | 40 | tr |
| Whole Wheat 100% (Freihofer's) | 1 slice | 75 | 0 |
| Whole Wheat 100% Stone Ground (Monks' Bread) | 1 slice | 70 | 0 |
| whole wheat | 1 slice | 56 | 1 |

## BREAD COATING

| FOOD | PORTION | CALORIES | CHOLESTEROL |
|------|---------|----------|-------------|
| Oven Fry Extra Crispy Recipe for Chicken (General Foods) | ¼ pkg (1 oz) | 111 | 0 |
| Oven Fry Extra Crispy Recipe for Pork (General Foods) | ¼ pkg (1 oz) | 115 | 0 |
| Oven Fry Light Crispy Homestyle Recipe (General Foods) | ¼ pkg (1 oz) | 107 | 0 |
| Shake 'N Bake Country Mild Recipe | ¼ pkg (½ oz) | 65 | 0 |
| Shake 'N Bake Italian Herb Recipe | ¼ pkg (½ oz) | 75 | tr |
| Shake 'N Bake Original Barbecue Recipe for Chicken | ¼ pkg (½ oz) | 90 | 0 |
| Shake 'N Bake Original Barbecue Recipe for Pork | ¼ pkg (½ oz) | 75 | 0 |
| Shake 'N Bake Original Recipe for Chicken | ¼ pkg (½ oz) | 75 | 0 |
| Shake 'N Bake Original Recipe for Fish | ¼ pkg (½ oz) | 74 | 0 |
| Shake 'N Bake Original Recipe for Pork | ¼ pkg (½ oz) | 80 | 0 |

| FOOD | PORTION | CALORIES | CHOLESTEROL |
|------|---------|----------|-------------|

## BREAD CRUMBS

| FOOD | PORTION | CALORIES | CHOLESTEROL |
|------|---------|----------|-------------|
| Contadina Seasoned | 1 rounded Tbsp | 35 | tr |
| Contadina Seasoned | 1 cup | 426 | tr |

## BREADFRUIT

| FOOD | PORTION | CALORIES | CHOLESTEROL |
|------|---------|----------|-------------|
| breadfruit | ¼ small | 99 | 0 |
| breadfruit | 3.5 oz | 109 | 0 |
| seeds; roasted | 1 oz | 59 | 0 |

## BREADSTICK

| FOOD | PORTION | CALORIES | CHOLESTEROL |
|------|---------|----------|-------------|
| Cheese Breadsticks (Lance) | 2 | 20 | 0 |
| Dunking Sticks (Lance) | 1⅜ oz | 190 | 0 |
| Garlic Breadsticks (Lance) | 2 | 30 | 0 |
| Plain Breadsticks (Lance) | 2 | 30 | 0 |
| Sesame Breadsticks (Lance) | 2 | 30 | 0 |
| breadstick | 1 med | 19 | 0 |
| onion poppyseed (home recipe) | 1 | 64 | 10 |

## BREAKFAST BAR
(see also BREAKFAST DRINKS, NUTRITIONAL SUPPLEMENTS)

| FOOD | PORTION | CALORIES | CHOLESTEROL |
|------|---------|----------|-------------|
| Chocolate Chip (Carnation) | 1 bar (1.44 oz) | 200 | tr |
| Chocolate Crunch (Carnation) | 1 bar (1.34 oz) | 190 | tr |

| FOOD | PORTION | CALORIES | CHOLESTEROL |
|------|---------|----------|-------------|
| Oat Bran Fruit Bar (Health Valley) | 1.5 oz | 140 | 0 |
| Peanut Butter Crunch (Carnation) | 1 bar (1.35 oz) | 190 | tr |
| Peanut Butter w/ Chocolate Chips (Carnation) | 1 bar (1.39 oz) | 200 | tr |

## BREAKFAST DRINKS
(*see also* BREAKFAST BAR, NUTRITIONAL SUPPLEMENTS)

| FOOD | PORTION | CALORIES | CHOLESTEROL |
|------|---------|----------|-------------|
| Chocolate Instant Breakfast (Carnation) | 1 pkg (1.25 oz) | 130 | 3 |
| Chocolate Instant Breakfast; as prep w/ whole milk (Carnation) | 1 pkg + 8 oz milk | 280 | 36 |
| Chocolate Instant Breakfast; as prep w/ skim milk (Carnation) | 1 pkg + 8 oz milk | 220 | 8 |
| Chocolate Instant Breakfast No Sugar Added (Carnation) | 1 pkg (.69 oz) | 70 | 2 |
| Chocolate Instant Breakfast No Sugar Added; as prep w/ skim milk (Carnation) | 1 pkg + 8 oz milk | 160 | 7 |
| Chocolate Malt Instant Breakfast (Carnation) | 1 pkg (1.24 oz) | 130 | 3 |
| Chocolate Malt Instant Breakfast; as prep w/ whole milk (Carnation) | 1 pkg + 8 oz milk | 280 | 36 |

| FOOD | PORTION | CALORIES | CHOLESTEROL |
| --- | --- | --- | --- |
| Chocolate Malt Instant Breakfast; as prep w/ skim milk (Carnation) | 1 pkg + 8 oz milk | 220 | 8 |
| Chocolate Malt Instant Breakfast No Sugar Added (Carnation) | 1 pkg (.71 oz) | 70 | 1 |
| Chocolate Malt Instant Breakfast No Sugar Added; as prep w/ skim milk (Carnation) | 1 pkg + 8 oz milk | 160 | 6 |
| Coffee Instant Breakfast (Carnation) | 1 pkg (1.26 oz) | 130 | 4 |
| Coffee Instant Breakfast; as prep w/ skim milk (Carnation) | 1 pkg + 8 oz milk | 220 | 9 |
| Coffee Instant Breakfast; as prep w/ whole milk (Carnation) | 1 pkg + 8 oz milk | 280 | 37 |
| Eggnog Instant Breakfast (Carnation) | 1 pkg (1.2 oz) | 130 | 15 |
| Eggnog Instant Breakfast; as prep w/ skim milk (Carnation) | 1 pkg + 8 oz milk | 220 | 20 |
| Eggnog Instant Breakfast; as prep w/ whole milk (Carnation) | 1 pkg + 8 oz milk | 280 | 48 |
| Strawberry Instant Breakfast (Carnation) | 1 pkg (1.25 oz) | 130 | 4 |
| Strawberry Instant Breakfast No Sugar Added (Carnation) | 1 pkg (.68 oz) | 70 | 3 |
| Strawberry Instant Breakfast; as prep w/ skim milk (Carnation) | 1 pkg + 8 oz milk | 220 | 9 |

| FOOD | PORTION | CALORIES | CHOLESTEROL |
|------|---------|----------|-------------|
| Strawberry Instant Breakfast; as prep w/ whole milk (Carnation) | 1 pkg + 8 oz milk | 280 | 37 |
| Strawberry Instant Breakfast No Sugar Added; as prep w/ skim milk (Carnation) | 1 pkg + 8 oz milk | 160 | 8 |
| Vanilla Instant Breakfast No Sugar Added (Carnation) | 1 pkg (.67 oz) | 70 | 3 |
| Vanilla Instant Breakfast No Sugar Added; as prep w/ skim milk (Carnation) | 1 pkg + 8 oz milk | 160 | 8 |
| Vanilla, Instant Breakfast (Carnation) | 1 pkg (1.23 oz) | 130 | 4 |
| Vanilla, Instant Breakfast: as prep w/ skim milk (Carnation) | 1 pkg + 8 oz skim milk | 220 | 9 |
| Vanilla, Instant Breakfast; as prep w/ whole milk (Carnation) | 1 pkg + 8 oz milk | 280 | 37 |
| orange drink powder; as prep w/ water | 6 oz | 86 | 0 |
| orange drink, powder | 3 rounded tsp | 93 | 0 |

## BROAD BEANS

| | | | |
|------|---------|----------|-------------|
| **CANNED** | | | |
| broad beans | 1 cup | 183 | 0 |
| **DRIED** | | | |
| cooked | 1 cup | 186 | 0 |
| raw | 1 cup | 511 | 0 |

| FOOD | PORTION | CALORIES | CHOLESTEROL |
|------|---------|----------|-------------|
| **FRESH** | | | |
| cooked | 3½ oz | 56 | 0 |
| raw | 1 cup | 79 | 0 |

## BROCCOLI

| FOOD | PORTION | CALORIES | CHOLESTEROL |
|------|---------|----------|-------------|
| **FRESH** | | | |
| raw; chopped | ½ cup | 12 | 0 |
| whole; cooked | ½ cup | 23 | 0 |
| **FROZEN** | | | |
| Baby Spears (Birds Eye) | ⅔ cup | 29 | 0 |
| Broccoli (Health Valley) | 3 oz | 24 | 0 |
| Broccoli Vegetable Crisp (Ore Ida) | 3 oz | 190 | 5 |
| Broccoli w/ Cheese Sauce (Birds Eye) | ½ cup | 115 | 6 |
| Broccoli w/ Creamy Italian Cheese Sauce (Birds Eye) | ½ cup | 90 | 14 |
| Chopped (Birds Eye) | ⅔ cup | 26 | 0 |
| Cut (Hanover) | ½ cup | 25 | 0 |
| Cuts (Birds Eye) | ⅔ cup | 25 | 0 |
| Florets (Birds Eye) | ⅔ cup | 26 | 0 |
| Florets (Hanover) | ½ cup | 30 | 0 |
| Spears (Birds Eye) | ⅔ cup | 26 | 0 |

| FOOD | PORTION | CALORIES | CHOLESTEROL |
|------|---------|----------|-------------|
| frzn; cooked | ½ cup | 25 | 0 |
| frzn; not prep | 10 oz pkg | 75 | 0 |
| spears; cooked | ½ cup | 69 | 0 |
| spears; not prep | 10 oz pkg | 84 | 0 |

## BROWNIE

| FOOD | PORTION | CALORIES | CHOLESTEROL |
|------|---------|----------|-------------|
| Estee Brownie Mix; as prep | 1 (2"x2") | 45 | 30 |
| Lance Brownie | 1 pkg (1¾ oz) | 200 | 5 |
| Little Debbie Fudge Brownies | 1 pkg (2 oz) | 240 | tr |
| Little Debbie Fudge Brownies | 1 pkg (2.9 oz) | 350 | tr |
| brownie w/ nuts (home recipe) | 1 (.8 oz) | 97 | 15 |

## BRUSSELS SPROUTS

| FOOD | PORTION | CALORIES | CHOLESTEROL |
|------|---------|----------|-------------|
| **FRESH** | | | |
| cooked | ½ cup | 30 | 0 |
| raw | ½ cup | 19 | 0 |
| **FROZEN** | | | |
| Baby Brussels Sprouts w/ Cheese Sauce (Birds Eye) | ½ cup | 113 | 5 |
| Brussels Sprouts (Birds Eye) | ½ cup | 37 | 0 |
| Brussels Sprouts (Hanover) | ½ cup | 40 | 0 |
| frzn; cooked | ½ cup | 33 | 0 |
| frzn; not prep | 10 oz | 116 | 0 |

| FOOD | PORTION | CALORIES | CHOLESTEROL |
|------|---------|----------|-------------|

# BULGUR

| bulgur; not prep | 1 cup | 605 | 0 |

# BURBOT (FISH)

**FRESH**

| raw | 1 fillet (4.1 oz) | 104 | 69 |
| raw | 3 oz | 76 | 51 |

# BURDOCK ROOT

| cooked | 1 cup | 110 | 0 |
| raw | 1 cup | 85 | 0 |

# BUTTER
(*see also* BUTTER BLENDS, BUTTER SUBSTITUTE, MARGARINE)

**REGULAR**

| Land O'Lakes, Lightly Salted | 1 Tbsp | 100 | 30 |
| Land O'Lakes, Unsalted | 1 Tbsp | 100 | 30 |
| butter | 4 oz | 813 | 248 |
| butter | 1 pat | 36 | 11 |
| butter | 1 stick | 813 | 248 |
| butter | 1 tsp | 36 | 11 |
| butter oil | 1 cup | 1795 | 524 |
| butter oil | 1 Tbsp | 112 | 33 |
| clarified butter | 3½ oz | 876 | 256 |

**WHIPPED**

| Land O'Lakes, Lightly Salted | 1 Tbsp | 60 | 20 |
| Land O'Lakes, Unsalted | 1 Tbsp | 60 | 20 |
| butter | 1 tsp | 27 | 8 |
| butter | 4 oz | 542 | 165 |

| FOOD | PORTION | CALORIES | CHOLESTEROL |
|------|---------|----------|-------------|

## BUTTER BEANS

| | | | |
|------|---------|----------|-------------|
| CANNED | | | |
| Butter Beans (Hanover) | ½ cup | 80 | 0 |
| Butter Beans in Sauce (Hanover) | ½ cup | 100 | 0 |
| Butter Beans Tender Cooked (S&W) | ½ cup | 100 | 0 |

## BUTTER BLENDS
(*see also* BUTTER, BUTTER SUBSTITUTE, MARGARINE)

| | | | |
|------|---------|----------|-------------|
| REGULAR | | | |
| Blue Bonnet | 1 Tbsp | 90 | 5 |
| Blue Bonnet, Unsalted | 1 Tbsp | 90 | 5 |
| Country Morning Blend, Lightly Salted | 1 Tbsp | 100 | 10 |
| Country Morning Blend, Unsalted | 1 Tbsp | 100 | 10 |
| SOFT | | | |
| Blue Bonnet | 1 Tbsp | 90 | 5 |
| Country Morning Blend, Lightly Salted | 1 Tbsp | 90 | 10 |
| Country Morning Blend, Unsalted | 1 Tbsp | 90 | 10 |

## BUTTER SUBSTITUTE
(*see also* BUTTER, BUTTER BLENDS, MARGARINE)

| | | | |
|------|---------|----------|-------------|
| Butter Buds | ⅛ oz | 12 | 0 |
| Butter Buds Sprinkles | ½ tsp | 4 | 0 |
| Molly McButter All Natural Butter Flavor Sprinkles | ½ tsp | 4 | 0 |

| FOOD | PORTION | CALORIES | CHOLESTEROL |
|------|---------|----------|-------------|
| Molly McButter Natural Sour Cream & Butter Flavor Sprinkles | ½ tsp | 4 | 0 |

## BUTTERFISH

| | | | |
|------|---------|----------|-------------|
| raw | 3 oz | 124 | 55 |
| raw | 1 fillet (1.1 oz) | 47 | 21 |

## BUTTERNUTS

| | | | |
|------|---------|----------|-------------|
| dried | 1 oz | 174 | 0 |

## CABBAGE

**FRESH**

| | | | |
|------|---------|----------|-------------|
| chinese cabbage (pak-choi), raw; shredded | 1 cup | 9 | 0 |
| chinese cabbage (pe-tsai), raw; shredded | 1 cup | 12 | 0 |
| chinese cabbage (pe-tsai); shredded, cooked | 1 cup | 16 | 0 |
| chinese cabbage; shredded, cooked | ½ cup | 10 | 0 |
| coleslaw | ½ cup | 42 | 0 |
| green, raw; shredded | ½ cup | 8 | 0 |
| green; shredded, cooked | ½ cup | 16 | 0 |
| red, raw; shredded | ½ cup | 10 | 0 |
| red; shredded, cooked | ½ cup | 16 | 0 |
| savoy, raw; shredded | ½ cup | 10 | 0 |
| savoy; shredded, cooked | ½ cup | 18 | 0 |

**HOME RECIPE**

| | | | |
|------|---------|----------|-------------|
| stuffed cabbage | 1 (6 oz) | 373 | 95 |

| FOOD | PORTION | CALORIES | CHOLESTEROL |
|------|---------|----------|-------------|

# CAKE
(*see also* BROWNIE, COOKIE, DANISH PASTRY, DOUGHNUT, PIE)

### FROSTING/ICING

| FOOD | PORTION | CALORIES | CHOLESTEROL |
|------|---------|----------|-------------|
| Frosting Mix; as prep (Estee) | 1½ Tbsp | 50–60 | 0 |
| caramel (home recipe) | 1 cup | 895 | 0 |
| chocolate (home recipe) | 1 cup | 1123 | 75 |
| coconut fluff (home recipe) | 1 cup | 533 | 77 |
| white boiled (home recipe) | 1 cup | 247 | 0 |
| white uncooked (home recipe) | 1 cup | 813 | 60 |

### FROZEN

| FOOD | PORTION | CALORIES | CHOLESTEROL |
|------|---------|----------|-------------|
| Cheese Cherry French Cream (Sara Lee) | 1 piece (3 oz) | 254 | 68 |
| Pound Cake Cholesterol Free (Pepperidge Farm) | 1 slice (1 oz) | 110 | 0 |
| eclair w/ chocolate icing & custard filling, frzn | 1 | 205 | 35 |

### HOME RECIPE

| FOOD | PORTION | CALORIES | CHOLESTEROL |
|------|---------|----------|-------------|
| apple cake | 1.5 oz piece | 145 | 21 |
| baklava | 1 oz | 126 | 23 |
| Boston cream | ⅛ of 9″ cake | 433 | 158 |
| carrot w/ cream cheese icing | 1 cake, 10″ diam tube | 6175 | 1183 |
| carrot w/ cream cheese icing | 1/16 of cake | 385 | 74 |
| chocolate cupcake | 1 (1.1 oz) | 103 | 21 |

| FOOD | PORTION | CALORIES | CHOLESTEROL |
|---|---|---|---|
| chocolate cupcake w/ chocolate icing | 1 (1.6 oz) | 175 | 32 |
| cobbler, peach | ½ cup | 201 | 35 |
| cream puff, shell only | 1 (2.3 oz) | 156 | 100 |
| hot cross bun | 1 (1.8 oz) | 172 | 39 |
| kuchen | 2¼"x2¼" (3.3 oz) | 315 | 84 |
| peanut butter | 1 piece (1.8 oz) | 211 | 22 |
| spice w/ caramel icing | ⅒ of 9" cake | 411 | 61 |
| sponge | ⅟₁₂ of 8½" cake | 135 | 48 |
| strudel | 1 piece (4.1 oz) | 272 | 39 |
| torte, chocolate | ⅟₁₆ of 8½" diam (3.2 oz) | 317 | 61 |
| white cupcake | 1 (1.1 oz) | 114 | 1 |
| white cupcake w/ white icing | 1 (1.6 oz) | 164 | 6 |
| yellow cupcake | 1 (1.1 oz) | 127 | 17 |
| yellow cupcake w/ chocolate icing | 1 (1.6 oz) | 186 | 28 |
| MIX<br>Angel Food; as prep (Duncan Hines) | ⅟₁₂ cake | 140 | 0 |
| Angel Food Chocolate (General Mills) | ⅟₁₂ cake | 150 | 0 |
| Angel Food Confetti (General Mills) | ⅟₁₂ cake | 160 | 0 |
| Angel Food Lemon Custard (General Mills) | ⅟₁₂ cake | 150 | 0 |

| FOOD | PORTION | CALORIES | CHOLESTEROL |
|---|---|---|---|
| Angel Food Strawberry (General Mills) | 1/12 cake | 150 | 0 |
| Angel Food Traditional (General Mills) | 1/12 cake | 130 | 0 |
| Angel Food White (General Mills) | 1/12 cake | 150 | 0 |
| Bisquick (General Mills) | 2 oz | 230 | 0 |
| Cheesecake No Bake Dessert; as prep (Jell-O) | 1/8 cake | 281 | 28 |
| Chocolate Lite Cake & Frosting Mix (Batter Lite) | 1/9 of cake | 110 | 0 |
| Chocolate; as prep (Estee) | 1/10 cake | 100 | 0 |
| Coffee Cake Easy Mix; as prep (Aunt Jemima) | 1/8 cake | 170 | 12 |
| White Lite Cake & Frosting Mix (Batter Lite) | 1/9 of cake | 110 | 0 |
| Yellow Cake Mix Microwave; as prep (Pillsbury) | 1/8 cake | 220 | 10 |
| yellow w/ chocolate frosting; as prep | 1 cake, 9" diam | 3735 | 576 |
| yellow w/ chocolate frosting; as prep | 1/16 of cake | 235 | 36 |
| READY-TO-USE Cheesecake La Creame Amaretto Almond (Formagg) | 2 oz | 115 | 0 |

| FOOD | PORTION | CALORIES | CHOLESTEROL |
|------|---------|----------|-------------|
| Cheesecake La Creame Pineapple (Formagg) | 2 oz | 115 | 0 |
| Cheesecake La Creame Plain (Formagg) | 2 oz | 115 | 0 |
| Cheesecake La Creame Strawberry (Formagg) | 2 oz | 115 | 0 |
| angel food | 1 cake, 9¾" diam | 1510 | 0 |
| angel food | 1/12 of cake | 125 | 0 |
| cheesecake | 1 cake, 9" diam | 3350 | 2053 |
| cheesecake | 1/12 of cake | 280 | 170 |
| cream puff w/ custard filling | 1 (4.6 oz) | 303 | 187 |
| crumb coffeecake | 1 cake, 7¾" × 5⅝" | 1385 | 279 |
| crumb coffeecake | 1/6 of cake | 230 | 47 |
| devil's food w/ chocolate frosting | 1 cake, 2" layers | 3755 | 598 |
| devil's food cupcake w/ chocolate frosting | 1 | 120 | 19 |
| devil's food w/ chocolate frosting | 1/16 of cake | 235 | 37 |
| fruitcake, dark | 1 cake, 7½"x2¼" tube | 5185 | 640 |
| fruitcake, dark | ⅔ slice | 165 | 20 |
| gingerbread | 1 cake, 8" sq | 1575 | 6 |

| FOOD | PORTION | CALORIES | CHOLESTEROL |
|------|---------|----------|-------------|
| gingerbread | ⅑ cake | 175 | 1 |
| pound | 1 loaf, 8½"x3½" | 1935 | 1100 |
| sheet cake w/ white frosting | ⅑ of cake | 445 | 70 |
| sheet cake w/ white frosting | 1 cake, 9" sq | 4020 | 636 |
| sheet cake w/o frosting | 1 cake, 9" sq | 2830 | 552 |
| sheet cake w/o frosting | ⅑ of cake | 315 | 61 |
| **SNACK** | | | |
| Apple Delights (Little Debbie) | 1 pkg (1.25 oz) | 140 | tr |
| Banana Slices (Little Debbie) | 1 pkg (3 oz) | 340 | tr |
| Banana Twins (Little Debbie) | 1 pkg (2.2 oz) | 250 | tr |
| Be My Valentine (Little Debbie) | 1 pkg (2.5 oz) | 330 | tr |
| Big Wheels (Hostess) | 2 | 345 | 14 |
| Caravella (Little Debbie) | 1 pkg (1.2 oz) | 170 | tr |
| Choc-O-Jel (Little Debbie) | 1 pkg (1.16 oz) | 150 | tr |
| Chocolate Cakes (Little Debbie) | 1 pkg (2.4 oz) | 320 | tr |
| Chocolate Twins (Little Debbie) | 1 pkg (2.2 oz) | 240 | tr |
| Christmas Tree Cakes (Little Debbie) | 1 pkg (1.6 oz) | 220 | tr |

| FOOD | PORTION | CALORIES | CHOLESTEROL |
|---|---|---|---|
| Coconut Crunch (Little Debbie) | 1 pkg (2 oz) | 320 | 1 |
| Coconut Rounds (Little Debbie) | 1 pkg (1.13 oz) | 150 | 1 |
| Crumb Cake (Hostess) | 2 cakes | 259 | 21 |
| Cupcake Chocolate (Hostess) | 2 cupcakes | 314 | 10 |
| Cupcake Orange (Hostess) | 2 cupcakes | 294 | 25 |
| Debbie Doodle Dandies (Little Debbie) | 1 pkg (2.5 oz) | 320 | tr |
| Dessert Cups (Little Debbie) | 1 pkg (.79 oz) | 80 | tr |
| Devil Cremes (Little Debbie) | 1 pkg (1.3 oz) | 160 | tr |
| Devil Slices (Little Debbie) | 1 pkg (3 oz) | 320 | tr |
| Devil Squares (Little Debbie) | 1 pkg (2.2 oz) | 270 | tr |
| Devil's Food Cupcake (Hostess) | 1 (1.5 oz) | 136 | 4 |
| Ding Dongs (Hostess) | 2 | 345 | 14 |
| Dutch Apple (Little Debbie) | 1 pkg (2.17 oz) | 230 | tr |
| Dutch Apple (Little Debbie) | 1 pkg (2.5 oz) | 270 | tr |
| Easter Bunny Cakes (Little Debbie) | 1 pkg (2.5 oz) | 320 | tr |
| Fancy Cakes (Little Debbie) | 1 pkg (2.6 oz) | 340 | tr |

| FOOD | PORTION | CALORIES | CHOLESTEROL |
|---|---|---|---|
| Fig Cake (Lance) | 2⅛ oz | 210 | 0 |
| Figaroos (Little Debbie) | 1 pkg (1.5 oz) | 160 | tr |
| Fudge Crispy (Little Debbie) | 1 pkg (2.08 oz) | 260 | tr |
| Fudge Rounds (Little Debbie) | 1 pkg (1.19 oz) | 150 | tr |
| Fudge Rounds (Little Debbie) | 1 pkg (2.75 oz) | 330 | tr |
| Golden Cremes (Little Debbie) | 1 pkg (1.4 oz) | 150 | tr |
| Golden Cremes (Little Debbie) | 1 pkg (2.5 oz) | 270 | tr |
| Hoho (Hostess) | 1 (1 oz) | 119 | 13 |
| Holiday Cakes Chocolate (Little Debbie) | 1 pkg (2.5 oz) | 320 | tr |
| Holiday Cakes Vanilla (Little Debbie) | 1 pkg (2.5 oz) | 320 | tr |
| Ice Cream Cups (Little Debbie) | 1 pkg (.15 oz) | 15 | tr |
| Jelly Rolls (Little Debbie) | 1 pkg (2.2 oz) | 250 | tr |
| Lemon Stix (Little Debbie) | 1 pkg (1.5 oz) | 220 | tr |
| Marshmallow Supremes (Little Debbie) | 1 pkg (1.1 oz) | 130 | tr |
| Mint Sprints (Little Debbie) | 1 pkg (1.33 oz) | 200 | tr |
| Nutty Bar (Little Debbie) | 1 pkg (2 oz) | 310 | tr |

| FOOD | PORTION | CALORIES | CHOLESTEROL |
|------|---------|----------|-------------|
| Nutty Bar (Little Debbie) | 1 pkg (2.5 oz) | 390 | tr |
| Nutty Wafers (Little Debbie) | 1 pkg (2 oz) | 310 | tr |
| Peanut Butter Bars (Little Debbie) | 1 pkg (1.83 oz) | 260 | tr |
| Peanut Butter Bars (Little Debbie) | 1 pkg (2.5 oz) | 370 | tr |
| Peanut Clusters (Little Debbie) | 1 pkg (1.5 oz) | 220 | tr |
| Pecan Twins (Little Debbie) | 1 pkg (2 oz) | 220 | tr |
| Pumpkin Delights (Little Debbie) | 1 pkg (1.1 oz) | 140 | tr |
| Snack Cakes Chocolate (Little Debbie) | 1 pkg (2.5 oz) | 320 | tr |
| Snack Cakes Chocolate (Little Debbie) | 1 pkg (3 oz) | 390 | tr |
| Snack Cakes Vanilla (Little Debbie) | 1 pkg (2.6 oz) | 330 | tr |
| Snack Cakes Vanilla (Little Debbie) | 1 pkg (3 oz) | 390 | tr |
| Snoball (Hostess) | 1 (1.5 oz) | 136 | 2 |
| Spice Cakes (Little Debbie) | 1 pkg (2.2 oz) | 270 | tr |
| Star Crunch (Little Debbie) | 1 pkg (1.08 oz) | 150 | tr |
| Swiss Cake Roll (Little Debbie) | 1 pkg (2.17 oz) | 270 | tr |
| Swiss Rolls (Little Debbie) | 1 pkg (2.25 oz) | 280 | tr |

| FOOD | PORTION | CALORIES | CHOLESTEROL |
| --- | --- | --- | --- |
| Turnover Apple, frzn (Lamb-Weston) | 3 oz | 230 | 10 |
| Turnover Blueberry, frzn (Lamb-Weston) | 3 oz | 260 | 10 |
| Turnover Cherry, frzn (Lamb-Weston) | 3 oz | 260 | 10 |
| Twinkie (Hostess) | 1 (1.5 oz) | 144 | 21 |
| toaster pastries | 1 (1.9 oz) | 210 | 0 |

## CANADIAN BACON

| FOOD | PORTION | CALORIES | CHOLESTEROL |
| --- | --- | --- | --- |
| Oscar Mayer | 1 slice (28 g) | 35 | 12 |
| Canadian bacon; grilled | 2 slices (1.7 oz) | 86 | 27 |
| Canadian bacon; unheated | 2 slices (1.9 oz) | 89 | 28 |

## CANDY

| FOOD | PORTION | CALORIES | CHOLESTEROL |
| --- | --- | --- | --- |
| 3 Musketeers Bar | 2.1 | 260 | 5 |
| Baby Ruth (Nabisco) | 1 oz | 130 | 0 |
| Bar None Candy Bar (Hershey) | 1.5 oz | 240 | 5 |
| Barat Bar | 1 (2 oz) | 340 | 0 |
| Bridge Mix (Nabisco) | 1 oz | 126 | tr |
| Butter Mints (Kraft) | 1 | 8 | 0 |
| Butterfinger | 1 oz | 130 | 0 |

| FOOD | PORTION | CALORIES | CHOLESTEROL |
|---|---|---|---|
| Caramels (Kraft) | 1 | 35 | 0 |
| Chocolate Fudgies (Kraft) | 1 | 35 | 0 |
| Chocolate Bar (Estee) | 2 squares | 60 | 2 |
| Chocolate Coated Raisins (Estee) | 6 pieces | 30 | tr |
| Chocolaty Peanut Bar (Lance) | 2 oz | 320 | 0 |
| Crunch 'N Munch Candied (Franklin) | 1.25 oz | 170 | 0 |
| Crunch 'N Munch Caramel | 1.25 oz | 160 | 13 |
| Crunch 'N Munch Maple Walnut (Franklin) | 1.25 oz | 160 | 6 |
| Crunch 'N Munch Toffee (Franklin) | 1.25 oz | 160 | 6 |
| Crunch Chocolate Bar (Estee) | 2 squares | 45 | 2 |
| Estee-ets (Estee) | 5 pieces | 35 | tr |
| Fruit and Nut Mix (Estee) | 4 pieces | 35 | tr |
| Gum Drops (Estee) | 4 pieces | 25 | 0 |
| Gummy Bears (Estee) | 4 pieces | 20 | 0 |
| Hard Candy (Estee) | 2 | 25 | 0 |
| Hard Candy Sugar Free (Louis Sherry) | 2 pieces | 25 | 0 |

| FOOD | PORTION | CALORIES | CHOLESTEROL |
|---|---|---|---|
| Hershey's Kisses | 9 pieces | 220 | 10 |
| Kit Kat Wafer (Hershey) | 1.625 oz | 250 | 10 |
| Krackel Chocolate Bar (Hershey) | 1.65 oz | 250 | 10 |
| Life Saver | 1 piece | 8 | 0 |
| Lollipops (Estee) | 2 | 12 | 0 |
| Lollipops Sugar Free (Louis Sherry) | 1 | 18 | 0 |
| M&M's, Peanut | 1.7 oz | 250 | 5 |
| M&M's, Plain | 1.7 oz | 240 | 8 |
| Mars Bar | 1.8 oz | 240 | 6 |
| Milk Chocolate Bar (Hershey) | 1.65 oz | 250 | 15 |
| Milk Way Bar | 2.2 oz | 290 | 9 |
| Mints (Estee) | 1 | 4 | 0 |
| Mr. GoodBar Chocolate Bar (Hershey) | 1.85 oz | 300 | 15 |
| Munch Bar | 1.4 oz | 220 | 6 |
| NECCO Mint Lozenges | 1 piece | 12 | 0 |
| Party Mints (Kraft) | 1 | 8 | 0 |
| Peanut Bar (Lance) | 1¾ oz | 260 | 0 |
| Peanut Brittle (Kraft) | 1 oz | 140 | 0 |
| Peanut Butter Cups (Estee) | 1 | 45 | tr |

| FOOD | PORTION | CALORIES | CHOLESTEROL |
|---|---|---|---|
| Peppermint Pattie Chocolate Covered (Nabisco) | 1 (½ oz) | 64 | tr |
| Reese's Pieces Candy (Hershey) | 1.95 oz | 270 | 5 |
| Rolo Caramels in Milk Chocolate (Hershey) | 9 pieces | 270 | 15 |
| Skittles | 2 oz | 320 | 0 |
| Skor Toffee Bar (Hershey) | 1.4 oz | 220 | 25 |
| Snickers Bar | 2.2 oz | 290 | 9 |
| Special Dark Sweet Chocolate Bar (Hershey) | 1.45 | 220 | 5 |
| Starburst Fruit Chews | 2 oz | 240 | 0 |
| Starburst Fruit Fruit Chews Strawberry | 2.07 oz | 240 | 0 |
| Thin Mint (Nabisco) | 1 (10 g) | 42 | 0 |
| Toffee (Kraft) | 1 | 30 | 0 |
| Tootsie Roll Miniature | 1 (6 g) | 24 | 0 |
| Twix Cookie Bar, Caramel | 2 bars (2 oz) | 140 | 3 |
| Twix Cookie Bar, Peanut Butter | 2 bars (1.8 oz) | 130 | tr |
| Velamints | 1 mint | 9 | 0 |
| Velamints Cocoamint | 1 mint | 8 | 0 |
| candy corn | ¼ cup | 182 | 0 |
| chocolate covered raisins | 1 oz | 121 | 2 |

| FOOD | PORTION | CALORIES | CHOLESTEROL |
|---|---|---|---|
| gum drop | 1 | 7 | 0 |
| hard candy ball | 1 | 19 | 0 |
| jelly beans | ¼ cup | 202 | 0 |
| licorice | 1 stick (10 g) | 35 | 0 |
| lollipop | 1 (1 oz) | 110 | 0 |
| malted milk balls, chocolate coated | 1 | 25 | 1 |
| mint fondant pattie | 1 (9 g) | 32 | 0 |
| peanut brittle | 1 oz | 120 | 0 |

## CANTALOUPE

FRESH
| | | | |
|---|---|---|---|
| Chiquita | 1 cup | 70 | 0 |
| cantaloupe | ½ | 94 | 0 |
| cubed | 1 cup | 57 | 0 |

## CARAMBOLA

FRESH
| | | | |
|---|---|---|---|
| carambola | 1 | 42 | 0 |

## CARDOON

FRESH
| | | | |
|---|---|---|---|
| cooked | 3½ oz | 22 | 0 |
| raw; shredded | 1 cup | 36 | 0 |

## CAROB

| | | | |
|---|---|---|---|
| carob flavor mix; as prep w/ whole milk | 8 oz | 195 | 33 |

| FOOD | PORTION | CALORIES | CHOLESTEROL |
|------|---------|----------|-------------|
| carob mix | 3 tsp | 45 | 0 |
| flour | 1 cup | 185 | 0 |
| flour | 1 Tbsp | 14 | 0 |

## CARP

FRESH

| | | | |
|------|---------|----------|-------------|
| cooked | 3 oz | 138 | 72 |
| cooked | 1 fillet (6 oz) | 276 | 143 |
| raw | 1 fillet (7.6 oz) | 276 | 143 |
| raw | 3 oz | 108 | 56 |
| roe, raw | 3½ oz | 130 | 360 |

## CARROT

CANNED

| | | | |
|------|---------|----------|-------------|
| Diced (Libby) | ½ cup | 20 | 0 |
| Diced (Seneca) | ½ cup | 20 | 0 |
| Diced Fancy (S&W) | ½ cup | 30 | 0 |
| Julienne French Style Fancy (S&W) | ½ cup | 30 | 0 |
| Sliced (Libby) | ½ cup | 20 | 0 |
| Sliced (Seneca) | ½ cup | 20 | 0 |
| Whole Tiny Fancy (S&W) | ½ cup | 30 | 0 |
| carrots | ½ cup | 17 | 0 |

| FOOD | PORTION | CALORIES | CHOLESTEROL |
|---|---|---|---|
| **FRESH** | | | |
| cooked | ½ cup | 35 | 0 |
| raw | 1 | 31 | 0 |
| **FROZEN** | | | |
| Crinkle Sliced (Hanover) | ½ cup | 35 | 0 |
| Whole Baby (Birds Eye) | ½ cup | 40 | 0 |
| carrots; cooked | ½ cup | 26 | 0 |
| sliced; not prep | ½ cup | 25 | 0 |
| **JUICE** | | | |
| carrot juice | 6 fl oz | 73 | 0 |

## CASABA

| | | | |
|---|---|---|---|
| **FRESH** | | | |
| cubed | 1 cup | 45 | 0 |

## CASHEWS

| | | | |
|---|---|---|---|
| Cashews (Beer Nuts) | 1 oz | 170 | 0 |
| Cashews (Lance) | 1⅛ oz | 190 | 0 |
| Cashews, Long Tube (Lance) | 1¼ oz | 200 | 0 |
| Dry Roasted (Planters) | 1 oz | 160 | 0 |
| Dry Roasted, Unsalted (Planters) | 1 oz | 160 | 0 |
| Fancy Oil Roasted (Planters) | 1 oz | 170 | 0 |

| FOOD | PORTION | CALORIES | CHOLESTEROL |
|---|---|---|---|
| Halves Oil Roasted, Unsalted (Planters) | 1 oz | 170 | 0 |
| Halves Oil Roasted (Planters) | 1 oz | 170 | 0 |
| Honey Roasted (Planters) | 1 oz | 170 | 0 |
| Honey Toasted (Lance) | 1⅛ oz | 200 | 0 |
| Honey Toasted Tube (Lance) | 1¹⁄₁₆ oz | 200 | 0 |
| Whole, Salted (Guy's) | 1 oz | 170 | 0 |
| cashew butter | 1 oz | 167 | 0 |
| cashew butter | 1 Tbsp | 94 | 0 |
| dry roasted | 1 oz | 163 | 0 |
| oil roasted | 1 oz | 163 | 0 |

## CASSAVA

FRESH
| raw | 3½ oz | 120 | 0 |
|---|---|---|---|

## CATFISH

FRESH
| channel, raw | 1 fillet (2.8 oz) | 92 | 46 |
|---|---|---|---|
| channel, raw | 3 oz | 99 | 49 |

HOME RECIPE
| channel; breaded & fried | 3 oz | 194 | 69 |
|---|---|---|---|
| channel; breaded & fried | 1 fillet (3.1 oz) | 199 | 70 |

| FOOD | PORTION | CALORIES | CHOLESTEROL |
|------|---------|----------|-------------|
| **CATSUP** | | | |
| Estee | 1 Tbsp | 6 | 0 |
| Health Valley | 1 Tbsp | 16 | 0 |
| Health Valley No Salt Added | 1 Tbsp | 16 | 0 |
| Smucker's | 1 tsp | 8 | 0 |
| Tillie Lewis Low Sodium, Low Calorie | 1 Tbsp | 8 | 0 |
| **CAULIFLOWER** | | | |
| FRESH | | | |
| cooked | ½ cup | 15 | 0 |
| raw | ½ cup | 12 | 0 |
| FROZEN | | | |
| Cauliflower (Birds Eye) | ⅔ cup | 23 | 0 |
| Cauliflower (Hanover) | ½ cup | 20 | 0 |
| Cauliflower Vegetable Crisp (Ore Ida) | 3 oz | 150 | 5 |
| Cauliflower in Cheddar Cheese Sauce (Budget Gourmet) | 5 oz | 110 | 25 |
| Cauliflower w/ Cheese Sauce (Birds Eye) | ½ cup | 113 | 6 |
| Florets (Hanover) | ½ cup | 20 | 0 |
| frzn; cooked | ½ cup | 17 | 0 |
| frzn; not prep | ½ cup | 16 | 0 |

| FOOD | PORTION | CALORIES | CHOLESTEROL |
|------|---------|----------|-------------|

## CAVIAR

| red granular | 1 Tbsp | 40 | 94 |
| red granular | 1 oz | 71 | 165 |
| sturgeon, granular | 1 Tbsp | 42 | 48 |

## CELERIC

**FRESH**

| cooked | 3½ oz | 25 | 0 |
| raw | ½ cup | 31 | 0 |

## CELERY

**FRESH**

| diced, cooked | ½ cup | 11 | 0 |
| raw | 1 stalk | 6 | 0 |

## CELTUCE

**FRESH**

| raw | 3½ oz | 22 | 0 |

## CEREAL
(*see also* GRANOLA)

Cup measurements represent approximately a 1 oz serving.

**COOKED**

| Barley Plus (Erewhon) | 1 oz | 110 | 0 |
| Brown Rice Cream (Erewhon) | 1 oz | 110 | 0 |
| Cream of Wheat Instant (Nabisco) | ¾ cup | 110 | 0 |

| FOOD | PORTION | CALORIES | CHOLESTEROL |
|---|---|---|---|
| Cream of Wheat Mix 'n Eat, flavored; not prep (Nabisco) | 1 pkg (1¼ oz) | 132 | 0 |
| Cream of Wheat Mix 'n Eat, plain; not prep (Nabisco) | 1 pkg (1 oz) | 103 | 0 |
| Cream of Wheat Quick (Nabisco) | ¾ cup | 110 | 0 |
| Cream of Wheat Regular (Nabisco) | ¾ cup | 114 | 0 |
| Farina Hot 'n Creamy; not prep (Quaker) | 1 oz | 101 | 0 |
| Hominy Quick Grits; uncooked (Albers) | ¼ cup | 150 | 0 |
| Maltex (Standard Milling) | ½ cup | 86 | 0 |
| Maypo 30 Second (Standard Milling) | ½ cup | 110 | 0 |
| Maypo Vermont Style (Standard Milling) | ½ cup | 90 | 0 |
| Oat Bran Hot Cereal (Health Valley) | 1 oz | 100 | 0 |
| Oat Bran w/ Toasted Wheat Germ (Erewhon) | 1 oz | 115 | 0 |
| Oat Bran; not prep (Quaker) | ⅓ cup | 90 | 0 |
| Oatmeal Instant Apple Cinnamon (Erewhon) | 1 oz | 145 | 0 |
| Oatmeal Instant Apple Raisin (Erewhon) | 1 oz | 150 | 0 |

| FOOD | PORTION | CALORIES | CHOLESTEROL |
|---|---|---|---|
| Oatmeal Instant Maple Spice (Erewhon) | 1 oz | 140 | 0 |
| Oatmeal Instant w/ Apples & Cinnamon; not prep (Quaker) | 1 pkg (1¼ oz) | 133 | 0 |
| Oatmeal Instant w/ Cinnamon & Spices; not prep (Quaker) | 1 pkg (1⅝ oz) | 176 | 0 |
| Oatmeal Instant w/ Cinnamon Spice; not prep (Ralston) | 1 pkg (1⅝ oz) | 176 | 0 |
| Oatmeal Instant w/ Maple & Brown Sugar; not prep (Quaker) | 1 pkg (1½ oz) | 161 | 0 |
| Oatmeal Instant w/ Maple & Brown Sugar; not prep (Ralston) | 1 pkg (1⅝ oz) | 175 | 0 |
| Oatmeal Instant; not prep (Quaker) | 1 pkg (½ oz) | 105 | 0 |
| Oatmeal Instant; not prep (Ralston) | 1 pkg (1 oz) | 110 | 0 |
| Oatmeal Quick or Old Fashioned; not prep (Quaker) | 1 cup | 307 | 0 |
| Oatmeal Quick or Regular; not prep (Quaker) | 1 cup | 442 | 0 |
| Oats, Old Fashioned; not prep (Roman Meal) | ⅓ cup (1 oz) | 100 | 0 |
| Oats, Quick; not prep (Roman Meal) | ⅓ cup (1 oz) | 100 | 0 |
| Oats, Quick & Regular (Ralston) | ⅔ cup | 110 | 0 |

| FOOD | PORTION | CALORIES | CHOLESTEROL |
|---|---|---|---|
| Oats, Wheat, Dates, Raisins, Almonds Cereal; not prep (Roman Meal) | ⅓ cup (1.3 oz) | 140 | 0 |
| Oats, Wheat, Honey, Coconut, Almonds Cereal; not prep (Roman Meal) | ⅓ cup (1.3 oz) | 150 | 0 |
| Oats, Wheat, Rye Flax Cereal; not prep (Roman Meal) | ⅓ cup (1 oz) | 90 | 0 |
| Original Cereal w/ Wheat, Rye, Bran, Flax; not prep (Roman Meal) | ⅓ cup (1 oz) | 80 | 0 |
| Pettijohns (Quaker) | ½ cup | 93 | 0 |
| Ralston Instant & Regular (Ralston) | ¾ cup | 110 | 0 |
| Total Oatmeal Apple Cinnamon Almond Instant (General Mills) | 1.5 oz pkg | 150 | 0 |
| Total Oatmeal Apple Cinnamon Instant (General Mills) | 1.25 oz pkg | 130 | 0 |
| Total Oatmeal Mixed Nut Instant (General Mills) | 1.3 oz pkg | 140 | 0 |
| Total Oatmeal Quick (General Mills) | 1 oz pkg | 90 | 0 |
| Total Oatmeal Regular Flavor Instant (General Mills) | 1 oz pkg | 90 | 0 |
| Wheat Hearts; as prep (General Mills) | ¾ cup | 110 | 0 |

| FOOD | PORTION | CALORIES | CHOLESTEROL |
|---|---|---|---|
| Wheatena (Standard Milling) | ½ cup | 79 | 0 |
| barley pearled light; not prep | 2 tsp (1 oz) | 99 | 0 |
| bulgur | ¼ cup | 63 | 0 |
| corn grits | ½ cup | 54 | 0 |
| corn grits, instant; as prep | 1 pkg (.8 oz) | 82 | 0 |
| corn grits, instant; not prep | 1 pkg (.8 oz) | 82 | 0 |
| corn grits, regular & quick; cooked | 1 cup | 146 | 0 |
| corn grits, regular & quick; not prep | 1 tbsp | 36 | 0 |
| corn grits, regular & quick; not prep | 1 cup | 579 | 0 |
| cornmeal, white or yellow | ½ cup | 60 | 0 |
| READY-TO-EAT 7-Grain Crunchy (Loma Linda) | ½ cup | 110 | 0 |
| 7-Grain No Sugar Added (Loma Linda) | 1 cup | 110 | 0 |
| All-Bran (Kellogg's) | ⅓ cup | 70 | 0 |
| All-Bran Fruit & Almonds (Kellogg's) | ⅔ cup | 100 | 0 |
| All-Bran with Extra Fiber (Kellogg's) | ½ cup | 60 | 0 |
| Alpha-Bits (Post) | 1 cup | 112 | 0 |
| Apple Cinnamon Squares (Kellogg's) | ½ cup | 90 | 0 |

| FOOD | PORTION | CALORIES | CHOLESTEROL |
|------|---------|----------|-------------|
| Apple Jacks (Kellogg's) | 1 cup | 110 | 0 |
| Apple Raisin Crisp (Kellogg's) | ⅔ cup | 130 | 0 |
| Aztec Corn and Amaranth (Erewhon) | 1 oz | 100 | 0 |
| BooBerry (General Mills) | 1 cup | 110 | 0 |
| Bran (Loma Linda) | ⅓ cup | 90 | 0 |
| Bran Buds (Kellogg's) | ⅓ cup | 70 | 0 |
| Bran Cereal w/ Raisins (Health Valley) | 1 oz | 70 | 0 |
| Bran Flakes (Kellogg's) | ⅔ cup | 90 | 0 |
| Brown Sugar & Honey Body Buddies (General Mills) | 1 cup | 110 | 0 |
| Cap'n Crunch (Quaker) | ¾ cup | 120 | 0 |
| Cap'n Crunch's Crunchberries (Quaker) | ¾ cup | 127 | 0 |
| Cheerios (General Mills) | 1¼ cup | 110 | 0 |
| Chex (Ralston) | ⅔ cup | 90 | 0 |
| Cinnamon Toast Crunch (General Mills) | 1 cup | 120 | 0 |
| Circus Fun (General Mills) | 1 cup | 110 | 0 |

| FOOD | PORTION | CALORIES | CHOLESTEROL |
| --- | --- | --- | --- |
| Clusters (General Mills) | ½ cup | 100 | 0 |
| Cocoa Krispies (Kellogg's) | ¾ cup | 110 | 0 |
| Cocoa Pebbles (Post) | ⅞ cup | 112 | 0 |
| Cocoa Puffs (General Mills) | 1 cup | 110 | 0 |
| Corn Flakes (Kellogg's) | 1 cup | 100 | 0 |
| Corn Flakes Blue (Health Valley) | 1 oz | 90 | 0 |
| Corn Pops (Kellogg's) | 1 cup | 110 | 0 |
| Country Corn Flakes (General Mills) | 1 cup | 110 | 0 |
| Cracklin' Oat Bran (Kellogg's) | ½ cup | 110 | 0 |
| Crispix (Kellogg's) | 1 cup | 110 | 0 |
| Crispy Brown Rice (Erewhon) | 1 oz | 110 | 0 |
| Crispy Brown Rice Cereal, Low Sodium (Erewhon) | 1 oz | 110 | 0 |
| Crispy Critters (Post) | 1 cup | 112 | 0 |
| Crispy Wheats 'n Raisins (General Mills) | ¾ cup | 110 | 0 |
| Fiber 7 Flakes (Health Valley) | 1 oz | 100 | 0 |

| FOOD | PORTION | CALORIES | CHOLESTEROL |
|---|---|---|---|
| Fortified Oat Flakes (Post) | ⅔ cup | 105 | 0 |
| Frankenberry (General Mills) | 1 cup | 110 | 0 |
| Froot Loops (Kellogg's) | 1 cup | 110 | 0 |
| Frosted Flakes (Kellogg's) | ¾ cup | 110 | 0 |
| Frosted Krispies (Kellogg's) | ¾ cup | 110 | 0 |
| Frosted Mini-Wheats (Kellogg's) | 4 biscuits | 100 | 0 |
| Fruit & Fiber Dates Raisins & Walnuts (Post) | ½ cup | 89 | 0 |
| Fruit & Fiber Harvest Medley (Post) | ½ cup | 88 | 0 |
| Fruit & Fiber Mountain Trail (Post) | ½ cup | 87 | tr |
| Fruit & Fiber Peach Raisin Almond (Post) | ½ cup | 85 | 0 |
| Fruit & Fiber Tropical Fruit (Post) | ½ cup | 90 | 0 |
| Fruit 'n Wheat (Erewhon) | 1 oz | 100 | 0 |
| Fruitful Bran (Kellogg's) | ⅔ cup | 110 | 0 |
| Fruity Marshmallow Krispies (Kellogg's) | 1¼ cups | 140 | 0 |
| Fruity Pebbles (Post) | ⅞ cup | 112 | 0 |

| FOOD | PORTION | CALORIES | CHOLESTEROL |
|---|---|---|---|
| Golden Grahams (General Mills) | ¾ cup | 110 | 0 |
| Grape-Nuts (Post) | ¼ cup | 104 | 0 |
| Grape-Nuts Flakes (Post) | ⅞ cup | 104 | 0 |
| Healthy Crunch w/ Almonds & Dates (Health Valley) | 1 oz | 110 | 0 |
| Healthy Crunch w/ Apples & Cinnamon (Health Valley) | 1 oz | 110 | 0 |
| Heartland Natural (Pet) | ¼ cup | 112 | 0 |
| Honey Buc Wheat Crisp (General Mills) | ¾ cup | 110 | 0 |
| Honey Nut Cheerios (General Mills) | 1 cup | 110 | 0 |
| Honey Smacks (Kellogg's) | ¾ cup | 110 | 0 |
| Honeycomb (Post) | 1⅓ cups | 110 | 0 |
| Ice Cream Cones Chocolate Chip (General Mills) | ¾ cup | 110 | 0 |
| Ice Cream Cones Vanilla (General Mills) | ¾ cup | 110 | 0 |
| Just Right Nugget & Flake (Kellogg's) | ⅔ cup | 100 | 0 |
| Just Right Fruit Nut & Flake (Kellogg's) | ¾ cup | 140 | 0 |
| Kaboom (General Mills) | 1 cup | 110 | 0 |

| FOOD | PORTION | CALORIES | CHOLESTEROL |
|------|---------|----------|-------------|
| Lucky Charms (General Mills) | 1 cup | 110 | 0 |
| Muesli (Ralston) | ½ cup | 160 | 0 |
| Muesli Unsweetened (Kentaur) | 1.2 oz | 120 | 0 |
| Muesli Sweetened (Kentaur) | 1.2 oz | 120 | 0 |
| Mueslix Bran (Kellogg's) | ½ cup | 130 | 0 |
| Mueslix Five Grain (Kellogg's) | ½ cup | 150 | 0 |
| Natural Bran Flakes (Post) | ⅔ cup | 87 | 0 |
| Natural Raisin Bran (Post) | ½ cup | 83 | 0 |
| Natural Sugar & Honey Body Buddies (General Mills) | 1 cup | 110 | 0 |
| Nut & Honey Crunch (Kellogg's) | ⅔ cup | 110 | 0 |
| Nutri-Grain Almond Raisin (Kellogg's) | ⅔ cup | 140 | 0 |
| Nutri-Grain Corn (Kellogg's) | ½ cup | 100 | 0 |
| Nutri-Grain Nuggets (Kellogg's) | ¼ cup | 90 | 0 |
| Nutri-Grain Wheat (Kellogg's) | ⅔ cup | 100 | 0 |
| Nutri-Grain Wheat & Raisins (Kellogg's) | ⅔ cup | 130 | 0 |
| Nutrific (Kellogg's) | 1 cup | 120 | 0 |

| FOOD | PORTION | CALORIES | CHOLESTEROL |
|---|---|---|---|
| Oat Bran Flakes (Health Valley) | 1 oz | 110 | 0 |
| Oat Bran Flakes w/ Almonds & Dates (Health Valley) | 1 oz | 100 | 0 |
| Oat Bran Flakes w/ Raisins (Health Valley) | 1 oz | 100 | 0 |
| Oat Bran O'S (Health Valley) | 1 oz | 90 | 0 |
| Oat Bran O'S Fruit & Nuts (Health Valley) | 1 oz | 90 | 0 |
| Pac-Man (General Mills) | 1 cup | 110 | 0 |
| Post Toasties (Post) | 1¼ cup | 108 | 0 |
| Pro Grain (Kellogg's) | ¾ cup | 100 | 0 |
| Product 19 (Kellogg's) | 1 cup | 100 | 0 |
| Puffed Corn (Health Valley) | ½ oz | 50 | 0 |
| Puffed Rice (Health Valley) | ½ oz | 50 | 0 |
| Puffed Rice (Quaker) | 1 cup | 40 | 0 |
| Puffed Wheat (Health Valley) | ½ oz | 50 | 0 |
| Puffed Wheat (Quaker) | 1 cup | 35 | 0 |
| Quisp (Quaker) | 1⅛ cup | 121 | 0 |
| Raisin Grape-Nuts (Post) | ¼ cup | 101 | 0 |

| FOOD | PORTION | CALORIES | CHOLESTEROL |
|---|---|---|---|
| Raisin Bran (Erewhon) | 1 oz | 100 | 0 |
| Raisin Bran (Kellogg's) | ¾ cup | 120 | 0 |
| Raisin Bran (Quaker) | ½ cup | 90 | 0 |
| Raisin Bran (Skinner's) | 1 oz | 100 | 0 |
| Raisin Bran Flakes (Health Valley) | 1 oz | 100 | 0 |
| Raisin Bran, No Salt Added (Skinner's) | 1 oz | 100 | 0 |
| Raisin Squares (Kellogg's) | ½ cup | 90 | 0 |
| Rice Crispy (Ralston) | 1 cup | 110 | 0 |
| Rice Krispies (Kellogg's) | 1 cup | 110 | 0 |
| Rice Toasties (Post) | ¾ oz | 81 | 2 |
| Ruskets Biscuits (Loma Linda) | 2 biscuits | 110 | 0 |
| Shredded Wheat (Nabisco) | 1 biscuit | 84 | 0 |
| Shredded Wheat (Sunshine) | 1 biscuit | 90 | 0 |
| Shredded Wheat Bite Size (Sunshine) | ⅔ cup | 110 | 0 |
| Shredded Wheat Spoon Size (Nabisco) | ⅔ cup | 102 | 0 |
| Special K (Kellogg's) | 1 cup | 110 | 0 |

| FOOD | PORTION | CALORIES | CHOLESTEROL |
| --- | --- | --- | --- |
| Sporting (Kentaur) | 1.47 oz | 140 | 0 |
| Sprouts 7 w/ Raisins (Health Valley) | 1 oz | 90 | 0 |
| Stoned Wheat Flakes (Health Valley) | 1 oz | 100 | 0 |
| Strawberry Squares (Kellogg's) | ½ cup | 90 | 0 |
| Sugar Frosted Flakes (Ralston) | ¾ cup | 110 | 0 |
| Sugar Sparkled Flakes (Post) | ¾ cup | 108 | 0 |
| Super Golden Crisp (Post) | ⅞ cup | 104 | 0 |
| Swiss Breakfast Raisin Nut (Health Valley) | 1 oz | 100 | 0 |
| Swiss Breakfast Tropical Fruit (Health Valley) | 1 oz | 100 | 0 |
| Team (Nabisco) | 1 cup | 110 | 0 |
| Total (General Mills) | 1 cup | 110 | 0 |
| Total Corn Flakes (General Mills) | 1 cup | 110 | 0 |
| Trix (General Mills) | 1 cup | 110 | 0 |
| Uncle Sam Cereal (US Mills) | 1 oz | 110 | 0 |
| Wheat Bran Millers Flakes (Health Valley) | 1 oz | 70 | 0 |
| Wheat Flakes (Erewhon) | 1 oz | 100 | 0 |

| FOOD | PORTION | CALORIES | CHOLESTEROL |
|------|---------|----------|-------------|
| **Wheat Germ** (Kretschmer) | ¼ cup | 110 | 0 |
| **Wheaties** (General Mills) | 1 cup | 110 | 0 |
| **WITH 1% MILK** **Cheerios** (General Mills) | 1 cup + ½ cup milk | 160 | 5 |
| **Crispy Wheats 'n Raisins** (General Mills) | ¾ cup + ½ cup milk | 160 | 5 |
| **Honey Buc Wheat Crisp** (General Mills) | ¾ cup + ½ cup milk | 160 | 5 |
| **Honey Nut Cheerios** (General Mills) | 1 cup + ½ cup milk | 160 | 5 |
| **Total Corn Flakes** (General Mills) | 1 cup + ½ cup milk | 160 | 3 |
| **Total** (General Mills) | 1 cup + ½ cup milk | 160 | 5 |
| **Trix** (General Mills) | 1½ cup + ½ cup milk | 160 | 3 |
| **Wheaties** (General Mills) | 1 cup + ½ cup milk | 160 | 5 |
| **WITH 2% MILK** **Alpha-Bits** (Post) | 1 cup + ½ cup milk | 172 | 9 |

| FOOD | PORTION | CALORIES | CHOLESTEROL |
|------|---------|----------|-------------|
| BooBerry<br>(General Mills) | 1 cup +<br>½ cup<br>milk | 170 | 9 |
| Cinnamon Toast Crunch<br>(General Mills) | 1 cup +<br>½ cup<br>milk | 180 | 9 |
| Cocoa Puffs<br>(General Mills) | 1 cup +<br>½ cup<br>milk | 170 | 9 |
| Frankenberry<br>(General Mills) | 1 cup +<br>½ cup<br>milk | 170 | 9 |
| Fruity Pebbles<br>(Post) | ⅞ cup +<br>½ cup<br>milk | 173 | 9 |
| Honeycomb<br>(Post) | 1⅓ cups<br>+ ½ cup<br>milk | 171 | 9 |
| Oats, Old Fashioned; as prep<br>(Roman Meal) | ⅓ cup +<br>½ cup<br>milk | 160 | 10 |
| Oats, Quick; as prep<br>(Roman Meal) | ⅓ cup +<br>½ cup<br>milk | 160 | 10 |
| Oats, Wheat, Dates, Raisins,<br>Almonds Cereal; as prep<br>(Roman Meal) | ⅓ cup +<br>½ cup<br>milk | 170 | 5 |
| Oats, Wheat, Honey,<br>Coconut, Almonds Cereal; as<br>prep<br>(Roman Meal) | ⅓ cup +<br>½ cup<br>milk | 190 | 5 |
| Oats, Wheat, Rye Flax Cereal;<br>as prep<br>(Roman Meal) | ⅓ cup +<br>½ cup<br>milk | 120 | 5 |

| FOOD | PORTION | CALORIES | CHOLESTEROL |
|---|---|---|---|
| Original Cereal w/ Wheat, Rye, Bran, Flax; as prep (Roman Meal) | ⅓ cup + ½ cup milk | 120 | 5 |
| Pac-Man (General Mills) | 1 cup + ½ cup milk | 170 | 9 |
| Shredded Wheat (Sunshine) | 1 biscuit + ½ cup milk | 150 | 9 |
| Shredded Wheat Bite Size (Sunshine) | ⅔ cup + ½ cup milk | 170 | 9 |
| Total Oatmeal Apple Cinnamon Almond Instant (General Mills) | 1.5 oz pkg + ½ cup milk | 210 | 9 |
| Total Oatmeal Apple Cinnamon Instant (General Mills) | 1.25 oz pkg + ½ cup milk | 190 | 9 |
| Total Oatmeal Quick (General Mills) | 1 oz pkg + ½ cup milk | 150 | 9 |
| Total Oatmeal Regular Flavor Instant (General Mills) | 1 oz pkg + ½ cup milk | 150 | 9 |
| **WITH SKIM MILK** BooBerry (General Mills) | 1 cup + ½ cup milk | 150 | 3 |
| Brown Sugar & Honey Body Buddies (General Mills) | 1 cup + ½ cup milk | 150 | 3 |
| Cheerios (General Mills) | 1 cup + ½ cup milk | 150 | 5 |

| FOOD | PORTION | CALORIES | CHOLESTEROL |
|------|---------|----------|-------------|
| Circus Fun (General Mills) | 1 cup + ½ cup milk | 150 | 3 |
| Clusters (General Mills) | ½ cup + ½ cup milk | 140 | 3 |
| Cocoa Puffs (General Mills) | 1 cup + ½ cup milk | 150 | 3 |
| Count Chocula (General Mills) | 1 cup + ½ cup milk | 150 | 3 |
| Country Corn Flakes (General Mills) | 1 cup + ½ cup milk | 150 | 3 |
| Crispy Wheats 'n Raisins (General Mills) | ¾ cup + ½ cup milk | 150 | 3 |
| Frankenberry (General Mills) | 1 cup + ½ cup milk | 150 | 3 |
| Fruit & Fiber Harvest Medley (Post) | ½ cup + ½ cup milk | 131 | 2 |
| Fruit & Fiber Peach Raisin Almond (Post) | ½ cup + ½ cup milk | 129 | 2 |
| Golden Grahams (General Mills) | ¾ cup + ½ cup milk | 150 | 3 |
| Grape-Nuts (Post) | ¼ cup + ½ cup milk | 148 | 2 |
| Honey Buc Wheat Crisp (General Mills) | ¾ cup + ½ cup milk | 150 | 3 |

| FOOD | PORTION | CALORIES | CHOLESTEROL |
|---|---|---|---|
| Honey Nut Cheerios (General Mills) | 1 cup + ½ milk | 150 | 3 |
| Ice Cream Cones Chocolate Chip (General Mills) | ¾ cup + ½ cup milk | 150 | 3 |
| Ice Cream Cones Vanilla (General Mills) | ¾ cup + ½ cup milk | 150 | 3 |
| Kaboom (General Mills) | 1 cup + ½ cup milk | 150 | 3 |
| Lucky Charms (General Mills) | 1 cup + ½ cup milk | 150 | 3 |
| Muesli (Ralston) | ½ cup + ½ cup milk | 200 | 3 |
| Natural Raisin Bran (Post) | ½ cup + ½ cup milk | 127 | 2 |
| Natural Sugar & Honey Body Buddies (General Mills) | 1 cup + ½ cup milk | 150 | 3 |
| Oat Bran; as prep (Quaker) | ⅓ cup + ½ cup milk | 140 | 3 |
| Oatmeal Raisin Crisp (General Mills) | ½ cup + ½ cup milk | 150 | 3 |
| Pac-Man (General Mills) | 1 cup + ½ cup milk | 150 | 3 |
| Raisin Grape-Nuts (Post) | ¼ cup + ½ cup milk | 144 | 2 |

| FOOD | PORTION | CALORIES | CHOLESTEROL |
|------|---------|----------|-------------|
| Shredded Wheat (Sunshine) | 1 biscuit + ½ cup milk | 135 | 3 |
| Shredded Wheat Bite Size (Sunshine) | ⅔ cup + ½ cup milk | 200 | 3 |
| Total (General Mills) | 1 cup + ½ cup milk | 150 | 3 |
| Total Corn Flakes (General Mills) | 1 cup + ½ cup milk | 150 | 3 |
| Total Oatmeal Apple Cinnamon Almond Instant (General Mills) | 1.5 oz pkg + ½ cup milk | 190 | 3 |
| Total Oatmeal Apple Cinnamon Instant (General Mills) | 1.25 oz pkg + ½ cup milk | 170 | 3 |
| Total Oatmeal Mixed Nut Instant (General Mills) | 1.3 oz pkg + ½ cup milk | 180 | 3 |
| Total Oatmeal Quick (General Mills) | 1 oz pkg + ½ cup milk | 130 | 3 |
| Total Oatmeal Regular Flavor Instant (General Mills) | 1 oz pkg + ½ cup milk | 130 | 3 |
| Trix (General Mills) | 1 cup + ½ cup milk | 150 | 3 |
| Trix (General Mills) | 1½ cup + ½ cup milk | 150 | 3 |

| FOOD | PORTION | CALORIES | CHOLESTEROL |
|------|---------|----------|-------------|
| Wheaties<br>(General Mills) | 1 cup +<br>½ cup<br>milk | 150 | 3 |
| **WITH WHOLE MILK** | | | |
| Brown Sugar & Honey Body<br>Buddies<br>(General Mills) | 1 cup +<br>½ cup<br>milk | 185 | 17 |
| Circus Fun<br>(General Mills) | 1 cup +<br>½ cup<br>milk | 185 | 17 |
| Clusters<br>(General Mills) | ½ cup +<br>½ cup<br>milk | 175 | 17 |
| Country Corn Flakes<br>(General Mills) | 1 cup +<br>½ cup<br>milk | 185 | 17 |
| Fortified Oat Flakes<br>(Post) | ⅔ cup +<br>½ cup<br>milk | 181 | 17 |
| Golden Grahams<br>(General Mills) | ¾ cup +<br>½ cup<br>milk | 185 | 17 |
| Ice Cream Cones Chocolate<br>Chip<br>(General Mills) | ¾ cup +<br>½ cup<br>milk | 185 | 17 |
| Ice Cream Cones Vanilla<br>(General Mills) | ¾ cup +<br>½ cup<br>milk | 185 | 17 |
| Kaboom<br>(General Mills) | 1 cup +<br>½ cup<br>milk | 185 | 17 |
| Lucky Charms<br>(General Mills) | 1 cup +<br>½ cup<br>milk | 185 | 17 |

| FOOD | PORTION | CALORIES | CHOLESTEROL |
|------|---------|----------|-------------|
| Oatmeal Raisin Crisp (General Mills) | ½ cup + ½ cup milk | 185 | 17 |
| Shredded Wheat (Sunshine) | 1 biscuit + ½ cup milk | 165 | 17 |
| Shredded Wheat Bite Size (Sunshine) | ⅔ cup + ½ cup milk | 225 | 17 |
| Sugar Sparkled Flakes (Post) | ¾ cup + ½ cup milk | 184 | 17 |
| Total Oatmeal Mixed Nut Instant (General Mills) | 1.3 oz pkg + ½ cup milk | 215 | 17 |
| Trix (General Mills) | 1 cup + ½ cup milk | 185 | 17 |

## CHAYOTE

| FRESH | | | |
|------|---------|----------|-------------|
| cooked, cut up | 1 cup | 38 | 0 |
| raw; cut up | 1 cup | 32 | 0 |

## CHEESE

(*see also* CHEESE DISHES, CHEESE SUBSTITUTE, COTTAGE CHEESE, CREAM CHEESE)

| NATURAL | | | |
|------|---------|----------|-------------|
| Blue (Kraft) | 1 oz | 100 | 30 |
| Blue (Sargento) | 1 oz | 100 | 21 |
| Blue Spread (Roka Brand) | 1 oz | 70 | 20 |

| FOOD | PORTION | CALORIES | CHOLESTEROL |
|---|---|---|---|
| Brick (Kraft) | 1 oz | 110 | 30 |
| Brick (Land O'Lakes) | 1 oz | 110 | 25 |
| Brick (Sargento) | 1 oz | 105 | 27 |
| Brie (Sargento) | 1 oz | 95 | 28 |
| Burger Cheese (Sargento) | 1 oz | 106 | 27 |
| Cajun (Sargento) | 1 oz | 110 | 28 |
| Camembert (Sargento) | 1 oz | 85 | 20 |
| Caraway (Kraft) | 1 oz | 100 | 30 |
| Cheddar (Alpine Lace) | 1 oz | 97 | 25 |
| Cheddar (Armour) | 1 oz | 110 | 30 |
| Cheddar (Kraft) | 1 oz | 110 | 30 |
| Cheddar (Land O'Lakes) | 1 oz | 110 | 30 |
| Cheddar (Sargento) | 1 oz | 114 | 30 |
| Cheddar New York (Sargento) | 1 oz | 114 | 30 |
| Cheddar Port Wine w/ Almonds, Cheese Log (Cracker Barrel) | 1 oz | 90 | 15 |
| Cheddar Sharp Nut Log (Sargento) | 1 oz | 97 | 18 |

| FOOD | PORTION | CALORIES | CHOLESTEROL |
|---|---|---|---|
| Cheddar Sharp w/ Almonds, Cheese Ball (Cracker Barrel) | 1 oz | 90 | 15 |
| Cheddar Sharp w/ Almonds, Cheese Log (Cracker Barrel) | 1 oz | 90 | 15 |
| Cheddar Shredded (Weight Watchers) | 1 oz | 80 | 28 |
| Cheddar Smokey w/ Almonds, Cheese Log (Cracker Barrel) | 1 oz | 90 | 15 |
| Cheddar, Lower Salt (Armour) | 1 oz | 110 | 30 |
| Cheddar-Jack Light Natural (Dorman's) | 1 oz | 90 | 23 |
| Colby (Alpine Lace) | 1 oz | 85 | 19 |
| Colby (Kraft) | 1 oz | 110 | 30 |
| Colby (Land O'Lakes) | 1 oz | 110 | 25 |
| Colby (Sargento) | 1 oz | 112 | 27 |
| Colby-Jack (Sargento) | 1 oz | 109 | 27 |
| Edam (Holland Farm) | 1 oz | 97 | 25 |
| Edam (Kraft) | 1 oz | 90 | 20 |
| Edam (Land O'Lakes) | 1 oz | 110 | 25 |
| Edam (Sargento) | 1 oz | 101 | 25 |

| FOOD | PORTION | CALORIES | CHOLESTEROL |
|---|---|---|---|
| Farmer (Friendship) | 4 oz | 160 | 40 |
| Farmer (Holland Farm) | 1 oz | 102 | 26 |
| Farmer No Salt Added (Friendship) | 4 oz | 160 | 40 |
| Farmers Cheese (May-Bud) | 1 oz | 90 | 20 |
| Farmers Cheese (Sargento) | 1 oz | 102 | 26 |
| Farmers Cheese (White Clover) | 1 oz | 90 | 20 |
| Farmers Cheese (White Clover) | 1 oz | 81 | 18 |
| Feta (Sargento) | 1 oz | 75 | 25 |
| Feta (White Clover) | 1 oz | 90 | 20 |
| Finland Swiss (Sargento) | 1 oz | 107 | 26 |
| Fior di Latte (Polly-O) | 1 oz | 80 | 20 |
| Fontina (Sargento) | 1 oz | 110 | 33 |
| Gorgonzola (Sargento) | 1 oz | 100 | 21 |
| Gouda (Holland Farm) | 1 oz | 103 | 27 |
| Gouda (Kraft) | 1 oz | 110 | 30 |
| Gouda (Land O'Lakes) | 1 oz | 110 | 30 |

| FOOD | PORTION | CALORIES | CHOLESTEROL |
|---|---|---|---|
| Gouda (Sargento) | 1 oz | 101 | 32 |
| Grated (Polly-O) | 1 oz | 130 | 25 |
| Gruyere (Sargento) | 1 oz | 117 | 31 |
| Havarti (Casino) | 1 oz | 120 | 35 |
| Havarti (Sargento) | 1 oz | 118 | 31 |
| Hoop (Friendship) | 4 oz | 84 | 8 |
| Italian Style Grated Cheese (Sargento) | 1 oz | 108 | 26 |
| Jack Slim Light Natural (Dorman's) | 1 oz | 90 | 22 |
| Jarlsberg (Sargento) | 1 oz | 100 | 16 |
| Limburger (Sargento) | 1 oz | 93 | 26 |
| Limburger Natural Little Gem Size (Mohawk Valley) | 1 oz | 90 | 25 |
| Lorraine (Universal Food) | 1 oz | 100 | 25 |
| Monterey Jack (Alpine Lace) | 1 oz | 80 | 14 |
| Monterey Jack (Armour) | 1 oz | 110 | 30 |
| Monterey Jack (Holland Farm) | 1 oz | 102 | 27 |
| Monterey Jack (Kraft) | 1 oz | 110 | 30 |

| FOOD | PORTION | CALORIES | CHOLESTEROL |
|---|---|---|---|
| Monterey Jack (Land O'Lakes) | 1 oz | 110 | 20 |
| Monterey Jack Lower Salt (Armour) | 1 oz | 110 | 30 |
| Monterey Jack w/ Jalapeno Peppers (Kraft) | 1 oz | 110 | 30 |
| Monterey Jack w/ Peppers Mild (Kraft) | 1 oz | 110 | 30 |
| Mozzarella (Alpine Lace) | 1 oz | 72 | 15 |
| Mozzarella (M.H. Greenbaum, Inc.) | 3½ oz | 334 | 59 |
| Mozzarella Lite Sandwich Slices (Polly-O) | 1 oz | 70 | 15 |
| Mozzarella Low-Moisture (Casino) | 1 oz | 90 | 25 |
| Mozzarella Low-Moisture Part-Skim (Sargento) | 1 oz | 79 | 15 |
| Mozzarella Low-Moisture Whole Milk (Sargento) | 1 oz | 90 | 25 |
| Mozzarella Low-Sodium Light (Dorman's) | 1 oz | 80 | 15 |
| Mozzarella Part-Skim (Polly-O) | 1 oz | 80 | 15 |
| Mozzarella Part-Skim Shredded (Polly-O) | 1 oz | 80 | 15 |
| Mozzarella Part-Skim Low-Moisture (Kraft) | 1 oz | 80 | 15 |

| FOOD | PORTION | CALORIES | CHOLESTEROL |
|------|---------|----------|-------------|
| Mozzarella Part-Skim (Land O'Lakes) | 1 oz | 80 | 15 |
| Mozzarella Part-Skim Low-Moisture String Cheese w/ Jalapeno Peppers (Kraft) | 1 oz | 80 | 20 |
| Mozzarella Smoked (Polly-O) | 1 oz | 85 | 25 |
| Mozzarella Whole Milk (Polly-O) | 1 oz | 90 | 20 |
| Mozzarella Whole Milk Sandwich Slices (Polly-O) | 1 oz | 90 | 20 |
| Mozzarella Whole Milk Shredded (Polly-O) | 1 oz | 90 | 20 |
| Mozzarella w/ Pizza Spices (Sargento) | 1 oz | 79 | 15 |
| Muenster (Alpine Lace) | 1 oz | 104 | 25 |
| Muenster (Holland Farm) | 1 oz | 102 | 27 |
| Muenster (Kraft) | 1 oz | 110 | 30 |
| Muenster (Land O'Lakes) | 1 oz | 100 | 25 |
| Muenster Red Rind (Sargento) | 1 oz | 104 | 27 |
| Nacho (Sargento) | 1 oz | 106 | 27 |
| Naturally Slender (Northfield) | 1 oz | 90 | 10 |
| Parmesan & Romano Grated (Sargento) | 1 oz | 111 | 24 |

| FOOD | PORTION | CALORIES | CHOLESTEROL |
|---|---|---|---|
| Parmesan Fresh (Sargento) | 1 oz | 111 | 19 |
| Parmesan Grated (Kraft) | 1 oz | 130 | 30 |
| Parmesan Grated (Polly-O) | 1 oz | 130 | 20 |
| Parmesan Grated (Sargento) | 1 oz | 129 | 22 |
| Parmesan Natural (Kraft) | 1 oz | 110 | 20 |
| Port Wine Nut Log (Sargento) | 1 oz | 97 | 18 |
| Provolone (Alpine Lace) | 1 oz | 85 | 20 |
| Provolone (Kraft) | 1 oz | 100 | 25 |
| Provolone (Land O'Lakes) | 1 oz | 100 | 20 |
| Provolone (Sargento) | 1 oz | 100 | 20 |
| Provolone Low Sodium Light Natural (Dorman's) | 1 oz | 90 | 20 |
| Queso Blanco (Sargento) | 1 oz | 104 | 27 |
| Queso de Papa (Sargento) | 1 oz | 114 | 30 |
| Ricotta Lite (Polly-O) | 2 oz | 80 | 10 |
| Ricotta Lite (Sargento) | 1 oz | 25 | 14 |

| FOOD | PORTION | CALORIES | CHOLESTEROL |
|---|---|---|---|
| Ricotta Part-Skim (Polly-O) | 2 oz | 90 | 20 |
| Ricotta Part-Skim (Sargento) | 1 oz | 32 | 10 |
| Ricotta Part-Skim No Salt (Polly-O) | 2 oz | 90 | 20 |
| Ricotta Whole Milk (Polly-O) | 2 oz | 100 | 35 |
| Ricotta Whole Milk (Sargento) | 1 oz | 53 | 15 |
| Ricotta Whole Milk & Whey (Sargento) | 1 oz | 40 | 13 |
| Ricotta Whole Milk No Salt (Polly-O) | 2 oz | 100 | 35 |
| Romano (Sargento) | 1 oz | 110 | 29 |
| Romano Grated (Casino) | 1 oz | 130 | 30 |
| Romano Grated (Polly-O) | 1 oz | 130 | 30 |
| Romano Natural (Casino) | 1 oz | 100 | 30 |
| Scamorze Part-Skim Low-Moisture (Kraft) | 1 oz | 80 | 15 |
| Smokestick (Sargento) | 1 oz | 103 | 24 |
| String Cheese (Polly-O) | 1 oz | 90 | 15 |
| String Cheese (Sargento) | 1 oz | 79 | 15 |

| FOOD | PORTION | CALORIES | CHOLESTEROL |
|---|---|---|---|
| String Cheese Smoked (Sargento) | 1 oz | 79 | 15 |
| Swiss (Alpine Lace) | 1 oz | 100 | 25 |
| Swiss (Kraft) | 1 oz | 110 | 25 |
| Swiss (Land O'Lakes) | 1 oz | 110 | 25 |
| Swiss (M.H. Greenbaum, Inc.) | 1 oz | 106 | 20 |
| Swiss (Sargento) | 1 oz | 107 | 26 |
| Swiss Almond Nut Log (Sargento) | 1 oz | 94 | 21 |
| Swiss, Aged (Kraft) | 1 oz | 110 | 25 |
| Taco (Sargento) | 1 oz | 109 | 27 |
| Taco Shredded (Kraft) | 1 oz | 110 | 30 |
| Tilsiter (Sargento) | 1 oz | 96 | 29 |
| Tybo Red Wax (Sargento) | 1 oz | 98 | 23 |
| blue | 1 oz | 100 | 21 |
| blue, crumbled | 1 cup | 477 | 102 |
| brick | 1 oz | 105 | 27 |
| Brie | 1 oz | 95 | 28 |
| Camembert | 1 oz | 85 | 20 |
| Cheddar | 1 oz | 114 | 30 |
| Cheshire | 1 oz | 110 | 29 |

| FOOD | PORTION | CALORIES | CHOLESTEROL |
|---|---|---|---|
| Colby | 1 oz | 112 | 27 |
| Edam | 1 oz | 101 | 25 |
| feta | 1 oz | 75 | 25 |
| fontina | 1 oz | 110 | 33 |
| Gouda | 1 oz | 101 | 32 |
| Gruyere | 1 oz | 117 | 31 |
| Limburger | 1 oz | 93 | 26 |
| mozzarella | 1 oz | 80 | 22 |
| mozzarella | 1 lb | 1276 | 356 |
| mozzarella, low-moisture | 1 oz | 90 | 25 |
| mozzarella, low-moisture, part-skim | 1 oz | 79 | 15 |
| mozzarella, part-skim | 1 oz | 72 | 16 |
| Muenster | 1 oz | 104 | 27 |
| Parmesan, grated | 1 Tbsp | 23 | 4 |
| Parmesan, grated | 1 oz | 129 | 22 |
| Parmesan, hard | 1 oz | 111 | 19 |
| Port du Salut | 1 oz | 100 | 35 |
| provolone | 1 oz | 100 | 20 |
| ricotta, part-skim | ½ cup | 171 | 38 |
| ricotta, part-skim | 1 cup | 340 | 76 |
| ricotta, whole milk | ½ cup | 216 | 63 |
| ricotta, whole milk | 1 cup | 428 | 124 |
| Romano | 1 oz | 110 | 29 |
| Roquefort | 1 oz | 105 | 26 |
| Swiss | 1 oz | 107 | 26 |
| Tilsit | 1 oz | 96 | 29 |

| FOOD | PORTION | CALORIES | CHOLESTEROL |
|---|---|---|---|
| yogurt cheese (home recipe) | 1 oz | 20 | 7 |
| PROCESSED American (Alpine Lace) | 1 oz | 80 | 20 |
| Borden Lite Line American | 1 oz | 50 | 10 |
| Borden Lite Line American Sodium Lite | 1 oz | 70 | 10 |
| Borden Lite Line Cheddar Sharp, Natural Shredded Reduced Fat Cheese | 1 oz | 80 | 15 |
| Cheez 'N Bacon Singles Pasteurized Process Cheese | 1 oz | 90 | 20 |
| Cheez Whiz | 1 oz | 80 | 20 |
| Cheez Whiz Hot Mexican | 1 oz | 80 | 15 |
| Cheez Whiz Mild Mexican | 1 oz | 80 | 15 |
| Cheez Whiz Pimento | 1 oz | 80 | 15 |
| Cheez Whiz w/ Jalapeno Peppers | 1 oz | 80 | 15 |
| Churney Maple Walnut Cheese Fudge | 1 oz | 118 | 7 |
| Churney Mint Cheese Fudge w/ Walnuts | 1 oz | 117 | 7 |
| Churney Cheese Fudge w/ Walnuts | 1 oz | 120 | 7 |
| Churney Diet Snack Cheddar Flavored | 1 oz | 70 | 10 |
| Churney Diet Snack Port Wine Flavored | 1 oz | 70 | 10 |
| Cracker Barrel Extra Sharp Cheddar Cold Pack Cheese Food | 1 oz | 90 | 20 |

| FOOD | PORTION | CALORIES | CHOLESTEROL |
|---|---|---|---|
| Cracker Barrel Port Wine Cheddar Cold Pack Cheese Food | 1 oz | 90 | 20 |
| Cracker Barrel Sharp Cheddar Cold Pack Cheese Food | 1 oz | 90 | 20 |
| Cracker Barrel w/ Bacon Cold Pack Cheese Food | 1 oz | 90 | 20 |
| Deluxe Pasteurized Process American Cheese (slices) | 1 oz | 110 | 25 |
| Deluxe Pasteurized Process American Cheese (loaf) | 1 oz | 110 | 25 |
| Deluxe Pasteurized Process Pimento Cheese Slices | 1 oz | 100 | 25 |
| Deluxe Pasteurized Process Swiss Cheese Slices | 1 oz | 90 | 25 |
| Dorman's Light Lo-Chol Low Cholesterol | 1 oz | 70 | 3 |
| Fineform | 1 oz | 70 | 8 |
| Formagg American Swiss Slices | ¾ oz | 70 | 0 |
| Formagg American White Slices | ¾ oz | 70 | 0 |
| Formagg American Yellow Slices | ¾ oz | 70 | 0 |
| Formagg Cheddar | 1 oz | 70 | 0 |
| Formagg Grated Italian Pasta Topping | 1 oz | 100 | 0 |
| Formagg Monterey Jack | 1 oz | 70 | 0 |
| Formagg Monterey Jack Jalapeno Flavored | 1 oz | 70 | 0 |
| Formagg Mozzarella | 1 oz | 70 | 0 |

| FOOD | PORTION | CALORIES | CHOLESTEROL |
|---|---|---|---|
| Formagg Pizza Topper | 1 oz | 70 | 0 |
| Formagg Provolone | 1 oz | 70 | 0 |
| Formagg Ricotta | 1 oz | 130 | 0 |
| Formagg Shredded Cheddar | 1 oz | 70 | 0 |
| Formagg Shredded Mozzarella | 1 oz | 70 | 0 |
| Formagg Shredded Parmesan | 1 oz | 70 | 0 |
| Formagg Shredded Provolone | 1 oz | 70 | 0 |
| Formagg Shredded Salad Topping | 1 oz | 70 | 0 |
| Formagg Shredded Swiss | 1 oz | 70 | 0 |
| Formagg Swiss | 1 oz | 70 | 0 |
| Gruyere (M.H.Greenbaum, Inc.) | 1 oz | 94 | 44 |
| Gruyere, Hot Pepper (M.H. Greenbaum, Inc.) | 1 oz | 93 | 44 |
| Harvest Moon Brand Pasteurized Process Cheese | 1 oz | 50 | 10 |
| Harvest Moon Brand American Flavored Pasteurized Process Cheese | 1 oz | 70 | 15 |
| Kraft American Pasteurized Process Cheese Spread | 1 oz | 80 | 20 |
| Kraft American Singles Pasteurized Process Cheese (colored) | 1 oz | 90 | 20 |
| Kraft American Singles Pasteurized Process Cheese (white) | 1 oz | 90 | 20 |
| Kraft Jalapeno Pasteurized Process Cheese Spread | 1 oz | 80 | 20 |

| FOOD | PORTION | CALORIES | CHOLESTEROL |
|---|---|---|---|
| Kraft Jalapeno Pepper Spread | 1 oz | 70 | 15 |
| Kraft Jalapeno Singles Pasteurized Process Cheese | 1 oz | 90 | 25 |
| Kraft Monterey Jack Singles Pasteurized Process Cheese | 1 oz | 90 | 25 |
| Kraft Olives & Pimento Spread | 1 oz | 60 | 15 |
| Kraft Pasteurized Process Cheese Spread w/ Bacon | 1 oz | 80 | 20 |
| Kraft Pasteurized Process Cheese Spread w/ Garlic | 1 oz | 80 | 15 |
| Kraft Pasteurized Process Cheese Food w/ Bacon | 1 oz | 90 | 20 |
| Kraft Pasteurized Process Cheese Food w/ Garlic | 1 oz | 90 | 20 |
| Kraft Pimento Singles Pasteurized Process Cheese | 1 oz | 90 | 20 |
| Kraft Pimento Spread | 1 oz | 70 | 15 |
| Kraft Pineapple Spread | 1 oz | 70 | 15 |
| Kraft Relish Spread | 1 oz | 70 | 15 |
| Kraft Sharp Singles Pasteurized Process Cheese | 1 oz | 100 | 25 |
| Kraft Swiss Singles Pasteurized Process Cheese | 1 oz | 90 | 25 |
| Lactaid | 1 slice (⅔ oz) | 62 | 18 |
| Land O'Lakes, American | 1 oz | 110 | 25 |
| Land O'Lakes, American/ Swiss | 1 oz | 100 | 25 |

| FOOD | PORTION | CALORIES | CHOLESTEROL |
|---|---|---|---|
| Land O'Lakes, Golden Velvet Cheese Spread | 1 oz | 80 | 15 |
| Land O'Lakes, Jalapeno Cheese Food | 1 oz | 90 | 20 |
| Land O'Lakes, LaCheddar Cheese Food | 1 oz | 90 | 20 |
| Land O'Lakes, Onion Cheese Food | 1 oz | 90 | 15 |
| Land O'Lakes, Pepperoni Cheese Food | 1 oz | 90 | 20 |
| Land O'Lakes, Salami Cheese Food | 1 oz | 100 | 20 |
| Lifetime Swiss | 1 oz | 60 | 9 |
| Light N'Lively Singles American Flavor Pasteurized Process Cheese | 1 oz | 70 | 15 |
| Light N'Lively Singles Sharp Cheddar Flavored Pasteurized Process Cheese | 1 oz | 70 | 15 |
| Light N'Lively Singles Swiss Flavored Pasteurized Process Cheese | 1 oz | 70 | 15 |
| Lunch Wagon Pizza Topping Made w/ Vegetable Oil | 1 oz | 80 | 0 |
| Lunch Wagon Sandwich Slices Make w/ Vegetable Oil | 1 oz | 80 | 5 |
| Michael's Country Gourmet Spread French Onion | 1 oz | 48 | 19 |
| Michael's Country Gourmet Spread Garden Vegetable | 1 oz | 48 | 19 |
| Michael's Country Gourmet Spread Garlic & Herbs | 1 oz | 48 | 19 |

| FOOD | PORTION | CALORIES | CHOLESTEROL |
|------|---------|----------|-------------|
| Mohawk Valley Limburger Pasteurized Process Cheese Spread | 1 oz | 70 | 20 |
| Old English Sharp Pasteurized Process Cheese Spread | 1 oz | 90 | 20 |
| Old English Sharp Pasteurized Process American Cheese (slices) | 1 oz | 110 | 30 |
| Old English Sharp Pasteurized Process American Cheese (loaf) | 1 oz | 110 | 30 |
| Sargento American Hot Pepper | 1 oz | 106 | 27 |
| Sargento American Sharp Spread | 1 oz | 106 | 27 |
| Sargento American w/ Pimento | 1 oz | 106 | 27 |
| Sargento Imitation Cheddar | 1 oz | 85 | 2 |
| Sargento Imitation Mozzarella | 1 oz | 80 | 2 |
| Sargento Process Brick | 1 oz | 95 | 25 |
| Sargento Process Swiss | 1 oz | 95 | 24 |
| Skitoast | 1 oz | 65 | 28 |
| Smokelle Pasteurized Process Cheese Food | 1 oz | 100 | 20 |
| Squeez-A-Snak Garlic Flavor Pasteurized Process Cheese Spread | 1 oz | 90 | 20 |
| Squeez-A-Snak Hickory Smoke Flavor Pasteurized Process Cheese Spread | 1 oz | 80 | 20 |

| FOOD | PORTION | CALORIES | CHOLESTEROL |
|---|---|---|---|
| Squeez-A-Snak Pasteurized Process Cheese Spread w/ Bacon | 1 oz | 90 | 20 |
| Squeez-A-Snak Sharp Pasteurized Process Cheese Spread | 1 oz | 80 | 20 |
| Velveeta Hot Mexican Pasteurized Process Cheese Spread | 1 oz | 80 | 20 |
| Velveeta Mild Mexican Pasteurized Process Cheese Spread | 1 oz | 80 | 20 |
| Velveeta Pasteurized Process Cheese Spread | 1 oz | 80 | 20 |
| Velveeta Pasteurized Process Cheese Spread Slices | 1 oz | 90 | 20 |
| Velveeta Pimento Pasteurized Process Cheese Spread | 1 oz | 80 | 20 |
| Weight Watchers Swiss Flavor | 1 oz | 50 | 8 |
| American | 1 oz | 106 | 27 |
| American, cheese food | 1 oz | 93 | 18 |
| American, cheese food, cold pack | 1 oz | 94 | 18 |
| American, cheese spread | 1 oz | 82 | 16 |
| pimento | 1 oz | 106 | 27 |
| Swiss | 1 oz | 95 | 24 |
| Swiss, cheese food | 1 oz | 92 | 23 |

## CHEESE DISHES

| | | | |
|---|---|---|---|
| fondue (home recipe) | ½ cup | 303 | 62 |

| FOOD | PORTION | CALORIES | CHOLESTEROL |
|---|---|---|---|
| **CHEESE SUBSTITUTE** | | | |
| American & Caraway Cheese Subsititute (Delicia) | 1 oz | 80 | 0 |
| American Cheese Substitute (Delicia) | 1 oz | 80 | 0 |
| American w/ Hot Peppers Cheese Substitute (Delicia) | 1 oz | 80 | 0 |
| Cheezola | 1 oz | 89 | 1 |
| Count Down (Fisher) | 1 oz | 89 | 1 |
| Count Down Smokey Flavor (Fisher) | 1 oz | 34 | 1 |
| Golden Image American Flavored Pasteurized Process Cheese | 1 oz | 90 | 5 |
| Golden Image Imitation Colby Cheese | 1 oz | 110 | 5 |
| Golden Image Imitation Mild Cheddar Cheese | 1 oz | 110 | 5 |
| Hickory Smoked American Cheese Substitute (Delicia) | 1 oz | 80 | 0 |
| **CHERIMOYA** | | | |
| FRESH cherimoya | 1 | 515 | 0 |

| FOOD | PORTION | CALORIES | CHOLESTEROL |
|---|---|---|---|

## CHERRY

CANDIED
cherry | 1 cherry | 12 | 0

CANNED
Red Tart Pitted Cherries
(White House) | 3.5 oz | 43 | 0

cherries, sour, water packed | 1 cup | 87 | 0

cherries, sweet, in heavy
syrup | ½ cup | 107 | 0

maraschino | 1 | 12 | 0

sour, in heavy syrup | ½ cup | 116 | 0

sour, in light syrup | ½ cup | 94 | 0

sweet, in water | ½ cup | 57 | 0

sweet, juice pack | ½ cup | 68 | 0

FRESH
cherries, sweet | 10 | 49 | 0

FROZEN
cherries, sour, unsweetened | 1 cup | 72 | 0

cherries, sweetened | 1 cup | 232 | 0

JUICE
Black Cherry
(Smucker's) | 8 oz | 130 | 0

Mountain Cherry Pure & Light
(Dole) | 6 oz | 87 | 0

## CHESTNUTS

Chinese dried | 1 oz | 103 | 0

Chinese; cooked | 1 oz | 44 | 0

| FOOD | PORTION | CALORIES | CHOLESTEROL |
|---|---|---|---|
| Chinese; roasted | 1 oz | 68 | 0 |
| Japanese; cooked | 1 oz | 16 | 0 |
| Japanese; roasted | 1 oz | 57 | 0 |
| cooked | 1 oz | 37 | 0 |
| dried; peeled | 1 oz | 105 | 0 |
| roasted | 1 oz | 70 | 0 |
| roasted | 1 cup | 350 | 0 |

## CHEWING GUM

| | | | |
|---|---|---|---|
| Hubba Bubba, Original & Fruit | 1 stick | 23 | 0 |
| Hubba Bubba, Strawberry, Grape & Raspberry | 1 stick | 23 | 0 |
| Wrigley's | 1 stick | 10 | 0 |

## CHIA SEEDS

| | | | |
|---|---|---|---|
| dried | 1 oz | 134 | 0 |

## CHICKEN
(see also CHICKEN DISHES, CHICKEN SUBSTITUTE, DINNER, HOT DOGS)

| | | | |
|---|---|---|---|
| CANNED<br>Chicken Salad<br>(The Spreadables) | ¼ can | 100 | 16 |
| FRESH<br>Breast Boneless, Oven Stuffer; cooked<br>(Perdue) | 3 oz | 141 | 72 |
| Breast Boneless; cooked<br>(Perdue) | 3 oz | 141 | 72 |
| Breast Cutlets Thin-Sliced, Oven Stuffer; cooked<br>(Perdue) | 3 oz | 141 | 72 |

| FOOD | PORTION | CALORIES | CHOLESTEROL |
|---|---|---|---|
| Breast Quarters, meat only; cooked (Perdue) | 3 oz | 169 | 72 |
| Breast Split, meat only; cooked (Perdue) | 3 oz | 169 | 72 |
| Breast Whole, Oven Stuffer, meat only; cooked (Perdue) | 3 oz | 169 | 72 |
| Breast Whole, meat only; cooked (Perdue) | 3 oz | 169 | 72 |
| Cornish Game Hen Fresh Whole; cooked (Perdue) | 3 oz | 205 | 75 |
| Drumsticks, Oven Stuffer, meat only; cooked (Perdue) | 3 oz | 185 | 78 |
| Drumsticks, meat only; cooked (Perdue) | 3 oz | 185 | 78 |
| Leg Quarters, meat only; cooked (Perdue) | 3 oz | 199 | 79 |
| Oven Stuffer Roaster Whole, meat only; cooked (Perdue) | 3 oz | 205 | 75 |
| Thighs, Boneless Cutlets, Oven Stuffer; cooked (Perdue) | 3 oz | 176 | 76 |
| Thighs, Oven Stuffer, meat only; cooked (Perdue) | 3 oz | 212 | 80 |
| Thighs, meat only; cooked (Perdue) | 3 oz | 212 | 80 |

| FOOD | PORTION | CALORIES | CHOLESTEROL |
|------|---------|----------|-------------|
| Whole, Fresh Young, meat only; cooked (Perdue) | 3 oz | 205 | 75 |
| Wing Drumettes, meat only; cooked (Perdue) | 3 oz | 249 | 72 |
| Wingettes, Oven Stuffer, meat only; cooked (Perdue) | 3 oz | 249 | 72 |
| Wingettes, Oven Stuffer, meat only; cooked (Perdue) | 3 oz | 249 | 72 |
| Wings, meat only; cooked (Perdue) | 3 oz | 249 | 72 |
| back, meat & skin; flour coated, fried | ½ back (2.5 oz) | 238 | 64 |
| back, meat & skin; flour coated, fried | 1.5 oz | 146 | 39 |
| back, meat & skin; fried | 2.5 oz | 238 | 63 |
| back, meat & skin; fried | ½ back (4.2 oz) | 397 | 105 |
| back, meat & skin, raw | ½ back (3.5 oz) | 316 | 79 |
| back, meat & skin, raw | 2.1 oz | 188 | 47 |
| back, meat & skin; roasted | 1 oz | 96 | 28 |
| back, meat & skin; roasted | ½ back (1.9 oz) | 159 | 46 |
| back, meat & skin; stewed | ½ back (2.1 oz) | 158 | 48 |
| back, meat & skin; stewed | 1.3 oz | 93 | 28 |
| back, meat only, raw | 1 oz | 42 | 25 |
| back, meat only, raw | ½ back (1.8 oz) | 70 | 41 |

| FOOD | PORTION | CALORIES | CHOLESTEROL |
|---|---|---|---|
| back, meat only; fried | ½ back (2 oz) | 167 | 54 |
| back, meat only; fried | 1.2 oz | 101 | 32 |
| back, meat only; fried | ½ back (2 oz) | 167 | 54 |
| back, meat only; roasted | .7 oz | 57 | 21 |
| back, meat only; roasted | ½ back (1.4 oz) | 96 | 36 |
| back, meat only; stewed | ½ back (1.5 oz) | 88 | 36 |
| back, meat only; stewed | 1 oz | 45 | 22 |
| breast, meat only; fried | 1.8 oz | 97 | 47 |
| breast, meat only; fried | ½ breast (3 oz) | 161 | 78 |
| breast, meat only, raw | ½ breast (4 oz) | 129 | 68 |
| breast, meat only, raw | 2.5 oz | 78 | 41 |
| breast, meat only; roasted | ½ breast (3 oz) | 142 | 73 |
| breast, meat only; roasted | 1.8 oz | 86 | 44 |
| breast, meat only; stewed | 2 oz | 86 | 44 |
| breast, meat only; stewed | ½ breast (3.3 oz) | 144 | 73 |
| breast, meat & skin; roasted | ½ breast (3.4 oz) | 193 | 83 |
| breast, meat & skin; roasted | 2 oz | 115 | 49 |
| breast, meat & skin; stewed | 2.3 oz | 121 | 50 |
| breast, meat & skin; stewed | ½ breast (3.9 oz) | 202 | 83 |

| FOOD | PORTION | CALORIES | CHOLESTEROL |
|---|---|---|---|
| breast, meat & skin; batter dipped, fried | ½ breast (4.9 oz) | 364 | 119 |
| breast, meat & skin; batter dipped, fried | 2.9 oz | 218 | 72 |
| breast, meat & skin; flour coated, fried | 2.1 oz | 131 | 53 |
| breast, meat & skin; flour coated, fried | ½ breast (3.4 oz) | 218 | 88 |
| breast, meat & skin, raw | 3.1 oz | 150 | 55 |
| breast, meat & skin, raw | ½ breast (5.1 oz) | 250 | 92 |
| broiler or fryer, flesh & skin; roasted | ½ chicken (10.5 oz) | 715 | 263 |
| broiler or fryer, flesh & skin; roasted | 6.2 oz | 426 | 157 |
| broiler or fryer, flesh & skin; stewed | ½ chicken (11.7 oz) | 730 | 262 |
| broiler or fryer, flesh & skin; stewed | 1 lb | 437 | 157 |
| capon, flesh & skin, raw | ½ chicken (2.1 lbs) | 2257 | 720 |
| capon, flesh & skin, raw | 10.4 oz | 695 | 222 |
| capon, flesh & skin; roasted | 6.9 oz | 448 | 169 |
| capon, flesh & skin; roasted | ½ chicken (1.4 lbs) | 1457 | 549 |
| capon, flesh, skin, giblets & neck, raw | 1 chicken (4.7 lbs) | 4987 | 1882 |
| capon, flesh, skin, giblets & neck; roasted | 1 chicken (3.1 lbs) | 3211 | 1458 |
| capon, flesh, skin, giblets & neck; roasted | 7.6 oz | 494 | 224 |

| FOOD | PORTION | CALORIES | CHOLESTEROL |
|---|---|---|---|
| dark meat w/ skin; batter dipped, fried | ½ chicken (9.8 oz) | 828 | 247 |
| dark meat w/ skin; batter dipped, fried | 5.9 oz | 497 | 149 |
| dark meat w/ skin; flour coated, fried | 3.9 oz | 313 | 101 |
| dark meat w/ skin; flour coated, fried | ½ chicken (6.5 oz) | 523 | 169 |
| dark meat w/ skin, raw | 5.6 oz | 379 | 130 |
| dark meat w/ skin, raw | ½ chicken (9.3 oz) | 630 | 217 |
| dark meat w/ skin; roasted | ½ chicken (5.9 oz) | 423 | 152 |
| dark meat w/ skin; roasted | 3.5 oz | 256 | 92 |
| dark meat w/ skin; stewed | 3.9 oz | 256 | 90 |
| dark meat w/ skin; stewed | ½ chicken (6.5 oz) | 428 | 151 |
| dark meat w/o skin; fried | 1 cup | 334 | 135 |
| dark meat w/o skin; fried | 3.2 oz | 217 | 88 |
| dark meat w/o skin, raw | 3.8 oz | 136 | 87 |
| dark meat w/o skin, raw | ½ chicken (6.4 oz) | 227 | 146 |
| dark meat w/o skin; roasted | 2.8 oz | 166 | 75 |
| dark meat w/o skin; roasted | 1 cup | 286 | 130 |
| dark meat w/o skin; stewed | 1 cup | 269 | 123 |
| dark meat w/o skin; stewed | 3 oz | 165 | 76 |
| drumstick, meat & skin; batter dipped, fried | 1.5 oz | 115 | 37 |
| drumstick, meat & skin; batter dipped, fried | 2.6 oz | 193 | 62 |

| FOOD | PORTION | CALORIES | CHOLESTEROL |
|---|---|---|---|
| drumstick, meat & skin; flour coated, fried | 1 oz | 71 | 26 |
| drumstick, meat & skin; flour coated, fried | 1.7 oz | 120 | 44 |
| drumstick, meat & skin, raw | 2.6 oz | 117 | 59 |
| drumstick, meat & skin, raw | 1.5 oz | 71 | 35 |
| drumstick, meat & skin; roasted | 1.8 oz | 112 | 48 |
| drumstick, meat & skin; roasted | 1 oz | 67 | 28 |
| drumstick, meat & skin; stewed | 2 oz | 116 | 48 |
| drumstick, meat & skin; stewed | 1.2 oz | 69 | 28 |
| drumstick, meat only; fried | 1.5 oz | 82 | 40 |
| drumstick, meat only, raw | 1.3 oz | 44 | 28 |
| drumstick, meat only, raw | 2.2 oz | 74 | 48 |
| drumstick, meat only; roasted | 1.5 oz | 76 | 41 |
| drumstick, meat only; stewed | 1.6 oz | 78 | 40 |
| drumstick, meat only; stewed | 1 oz | 47 | 25 |
| flesh & skin, raw | ½ chicken (16.1 oz) | 990 | 347 |
| flesh & skin; flour coated, fried | ½ chicken (11 oz) | 844 | 283 |
| flesh & skin; flour coated, fried | 1 lb | 505 | 169 |
| flesh & skin; fried | ½ chicken (16.4 oz) | 1347 | 404 |
| flesh only; fried | 1 cup | 307 | 131 |

| FOOD | PORTION | CALORIES | CHOLESTEROL |
|---|---|---|---|
| flesh only; fried | 5.4 oz | 340 | 145 |
| flesh only; roasted | 5.1 oz | 278 | 130 |
| flesh only; roasted | 1 cup | 266 | 125 |
| flesh only; stewed | 1 cup | 248 | 116 |
| flesh only; stewed | 5.5 oz | 278 | 130 |
| flesh only, raw | ½ chicken (11.5 oz) | 392 | 231 |
| leg, meat & skin; batter dipped, fried | 5.5 oz | 431 | 142 |
| leg, meat & skin; batter dipped, fried | 3.3 oz | 259 | 85 |
| leg, meat & skin; flour coated, fried | 3.9 oz | 285 | 105 |
| leg, meat & skin; flour coated, fried | 2.4 oz | 170 | 63 |
| leg, meat & skin, raw | 5.6 oz | 312 | 138 |
| leg, meat & skin, raw | 3.5 oz | 189 | 83 |
| leg, meat & skin; roasted | 4 oz | 265 | 105 |
| leg, meat & skin; roasted | 2.4 oz | 160 | 64 |
| leg, meat & skin; stewed | 4.4 oz | 275 | 105 |
| leg, meat & skin; stewed | 2.6 oz | 165 | 63 |
| leg, meat only, raw | 4.6 oz | 156 | 104 |
| leg, meat only, raw | 2.7 oz | 94 | 62 |
| leg, meat only; fried | 3.3 oz | 195 | 93 |
| leg, meat only; fried | 2 oz | 116 | 55 |
| leg, meat only; roasted | 3.3 oz | 182 | 89 |
| leg, meat only; roasted | 2 oz | 109 | 53 |
| leg, meat only; stewed | 3.5 oz | 187 | 90 |

| FOOD | PORTION | CALORIES | CHOLESTEROL |
|---|---|---|---|
| leg, meat only; stewed | 2.1 oz | 111 | 53 |
| light meat w/ skin; battered dipped, fried | 4 oz | 312 | 94 |
| light meat w/ skin; battered dipped, fried | ½ chicken (6.6 oz) | 520 | 157 |
| light meat w/ skin; flour coated, fried | ½ chicken (4.7 oz) | 320 | 113 |
| light meat w/ skin; flour coated, fried | 2.7 oz | 192 | 68 |
| light meat w/ skin, raw | ½ chicken (6.8 oz) | 362 | 130 |
| light meat w/ skin, raw | 4.1 oz | 216 | 78 |
| light meat w/ skin; roasted | 2.8 oz | 175 | 67 |
| light meat w/ skin; roasted | ½ chicken (4.6 oz) | 293 | 111 |
| light meat w/ skin; stewed | ½ chicken (5.3 oz) | 302 | 111 |
| light meat w/ skin; stewed | 3.2 oz | 181 | 66 |
| light meat w/o skin; fried | 2.2 oz | 123 | 57 |
| light meat w/o skin; fried | 1 cup | 268 | 125 |
| light meat w/o skin, raw | ½ chicken (5.2 oz) | 168 | 85 |
| light meat w/o skin, raw | 3.1 oz | 100 | 51 |
| light meat w/o skin; roasted | 1 cup | 242 | 118 |
| light meat w/o skin; roasted | 2.2 oz | 110 | 54 |
| light meat w/o skin; stewed | 2.3 oz | 113 | 54 |
| light meat w/o skin; stewed | 1 cup | 223 | 107 |
| neck, meat & skin; batter dipped, fried | 1.8 oz | 172 | 47 |

| FOOD | PORTION | CALORIES | CHOLESTEROL |
|---|---|---|---|
| neck, meat & skin; flour coated, fried | 1.3 oz | 119 | 34 |
| neck, meat & skin, raw | 1.8 oz | 148 | 49 |
| neck, meat & skin; simmered | 1.3 oz | 95 | 27 |
| neck, meat only, raw | .7 oz | 31 | 17 |
| neck, meat only; fried | .8 oz | 50 | 23 |
| neck, meat only; simmered | .6 oz | 32 | 14 |
| roaster flesh & skin; roasted | ½ chicken (1.1 lbs) | 1071 | 365 |
| roaster, flesh & skin; roasted | 7.4 oz | 469 | 160 |
| skin only; roasted | from ½ chicken (2 oz) | 254 | 46 |
| skin only; roasted | 1.2 oz | 154 | 28 |
| skin only; stewed | 1.6 oz | 160 | 28 |
| skin only; stewed | from ½ chicken (2.5 oz) | 261 | 45 |
| skin only; flour coated, fried | 1 oz | 166 | 24 |
| skin only; flour coated, fried | from ½ chicken (2 oz) | 281 | 41 |
| skin only; fried | from ½ chicken (6.7 oz) | 748 | 140 |
| skin only; fried | 4 oz | 449 | 84 |
| skin only, raw | 1.6 oz | 164 | 51 |
| skin only, raw | from ½ chicken (2.8 oz) | 275 | 86 |

| FOOD | PORTION | CALORIES | CHOLESTEROL |
|---|---|---|---|
| stewing, flesh & skin; stewed | 6.2 oz | 507 | 140 |
| stewing, flesh & skin; stewed | ½ chicken (9.2 oz) | 744 | 205 |
| thigh, meat only, raw | 2.4 oz | 82 | 57 |
| thigh, meat only; fried | 1.8 oz | 113 | 53 |
| thigh, meat only; roasted | 1.8 oz | 109 | 49 |
| thigh, meat only; stewed | 1.9 oz | 107 | 49 |
| thigh, meat & skin, raw | 3.3 oz | 199 | 79 |
| thigh, meat & skin, raw | 2 oz | 120 | 48 |
| thigh, meat & skin; batter dipped, fried | 3 oz | 238 | 80 |
| thigh, meat & skin; batter dipped, fried | 1.8 oz | 144 | 48 |
| thigh, meat & skin; flour coated, fried | 2.2 oz | 162 | 60 |
| thigh, meat & skin; flour coated, fried | 1.3 oz | 99 | 37 |
| thigh, meat & skin; roasted | 2.2 oz | 153 | 58 |
| thigh, meat & skin; roasted | 1.3 oz | 91 | 34 |
| thigh, meat & skin; stewed | 2.4 oz | 158 | 57 |
| thigh, meat & skin; stewed | 1.4 oz | 95 | 35 |
| whole w/ giblets & neck | 1 chicken (2.3 lbs) | 2223 | 940 |
| whole w/ giblets & neck; batter dipped, fried | 1 chicken (2.3 lbs) | 2987 | 1054 |
| whole w/ giblets & neck; batter dipped, fried | 1 lb | 895 | 316 |
| whole w/ giblets & neck; flour coated, fried | 1 lb | 577 | 238 |
| whole w/ giblets & neck; flour coated, fried | 1 chicken (1.6 lbs) | 1928 | 795 |

| FOOD | PORTION | CALORIES | CHOLESTEROL |
|---|---|---|---|
| whole w/ giblets & neck; roasted | 1 chicken (1.5 lbs) | 1598 | 730 |
| whole w/ giblets & neck; roasted | 1 lb | 480 | 219 |
| whole w/ giblets & neck; stewed | 1 lb | 487 | 218 |
| whole w/ giblets & neck; stewed | 1 chicken (1.6 lbs) | 1625 | 726 |
| wing, meat & skin, raw | 1.7 oz | 109 | 38 |
| wing, meat & skin; batter dipped, fried | 1.7 oz | 159 | 39 |
| wing, meat & skin; flour coated, fried | 1.1 oz | 103 | 26 |
| wing, meat & skin; roasted | 1.2 oz | 99 | 29 |
| wing, meat & skin; stewed | 1.4 oz | 100 | 28 |
| wing, meat only, raw | 1 oz | 36 | 17 |
| wing, meat only; fried | .7 oz | 42 | 17 |
| wing, meat only; roasted | .7 oz | 43 | 18 |
| wing, meat only; stewed | .8 oz | 43 | 18 |
| **FROZEN PREPARED** | | | |
| Kibun Chicken Pasta Salad w/ dressing | ½ pkg | 220 | 15 |
| Kibun Chicken Pasta Salad w/o dressing | ½ pkg | 150 | 10 |
| MicroMagic Chicken Sandwich | 1 (4.5 oz) | 390 | 35 |
| Microwave Chefwich Chicken Parmigiana Sandwich | 1 (5 oz) | 380 | 24 |
| Weaver Breast Fillets | 3.5 oz | 195 | 84 |
| Weaver Breast Fillets Strips | 3.5 oz | 200 | 84 |

| FOOD | PORTION | CALORIES | CHOLESTEROL |
|---|---|---|---|
| Weaver Chicken Nuggets | 4 pieces | 240 | 74 |
| Weaver Mini-Drums Crispy | 3 oz | 205 | 51 |
| Weaver Mini-Drums Herbs 'n Spice | 3 oz | 205 | 51 |
| Weaver Rondelets Cheese | 3 oz | 215 | 33 |
| Weaver Rondelets Homestyle | 3 oz | 185 | 46 |
| Weaver Rondelets Italian | 3 oz | 200 | 44 |
| Weaver Rondelets Original | 3 oz | 185 | 46 |
| Weaver Thigh Fillets Strips | 3.5 oz | 240 | 95 |
| Weaver Batter Dipped Breast | 3.5 oz | 250 | 84 |
| Weaver Batter Dipped Thighs/ Drums | 3.5 oz | 245 | 89 |
| Weaver Batter Dipped Wings | 3.5 oz | 270 | 78 |
| Weaver Chicken Croquetts | 3.5 oz | 245 | 44 |
| Weaver Crispy Dutch Frye Breasts | 3.5 oz | 285 | 84 |
| Weaver Crispy Dutch Frye Thighs/Drums | 3.5 oz | 295 | 89 |
| Weaver Crispy Dutch Frye Wings | 3.5 oz | 360 | 78 |
| Weaver Crispy Light Fried Chicken | 2.9 oz | 160 | 70 |
| **READY-TO-USE** | | | |
| Bologna (Health Valley) | 3.5 oz | 300 | 49 |
| Bologna (Weaver) | 3.5 oz | 240 | 100 |
| Breast (Mr. Turkey) | 1 slice (1 oz) | 32 | 9 |

| FOOD | PORTION | CALORIES | CHOLESTEROL |
|---|---|---|---|
| Breast Deli Slice Browned & Roasted (Wampler Longacre) | 1 oz | 49 | 12 |
| Breast Deluxe Oven Roasted (Louis Rich) | 1 slice (28 g) | 30 | 13 |
| Breast Hickory Smoked (Weaver) | 3.5 oz | 125 | 68 |
| Breast Meat (Wampler Longacre) | 1 oz | 38 | 10 |
| Breast Oven Roasted (Oscar Mayer) | 1 slice (28 g) | 29 | 15 |
| Breast Oven Roasted (Weaver) | 3.5 oz | 120 | 68 |
| Breast Smoked (Louis Rich) | 1 slice (28 g) | 31 | 13 |
| Breast Smoked (Oscar Mayer) | 1 slice (28 g) | 26 | 15 |
| Chicken (Carl Buddig) | 1 oz | 50 | 12 |
| Cutlets, Perdue Done It! | 3 oz | 180 | 33 |
| Diced Breast Roll (Wampler Longacre) | 1 oz | 49 | 12 |
| Diced White Breast (Wampler Longacre) | 1 oz | 38 | 10 |
| Nuggets White Breaded Fully Cooked (Wampler Longacre) | 1 oz | 71 | 12 |
| Nuggets, Perdue Done It! | 3 oz | 179 | 45 |
| Roll (Dutch Family) | 1 oz | 61 | 21 |
| Roll (Wampler Longacre) | 1 oz | 65 | 22 |

| FOOD | PORTION | CALORIES | CHOLESTEROL |
| --- | --- | --- | --- |
| Roll Sliced (Wampler Longacre) | 1 oz | 63 | 19 |
| Salad (Wampler Longacre) | 1 oz | 65 | 9 |
| Tenders, Perdue Done It! | 3 oz | 159 | 51 |
| White Oven Roasted (Louis Rich) | 1 slice (28 g) | 39 | 14 |
| White Meat Roll (Weaver) | 3.5 oz | 130 | 43 |
| Wings Hot & Spicy, Perdue Done It! | 3 oz | 186 | 82 |
| chicken roll, light meat | 1 slice (28 g) | 45 | 14 |
| chicken roll, light meat | 1 pkg (6 oz) | 271 | 85 |
| poultry salad sandwich spread | 1 Tbsp | 109 | 4 |
| poultry salad sandwich spread | 1 oz | 238 | 9 |

## CHICKEN DISHES
(*see also* CHICKEN SUBSTITUTE, DINNER)

| HOME RECIPE | | | |
| --- | --- | --- | --- |
| chicken cacciatore | ¾ cup | 394 | 99 |
| chicken paprikash | 1½ cups | 296 | 90 |
| chicken & dumplings | ¾ cup | 256 | 109 |
| chicken & noodles | ¾ cup | 191 | 43 |
| chicken a la king | ¾ cup | 234 | 76 |

| FOOD | PORTION | CALORIES | CHOLESTEROL |
|------|---------|----------|-------------|
| **CHICKEN SUBSTITUTE** | | | |
| Chick Stiks, frzn (Worthington) | 3.5 oz | 232 | tr |
| Chick-Ketts, frzn (Worthington) | 3.5 oz | 199 | tr |
| Chik-Nuggets (Loma Linda) | 5 nuggets (3 oz) | 228 | 0 |
| Chik-Patties (Loma Linda) | 1 patty (3 oz) | 226 | 0 |
| Meatless Chicken (Loma Linda) | 2 slices (2 oz) | 93 | 0 |
| Meatless Chicken Supreme; mix not prep (Loma Linda) | ¼ cup | 50 | 0 |
| Meatless Fried Chicken (Loma Linda) | 1 piece (2 oz) | 180 | 0 |
| Meatless Fried Chicken w/ Gravy (Loma Linda) | 2 piece (3 oz) | 140 | 0 |
| Spicy-Chik Minidrums (Loma Linda) | 5 pieces (3 oz) | 230 | 0 |
| **CHICKPEAS** | | | |
| CANNED Chickpeas (Hanover) | ½ cup | 100 | 0 |
| Garbanzo Lite 50% Less Salt (S&W) | ½ cup | 110 | 0 |
| Garbanzo Premium Large (S&W) | ½ cup | 110 | 0 |
| chickpeas | 1 cup | 285 | 0 |

| FOOD | PORTION | CALORIES | CHOLESTEROL |
|------|---------|----------|-------------|
| DRIED<br>Garbanzo<br>(Hurst Brand) | 1 cup | 288 | 0 |
| cooked | 1 cup | 269 | 0 |
| raw | 1 cup | 729 | 0 |

## CHICORY

| | | | |
|------|---------|----------|-------------|
| FRESH<br>greens, raw | ½ cup | 21 | 0 |

## CHILI

| | | | |
|------|---------|----------|-------------|
| Chili Beans<br>(S&W) | ½ cup | 130 | 0 |
| Chili Con Carne<br>(Health Valley) | 4 oz | 170 | 0 |
| Chili Makin's Original<br>(S&W) | ½ cup | 100 | 0 |
| Lentil Chili<br>(Health Valley) | 4 oz | 110 | 0 |
| Mild Vegetarian w/ Beans<br>(Health Valley) | 4 oz | 120 | 0 |
| Oscar Mayer Chili Con Carne<br>Concentrate | 1 oz | 78 | 14 |
| Spicy Vegetarian w/ Beans<br>(Health Valley) | 4 oz | 120 | 0 |
| chili w/ beans | 1 cup | 286 | 43 |
| chili w/ beans (home recipe) | 1 cup | 399 | 61 |

## CHINESE CABBAGE
(*see* CABBAGE)

| FOOD | PORTION | CALORIES | CHOLESTEROL |
|---|---|---|---|

# CHINESE FOOD
(*see* ORIENTAL FOOD)

# CHIPS
(*see also* POPCORN, PRETZELS, SNACKS)

| FOOD | PORTION | CALORIES | CHOLESTEROL |
|---|---|---|---|
| **CORN** | | | |
| Corn Chips (Health Valley) | 1 oz | 160 | 0 |
| Corn Chips (Wise) | 1 oz | 160 | 0 |
| Corn Chips BBQ (Lance) | 1 pkg (1¾ oz) | 280 | 0 |
| Corn Chips Plain (Lance) | 1 pkg (1¾ oz) | 260 | 0 |
| Corn Chips w/ Cheese (Health Valley) | 1 oz | 160 | 2 |
| Corn Crunchies (Wise) | 1 oz | 160 | 0 |
| Corn Nacho Cheese Flavor Spirals Crispy Corn Twists (Wise) | 1 oz | 160 | 0 |
| Corn Toasted Spirals Crispy Corn Twists (Wise) | 1 oz | 160 | 0 |
| Fritos | 1 oz | 150 | 0 |
| Fritos Bar-B-Q | 1 oz | 150 | 0 |
| **POTATO** | | | |
| Eagle | 1 oz | 150 | 0 |
| Lay's | 1 oz | 150 | 0 |
| Lay's Jalapeno & Cheddar Flavored | 1 oz | 150 | 0 |

| FOOD | PORTION | CALORIES | CHOLESTEROL |
|------|---------|----------|-------------|
| Potato (Kelly's) | 1 oz | 150 | 0 |
| Potato (Lance) | 1 pkg (1⅛ oz) | 190 | 0 |
| Potato BBQ (Lance) | 1 pkg (1⅛ oz) | 190 | 0 |
| Potato Cajun Style (Lance) | 1 pkg (1 oz) | 160 | 0 |
| Potato Chips (Health Valley) | 1 oz | 160 | 0 |
| Potato Chips (New York Deli) | 1 oz | 160 | 0 |
| Potato Chips Barbecue Flavor Ripple (Wise) | 1 oz | 150 | 0 |
| Potato Chips Natural Flavor (Wise) | 1 oz | 160 | 0 |
| Potato Chips No Salt Added (Cottage Fries) | 1 oz | 160 | 0 |
| Potato Country Chips (Health Valley) | 1 oz | 160 | 0 |
| Potato Country Ripple (Health Valley) | 1 oz | 160 | 0 |
| Potato Dip Chips (Health Valley) | 1 oz | 160 | 0 |
| Potato Ripple (Lance) | 1 pkg (1⅛ oz) | 190 | 0 |
| Potato Rippled (Kelly's) | 1 oz | 150 | 0 |
| Potato Sour Cream & Onion (Lance) | 1 pkg (1⅛ oz) | 190 | 0 |
| Potato, Unsalted (Kelly's) | 1 oz | 150 | 0 |

| FOOD | PORTION | CALORIES | CHOLESTEROL |
|---|---|---|---|
| Ripple (Lance) | 1 oz | 160 | 0 |
| Ruffles | 1 oz | 150 | 0 |
| Ruffles Bar-B-Q Flavored | 1 oz | 150 | 0 |
| Ruffles Sour Cream & Onion Artificially Flavored | 1 oz | 150 | 0 |
| Sour Cream and Onion Ripple (Lance) | 1 oz | 170 | tr |
| potato | 10 chips | 105 | 0 |
| potato | 1 oz | 148 | 0 |
| potato sticks | 1 oz pkg | 148 | 0 |
| TORTILLA Doritos | 1 oz | 140 | 0 |
| Doritos Cool Ranch | 1 oz | 140 | 0 |
| Doritos Nacho Cheese Flavored | 1 oz | 140 | 0 |
| Tortilla Chips (La Famous) | 1 oz | 140 | 0 |
| Tortilla Chips Buenitos (Health Valley) | 1 oz | 130 | 0 |
| Tortilla Chips Nacho Cheese Flavor Round Bravos (Wise) | 1 oz | 150 | 0 |
| Tortilla Chips No Salt Added (La Famous) | 1 oz | 140 | 0 |
| Tortilla Jalapeno Cheese (Lance) | 1 pkg (1⅛ oz) | 160 | 0 |
| Tortilla Nacho (Lance) | 1 pkg (1⅛ oz) | 160 | 0 |

| FOOD | PORTION | CALORIES | CHOLESTEROL |
|------|---------|----------|-------------|

# CHITTERLINGS

**FRESH**
| | | | |
|------|---------|----------|-------------|
| pork, raw | 3 oz | 213 | 135 |
| pork; simmered | 3 oz | 258 | 122 |

# CHIVES

**DRIED**
| | | | |
|------|---------|----------|-------------|
| freeze-dried | 1 Tbsp | 1 | 0 |

**FRESH**
| | | | |
|------|---------|----------|-------------|
| raw | 1 tsp | 0 | 0 |

# CHOCOLATE
(*see also* CANDY, CAROB, COCOA, ICE CREAM TOPPINGS, MILK DRINKS)

**BAKING**
| | | | |
|------|---------|----------|-------------|
| German Sweet (Bakers) | 1 oz | 144 | tr |
| Semi-Sweet Chocolate (Bakers) | 1 oz | 136 | tr |
| Unsweetened (Bakers) | 1 oz | 142 | tr |
| Unsweetened Baking Chocolate (Hershey) | 1 oz | 190 | 5 |

**CHIPS**
| | | | |
|------|---------|----------|-------------|
| Chocolate Flavored Chips (Bakers) | ¼ cup | 196 | tr |
| German Sweet Chocolate Chips (Bakers) | ¼ cup | 203 | tr |
| Real Semi-Sweet Chocolate Chips (Bakers) | ¼ cup | 201 | tr |

| FOOD | PORTION | CALORIES | CHOLESTEROL |
|------|---------|----------|-------------|
| Semi-Sweet Chocolate Chips, miniature (Hershey) | ¼ cup | 220 | 10 |
| Semi-Sweet Chocolate Chips, regular (Hershey) | ¼ cup | 220 | 10 |
| **MIX** | | | |
| Hershey Instant Mix | 3 Tbsp | 80 | 0 |
| Ovaltine; as prep w/ whole milk | 8 oz | 227 | 34 |
| Quik Chocolate Flavor (Nestle) | 2 tsp | 90 | 0 |
| chocolate mix; as prep w/ whole milk | 9 oz | 226 | 33 |
| chocolate powder | 2–3 heaping tsp | 75 | 0 |
| **SYRUP** | | | |
| Estee | 1 Tbsp | 6 | 0 |
| Hershey's Chocolate Flavored | 2 Tbsp | 80 | 0 |
| chocolate | 1 cup | 653 | 0 |
| chocolate; as prep w/ whole milk | 9 oz | 232 | 33 |

# CHOCOLATE MILK
(*see* CHOCOLATE, COCOA, MILK DRINKS)

# CISCO

| | | | |
|------|---------|----------|-------------|
| smoked | 3 oz | 151 | 27 |
| smoked | 1 oz | 50 | 9 |

| FOOD | PORTION | CALORIES | CHOLESTEROL |
|------|---------|----------|-------------|

# CITRON

| | | | |
|------|---------|----------|-------------|
| candied | 1 oz | 89 | 0 |

# CLAM

**CANNED**

| | | | |
|------|---------|----------|-------------|
| Quahogs (American Original Foods) | 4 oz | 66 | 16 |
| meat only | 1 cup | 236 | 107 |
| meat only | 3 oz | 126 | 57 |

**FRESH**

| | | | |
|------|---------|----------|-------------|
| clam; cooked | 20 sm | 133 | 60 |
| clam; cooked | 3 oz | 126 | 57 |
| raw | 3 oz | 63 | 29 |
| raw | 9 lg | 133 | 60 |
| raw | 20 sm | 133 | 60 |

**HOME RECIPE**

| | | | |
|------|---------|----------|-------------|
| clam sauce | ½ cup | 274 | 87 |
| clam; breaded & fried | 3 oz | 171 | 52 |
| clam; breaded & fried | 20 sm | 379 | 115 |

# COCOA
(*see also* CHOCOLATE)

**MIX**

| | | | |
|------|---------|----------|-------------|
| Carnation Hot Cocoa 70 Calorie | 3 tsp (21 g) | 70 | 2 |
| Carnation Hot Cocoa Milk Chocolate | 1 pkg or 4 heaping tsp (1 oz) | 110 | 2 |

| FOOD | PORTION | CALORIES | CHOLESTEROL |
|---|---|---|---|
| Carnation Hot Cocoa Natural Mint | 1 pkg or 4 heaping tsp (1 oz) | 110 | 2 |
| Carnation Hot Cocoa Rich Chocolate | 1 pkg or 4 heaping tsp (1 oz) | 110 | 2 |
| Carnation Hot Cocoa Rich Chocolate w/ Marshmallows | 1 pkg or 4 heaping tsp (1 oz) | 110 | 2 |
| Carnation Hot Cocoa Sugar Free Mint | 1 pkg or 4 heaping tsp (15 g) | 50 | 2 |
| Carnation Hot Cocoa Sugar Free Rich Chocolate | 1 pkg or 4 heaping tsp (15 g) | 50 | 2 |
| Hershey's Cocoa | ⅓ cup | 120 | 0 |
| PREPARED Hills Bros. Hot Cocoa Sugar Free; as prep w/ water | 6 oz | 60 | 0 |
| Hills Bros. Hot Cocoa; as prep w/ water | 6 oz | 110 | 0 |
| hot cocoa | 1 cup | 218 | 33 |

## COCONUT

| FOOD | PORTION | CALORIES | CHOLESTEROL |
|---|---|---|---|
| Angel Flake Bag (Bakers) | ⅓ cup | 116 | 0 |
| Angel Flake Can (Bakers) | ⅓ cup | 114 | 0 |
| Premium Shred (Bakers) | ⅓ cup | 136 | 0 |
| coconut water | 1 Tbsp | 3 | 0 |
| coconut water | 1 cup | 46 | 0 |
| cream, canned | 1 Tbsp | 36 | 0 |

| FOOD | PORTION | CALORIES | CHOLESTEROL |
|---|---|---|---|
| cream, canned | 1 cup | 568 | 0 |
| dried, creamed | 1 oz | 194 | 0 |
| dried, sweetened, flaked | 1 cup | 351 | 0 |
| dried, sweetened, flaked | 7 oz pkg | 944 | 0 |
| dried, sweetened, flaked, canned | 1 cup | 341 | 0 |
| dried, sweetened, shredded | 7 oz pkg | 997 | 0 |
| dried, sweetened, shredded | 1 cup | 466 | 0 |
| dried, toasted | 1 oz | 168 | 0 |
| dried, unsweetened | 1 oz | 187 | 0 |
| milk, canned | 1 Tbsp | 30 | 0 |
| milk, canned | 1 cup | 445 | 0 |
| milk, frozen | 1 Tbsp | 30 | 0 |
| milk, frozen | 1 cup | 486 | 0 |
| raw | 1 piece | 159 | 0 |

## COD

| CANNED | | | |
|---|---|---|---|
| Atlantic | 3 oz | 89 | 47 |
| Atlantic | 1 can (11 oz) | 327 | 171 |
| **DRIED** | | | |
| Atlantic | 3 oz | 246 | 129 |
| **FRESH** | | | |
| Atlantic, raw | 3 oz | 70 | 37 |
| Atlantic, raw | 1 fillet (8.1 oz) | 190 | 99 |
| Atlantic; cooked | 1 fillet (6.3 oz) | 189 | 99 |

| FOOD | PORTION | CALORIES | CHOLESTEROL |
|---|---|---|---|
| Atlantic; cooked | 3 oz | 89 | 47 |
| Pacific, raw | 1 fillet (4.1 oz) | 95 | 43 |
| Pacific, raw | 3 oz | 70 | 31 |
| roe, raw | 3½ oz | 130 | 360 |
| FROZEN Au Poivre Style Cod (Icelandic) | 4 oz | 100 | 49 |
| Au Poivre Style Cod (Icelandic) | 6 oz | 150 | 74 |
| Bacon Crumb Flavor Cod (Icelandic) | 4 oz | 216 | 57 |
| Bacon Crumb Flavor Cod (Icelandic) | 6 oz | 324 | 86 |
| Bake 'N' Serve Light Cod (Icelandic) | 4 oz | 199 | 46 |
| Bake 'N' Serve Light Cod (Icelandic) | 6 oz | 300 | 70 |
| Blackened Style Cod (Icelandic) | 4 oz | 126 | 58 |
| Blackened Style Cod (Icelandic) | 6 oz | 189 | 86 |
| Cajun Style Cod (Icelandic) | 4 oz | 138 | 53 |
| Cajun Style Cod (Icelandic) | 6 oz | 208 | 80 |
| Fish in Sauce Danish Dill Cod (Icelandic) | 4 oz | 95 | 47 |
| Fish in Sauce Danish Dill Cod (Icelandic) | 6 oz | 142 | 71 |
| Scampi Style Cod (Icelandic) | 4 oz | 110 | 44 |

| FOOD | PORTION | CALORIES | CHOLESTEROL |
|---|---|---|---|
| Scampi Style Cod (Icelandic) | 6 oz | 166 | 66 |

## COFFEE
(*see also* COFFEE BEVERAGES, COFFEE SUBSTITUTE)

| | | | |
|---|---|---|---|
| INSTANT | | | |
| powder | 1 rounded tsp | 4 | 0 |
| powder w/ chicory | 1 rounded tsp | 6 | 0 |
| INSTANT, DECAFFEINATED | | | |
| powder | 1 rounded tsp | 4 | 0 |
| REGULAR | | | |
| coffee | 6 oz | 4 | 0 |

## COFFEE BEVERAGES
(*see also* COFFEE SUBSTITUTE)

| | | | |
|---|---|---|---|
| Cafe Amaretto International Coffee (General Foods) | 6 oz | 51 | tr |
| Cafe Francais International Coffee (General Foods) | 6 oz | 55 | tr |
| Cafe Francais Sugar Free International Coffee (General Foods) | 6 oz | 35 | tr |
| Cafe Irish Creme International Coffee (General Foods) | 6 oz | 55 | tr |

| FOOD | PORTION | CALORIES | CHOLESTEROL |
|---|---|---|---|
| Cafe Irish Creme Sugar Free International Coffee (General Foods) | 6 oz | 31 | tr |
| Cafe Vienna International Coffee (General Foods) | 6 oz | 59 | tr |
| Cafe Vienna Sugar Free International Coffee (General Foods) | 6 oz | 29 | tr |
| Irish Mocha Mint International Coffee (General Foods) | 6 oz | 51 | tr |
| Irish Mocha Mint Sugar Free International Coffee (General Foods) | 6 oz | 28 | tr |
| Orange Cappuccino International Coffee (General Foods) | 6 oz | 59 | tr |
| Orange Cappuccino Sugar Free International Coffee (General Foods) | 6 oz | 29 | tr |
| Suisse Mocha International Coffee (General Foods) | 6 oz | 53 | tr |
| Suisse Mocha Sugar Free International Coffee (General Foods) | 6 oz | 29 | tr |

## COFFEE SUBSTITUTE

| FOOD | PORTION | CALORIES | CHOLESTEROL |
|---|---|---|---|
| Postum Instant Coffee Flavored; as prep | 6 oz | 11 | 0 |
| Postum Instant; as prep | 6 oz | 11 | 0 |
| as prep w/ milk | 6 oz | 121 | 25 |
| powder | 1 tsp | 9 | 0 |

| FOOD | PORTION | CALORIES | CHOLESTEROL |
|---|---|---|---|

## COFFEE WHITENERS
(*see also* MILK SUBSTITUTE)

LIQUID

| | | | |
|---|---|---|---|
| Coffee Rich | 1 Tbsp | 20 | 0 |
| Coffee-Mate | 1 oz | 31 | 0 |
| Grand Union | 1 Tbsp | 24 | 0 |
| Mocha Mix | 1 Tbsp (½ oz) | 19 | 0 |
| non-dairy, frozen | ½ oz | 20 | 0 |

POWDER

| | | | |
|---|---|---|---|
| Coffee-Mate | 1 pkg (3 g) | 16 | 0 |
| Coffee-Mate | 1 tsp | 10 | 0 |
| non-dairy | 1 tsp | 11 | 0 |

## COLD CUTS
(*see* LUNCHEON MEATS/COLD CUTS)

## COLESLAW
(*see* CABBAGE, SALAD)

## COLLARDS

FRESH

| | | | |
|---|---|---|---|
| cooked | ½ cup | 13 | 0 |
| raw; chopped | 1 cup | 35 | 0 |

FROZEN

| | | | |
|---|---|---|---|
| frzn; cooked | ½ cup | 31 | 0 |
| frzn; not prep | 10 oz | 93 | 0 |

| FOOD | PORTION | CALORIES | CHOLESTEROL |
|------|---------|----------|-------------|

# COOKIE
(*see also* BROWNIE, CAKE, DOUGHNUT, PIE)

HOME RECIPE

| FOOD | PORTION | CALORIES | CHOLESTEROL |
|------|---------|----------|-------------|
| chocolate chip | 1 (.4 oz) | 59 | 5 |
| fortune cookie | 1 (½ oz) | 66 | tr |
| lemon bar | 1 (1 oz) | 110 | 37 |
| molasses | 1 (1.1 oz) | 138 | 25 |
| oatmeal w/ raisins | 1 (.5 oz) | 54 | 5 |
| peanut butter | 1 (.5 oz) | 61 | 5 |
| pumpkin bar | 1 (1.2 oz) | 151 | 25 |
| raspberry bar | 1 (.8 oz) | 76 | 6 |
| sugar | 1 (.4 oz) | 36 | 8 |

READY-TO-EAT

| FOOD | PORTION | CALORIES | CHOLESTEROL |
|------|---------|----------|-------------|
| Amaranth Graham Crackers (Health Valley) | 1.2 oz | 110 | 0 |
| Amaranth Jumbo (Health Valley) | .6 oz | 70 | 0 |
| Animal Crackers (Sunshine) | 14 | 120 | 0 |
| Apple Oatmeal Bar (Lance) | 1 pkg (1.65 oz) | 190 | 5 |
| Apple-Cinnamon (Lance) | 1 pkg (1 oz) | 120 | 0 |
| Baked Apple Bar (Sunbelt) | 1 pkg (1.31 oz) | 130 | tr |
| Blueberry (Lance) | 1 pkg (1 oz) | 120 | 0 |
| Bonnie (Lance) | 1 pkg (¾ oz) | 100 | 5 |

| FOOD | PORTION | CALORIES | CHOLESTEROL |
|---|---|---|---|
| Butter Flavored (Sunshine) | 4 | 120 | 5 |
| Chip-A-Roos (Sunshine) | 2 | 130 | 0 |
| Chips'n Middles (Sunshine) | 2 | 140 | 0 |
| Choc-O-Lunch (Lance) | 1 5/16 oz | 180 | 0 |
| Choc-O-Lunch (Lance) | 1 oz | 130 | 0 |
| Choc-O-Mint (Lance) | 1¼ oz | 180 | 0 |
| Chocolate Chip (Archway) | 1 | 60 | 5 |
| Chocolate Chip (Lance) | 1 pkg (1 oz) | 135 | 5 |
| Chocolate Chip Fudge (Lance) | 1 pkg (1 oz) | 130 | 0 |
| Chocolate Coated Snack Wafer (Estee) | 1 | 120 | <5 |
| Chocolate Creme Filled Wafer (Estee) | 1 | 20 | 0 |
| Chocolate Fudge Sandwich (Sunshine) | 2 | 150 | 0 |
| Chocolate Snack Wafer (Estee) | 1 | 80 | 0 |
| Cinnamon Jumbo (Health Valley) | ½ oz | 70 | 0 |
| Coated Graham (Lance) | 1 5/16 oz | 180 | 0 |
| Cup Custard (Sunshine) | 2 | 130 | 5 |

| FOOD | PORTION | CALORIES | CHOLESTEROL |
|---|---|---|---|
| Fig Bar (Keebler) | 1 | 71 | 12 |
| Fig Bar (Lance) | 1½ oz | 150 | 0 |
| Fig Bars (Sunshine) | 2 | 90 | 0 |
| Ginger Snaps (Sunshine) | 5 | 100 | 0 |
| Gingersnaps (Archway) | 1 | 35 | 0 |
| Golden Fruit Raisin Biscuits (Sunshine) | 2 | 150 | 0 |
| Graham Cinnamon (Sunshine) | 4 | 70 | 0 |
| Graham Honey (Sunshine) | 4 | 60 | 0 |
| Honey Graham (Health Valley) | 1 oz | 100 | 0 |
| Hydrox (Sunshine) | 3 | 160 | 0 |
| Lemon Coolers (Sunshine) | 5 | 140 | 0 |
| Mallopuffs (Sunshine) | 2 | 140 | 0 |
| Malt (Lance) | 1¼ oz | 190 | 0 |
| Molasses (Archway) | 1 | 100 | 10 |
| Nut-O-Lunch (Lance) | 1 oz | 140 | 0 |
| Oat Bran Animal Cookies (Health Valley) | 1 oz | 90 | 0 |

| FOOD | PORTION | CALORIES | CHOLESTEROL |
|---|---|---|---|
| Oat Bran Fruit Cookies (Health Valley) | 1 oz | 110 | 0 |
| Oat Bran Fruit Jumbos (Health Valley) | ½ oz | 70 | 0 |
| Oat Bran Graham Crackers (Health Valley) | 1.1 oz | 100 | 0 |
| Oat Bran Honey Jumbos (Health Valley) | ½ oz | 70 | 0 |
| Oatmeal (Archway) | 1 | 110 | 5 |
| Oatmeal (Lance) | 1 pkg (1 oz) | 130 | 0 |
| Oatmeal (Little Debbie) | 1 pkg (2.75 oz) | 340 | 1 |
| Oatmeal Country Style (Sunshine) | 2 | 110 | 0 |
| Oatmeal Date Filled (Archway) | 1 | 100 | 5 |
| Oatmeal Peanut Sandwich (Sunshine) | 2 | 140 | 0 |
| Oatmeal, Apple Filled (Archway) | 1 | 90 | 5 |
| Peanut Butter & Honey Wafers (Sunbelt) | 1 pkg (1.2 oz) | 160 | tr |
| Peanut Butter Creme Filled Wafer (Lance) | 1 pkg (1¾ oz) | 240 | 0 |
| Peanut Butter Jumbo (Health Valley) | ½ oz | 70 | 0 |
| Peanut Butter Wafers (Sunshine) | 3 | 120 | 0 |

| FOOD | PORTION | CALORIES | CHOLESTEROL |
|---|---|---|---|
| Pecan Crunch (Archway) | 1 | 35 | 0 |
| Pecan Sandie (Keebler) | 1 | 85 | 0 |
| Raisin Oatmeal (Archway) | 1 | 35 | 0 |
| Sandwich Cookies (Estee) | 1 | 44–50 | 0 |
| Select Assortment (Archway) | 1 | 60 | 5 |
| Sprinkles (Sunshine) | 2 | 130 | 0 |
| Strawberry (Lance) | 1 pkg (1 oz) | 120 | 0 |
| Strawberry Snack Wafer (Estee) | 1 | 80 | 0 |
| Sugar Wafers (Sunshine) | 3 | 130 | 0 |
| Tofu Cookies (Health Valley) | 1.2 oz | 130 | 0 |
| Van-O-Lunch (Lance) | 1 5/16 oz | 180 | 0 |
| Van-O-Lunch (Lance) | 1 oz | 140 | 0 |
| Vanilla Snack Wafer (Estee) | 1 | 80 | 0 |
| Vanilla Creme Filled Wafer (Estee) | 1 | 20 | 0 |
| Vanilla Wafers (Sunshine) | 6 | 130 | 5 |
| Vienna Finger Sandwich (Sunshine) | 2 | 140 | 0 |

| FOOD | PORTION | CALORIES | CHOLESTEROL |
|------|---------|----------|-------------|
| Wheat Free (Health Valley) | 1.5 oz | 160 | 0 |
| chocolate oatmeal | 1 (½ oz) | 66 | 5 |
| fig bar | 1 (½ oz) | 49 | 8 |
| gingersnap | 1 (¼ oz) | 30 | 2 |
| graham cracker | 4 pieces | 108 | 0 |
| graham cracker, chocolate covered | 2 pieces | 123 | tr |
| lady finger | 1 | 40 | 39 |
| macaroon | 1 (½ oz) | 54 | 0 |

## CORN

| FOOD | PORTION | CALORIES | CHOLESTEROL |
|------|---------|----------|-------------|
| CANNED | | | |
| Cream Style (Libby) | ½ cup | 80 | 0 |
| Cream Style (Owatonna) | ½ cup | 100 | 0 |
| Cream Style Premium Homestyle (S&W) | ½ cup | 105 | 0 |
| Whole Kernel (Libby) | ½ cup | 80 | 0 |
| Whole Kernel (Seneca) | ½ cup | 80 | 0 |
| Whole Kernel Natural Pack (Libby) | ½ cup | 80 | 0 |
| Whole Kernel Natural Pack (Seneca) | ½ cup | 80 | 0 |
| Whole Kernel Premium Homestyle (S&W) | ½ cup | 90 | 0 |

| FOOD | PORTION | CALORIES | CHOLESTEROL |
|---|---|---|---|
| Whole Kernel Vacuum Pack (Owatonna) | ½ cup | 100 | 0 |
| Whole Kernel in Brine (Owatonna) | ½ cup | 90 | 0 |
| corn | ½ cup | 93 | 0 |
| corn, sweet | ½ cup | 66 | 0 |
| corn, cream style | ½ cup | 93 | 0 |
| FRESH | | | |
| corn, sweet; cooked | 1 ear (2.5 oz) | 83 | 0 |
| sweet kernel, raw | ½ cup | 66 | 0 |
| FROZEN | | | |
| Cob Corn (Ore Ida) | 1 ear (5.3 oz) | 180 | 0 |
| Corn Cob (Birds Eye) | 1 ear (4.4 oz) | 120 | 0 |
| Corn Cob Little Ears (Birds Eye) | 2 ears (4.6 oz) | 126 | 0 |
| Corn Country Style (Budget Gourmet) | 5.57 oz | 140 | 15 |
| Corn on the Cob Natural Ears (Birds Eye) | 1 ear (5.7 oz) | 156 | 0 |
| Corn Sweet, in Butter Sauce (Budget Gourmet) | 5.5 oz | 190 | 15 |
| Kernels; cooked (Health Valley) | 5.8 oz | 134 | 0 |
| White Shoepeg (Hanover) | ½ cup | 80 | 0 |
| White Sweet (Hanover) | ½ cup | 80 | 0 |

| FOOD | PORTION | CALORIES | CHOLESTEROL |
|------|---------|----------|-------------|
| Whole Kernel Tendersweet (Birds Eye) | ½ cup | 82 | tr |
| Whole Kernel Cut (Birds Eye) | ½ cup | 82 | tr |
| Yellow Sweet (Hanover) | ½ cup | 80 | 0 |
| frzn; not prep | ½ cup | 67 | 0 |
| on the cob; cooked | 1 ear (2.2 oz) | 59 | 0 |
| on the cob; not prep | 1 ear (4.4 oz) | 123 | 0 |
| HOME RECIPE fritters | 1 (1 oz) | 62 | 12 |
| scalloped | ½ cup | 258 | 47 |

## CORN CHIPS
(see CHIPS)

## CORNMEAL

| | | | |
|------|---------|----------|-------------|
| Albers White | 1 oz | 100 | 0 |
| Albers Yellow | 1 oz | 100 | 0 |

## CORNSTARCH

| | | | |
|------|---------|----------|-------------|
| Argo | 1 Tbsp | 30 | 0 |
| Argo | 1 cup | 460 | 0 |
| Kingsford's | 1 Tbsp | 30 | 0 |
| Kingsford's | 1 cup | 460 | 0 |

## CORNISH HENS
(see CHICKEN)

| FOOD | PORTION | CALORIES | CHOLESTEROL |
|---|---|---|---|

## COTTAGE CHEESE

| FOOD | PORTION | CALORIES | CHOLESTEROL |
|---|---|---|---|
| **REDUCED CALORIE** | | | |
| Friendship 'N Fruit | 6 oz | 100 | 7 |
| Friendship Lactose Reduced, Lowfat | ½ cup | 90 | 5 |
| Friendship Large Curd Pot Style, Lowfat | ½ cup | 100 | 9 |
| Friendship, Lowfat | ½ cup | 90 | 5 |
| Friendship, Lowfat, No Salt Added | ½ cup | 90 | 5 |
| Land O'Lakes, 2% Fat | 4 oz | 100 | 10 |
| Light n' Lively, Lowfat, 1% | 4 oz | 80 | 15 |
| lowfat, 1% | 4 oz | 82 | 5 |
| lowfat, 1% | 1 cup | 164 | 10 |
| lowfat, 2% | 1 cup | 203 | 19 |
| lowfat, 2% | 4 oz | 101 | 9 |
| **REGULAR** | | | |
| Friendship w/ Pineapple | ½ cup | 140 | 17 |
| Friendship, California Style | ½ cup | 120 | 17 |
| Land O'Lakes | 4 oz | 120 | 15 |
| creamed | ½ cup | 109 | 16 |
| creamed | 1 cup | 217 | 31 |
| creamed, w/ fruit | 4 oz | 140 | 13 |
| dry curd | 1 cup | 123 | 10 |

## COWPEAS

| FOOD | PORTION | CALORIES | CHOLESTEROL |
|---|---|---|---|
| **CANNED** | | | |
| common | 1 cup | 184 | 0 |

| FOOD | PORTION | CALORIES | CHOLESTEROL |
|---|---|---|---|
| common w/ pork | ½ cup | 99 | 8 |
| **DRIED** | | | |
| catjang, raw | 1 cup | 572 | 0 |
| catjang; cooked | 1 cup | 200 | 0 |
| common, raw | 1 cup | 562 | 0 |
| common; cooked | 1 cup | 198 | 0 |
| **FROZEN** | | | |
| cowpeas | ½ cup | 112 | 0 |

# CRAB

| FOOD | PORTION | CALORIES | CHOLESTEROL |
|---|---|---|---|
| **CANNED** | | | |
| blue | 3 oz | 84 | 76 |
| blue | 1 cup | 133 | 120 |
| **FRESH** | | | |
| Alaska king, raw | 3 oz | 71 | 35 |
| Alaska king, raw | 1 leg (6 oz) | 144 | 72 |
| Alaska king, raw | 1 leg (4.7 oz) | 129 | 72 |
| Alaska king, raw | 3 oz | 82 | 45 |
| blue, raw | 3 oz | 74 | 66 |
| blue, raw | 1 crab (.7 oz) | 18 | 16 |
| blue; cooked | 3 oz | 87 | 85 |
| blue; cooked | 1 cup | 138 | 135 |
| dungeness, raw | 1 crab | 140 | 97 |

| FOOD | PORTION | CALORIES | CHOLESTEROL |
|---|---|---|---|
| dungeness, raw | 3 oz | 73 | 50 |
| queen, raw | 3 oz | 76 | 47 |
| **FROZEN**<br>Crab Crisp<br>(King & Prince) | 4 oz | 310 | 34 |
| Crab Del Rey<br>(King & Prince) | 2 oz | 102 | 31 |
| Crab Del Rey<br>(King & Prince) | 3 oz | 153 | 47 |
| Crab Del Rey<br>(King & Prince) | 4 oz | 205 | 63 |
| **HOME RECIPE**<br>deviled | ½ cup | 182 | 125 |
| imperial | ½ cup | 162 | 154 |
| stew | 1 cup | 208 | 73 |
| stuffed | ¾ cup | 129 | 123 |
| **READY-TO-USE**<br>crab cakes | 1 cake<br>(2.1 oz) | 93 | 90 |

# CRABAPPLE

| | | | |
|---|---|---|---|
| **FRESH**<br>raw; sliced | 1 cup | 83 | 0 |

# CRACKER CRUMBS

| | | | |
|---|---|---|---|
| Cracker Meal<br>(Lance) | 1 oz | 100 | 0 |
| Graham<br>(Sunshine) | 1 cup | 550 | 0 |
| cracker meal | 1 cup | 538 | 0 |

| FOOD | PORTION | CALORIES | CHOLESTEROL |
|---|---|---|---|

# CRACKERS
(*see also* CRACKER CRUMBS)

| FOOD | PORTION | CALORIES | CHOLESTEROL |
|---|---|---|---|
| 6 Calorie Wafer (Estee) | 1 | 6 | <5 |
| Bonnie (Lance) | 1³⁄₁₆ oz | 160 | 5 |
| Captain Wafers (Lance) | 2 crackers | 30 | 0 |
| Captain Wafers Very Low Sodium (Lance) | 2 crackers | 30 | 0 |
| Captain's Wafers w/ Cream Cheese & Chives (Lance) | 1⁵⁄₁₆ oz | 170 | 0 |
| Cheddar American Heritage (Sunshine) | 5 | 80 | 5 |
| Cheese Wheels (Health Valley) | 1 oz | 140 | 3 |
| Cheese n' Crackers (Handi-Snacks) | 1 pkg | 130 | 15 |
| Cheese-On-Wheat (Lance) | 1⁵⁄₁₆ oz | 180 | 0 |
| Cheez-It (Sunshine) | 12 | 70 | 0 |
| Dark Finn Crisp Bread (Ryvita) | 2 | 38 | 0 |
| Dark Rye Crisp Bread (Ryvita) | 1 | 26 | 0 |
| Dark w/ Caraway Seeds Finn Crisp Bread (Ryvita) | 2 | 38 | 0 |

| FOOD | PORTION | CALORIES | CHOLESTEROL |
|------|---------|----------|-------------|
| Gold-N-Chee Spicy (Lance) | 15 crackers | 70 | tr |
| Herb No Salt (Health Valley) | 1 oz | 120 | 0 |
| Hi Ho (Sunshine) | 4 | 80 | 0 |
| High Fiber Snackbread (Ryvita) | 1 | 14 | 0 |
| High Fiber Crisp Bread (Ryvita) | 1 | 23 | 0 |
| Krispy Saltine (Sunshine) | 5 | 60 | 0 |
| Krispy Unsalted Tops (Sunshine) | 5 | 60 | 0 |
| Lanchee (Lance) | 1¼ oz | 180 | 5 |
| Light Rye Crisp Bread (Ryvita) | 1 | 26 | 0 |
| Melba Toast Oblong (Lance) | 2 crackers | 30 | 0 |
| Melba Toast Round Garlic (Lance) | 2 crackers | 20 | 0 |
| Melba Toast Round Onion (Lance) | 2 crackers | 20 | 0 |
| Melba Toast Round Plain (Lance) | 2 crackers | 20 | 0 |
| Melba Toast Sesame (Lance) | 2 crackers | 25 | 0 |
| Nekot (Lance) | 1½ oz | 210 | 5 |
| Nip-Chee (Lance) | 1⁵⁄₁₆ oz | 180 | 5 |

| FOOD | PORTION | CALORIES | CHOLESTEROL |
|---|---|---|---|
| Original Wheat Snackbread (Ryvita) | 1 | 20 | 0 |
| Oyster (Nabisco) | 37 pieces | 124 | 0 |
| Oyster & Soup (Sunshine) | 16 | 60 | 0 |
| Oyster Crackers (Lance) | ½ oz | 70 | 0 |
| Parmesan American Heritage (Sunshine) | 4 | 70 | 0 |
| Party Crackers (Estee) | ½ oz | 40 | 0 |
| Peanut Butter Toasty Crackers (Little Debbie) | 1 pkg (.93 oz) | 140 | tr |
| Peanut Butter Toasty Crackers (Little Debbie) | 1 pkg (1.4 oz) | 200 | tr |
| Peanut Butter Wheat (Lance) | 1 5/16 oz | 190 | 0 |
| Peanut Butter 'n Cheese Crackers (Handi-Snacks) | 1 pkg | 190 | 0 |
| Pepato Flavor Tuscany Toast (Tuscany) | 1 oz | 93 | 0 |
| Pesto Flavor Tuscany Toast (Tuscany) | 1 oz | 96 | 3 |
| Pita Crisps (Tuscany) | 1 oz | 90 | 0 |
| Ritz (Nabisco) | 9 pieces | 149 | 0 |
| Rye Twins (Lance) | 2 crackers | 30 | 0 |
| Rye-Chee (Lance) | 1 7/16 oz | 190 | 5 |

| FOOD | PORTION | CALORIES | CHOLESTEROL |
|---|---|---|---|
| Rykrisp (Ralston) | 4 pieces | 91 | 0 |
| Saltines (Lance) | 2 | 25 | 0 |
| Saltines, Slug Pack (Lance) | 4 crackers | 50 | 0 |
| Sesame (Health Valley) | 1 oz | 130 | 0 |
| Sesame American Heritage (Sunshine) | 4 | 70 | 0 |
| Sesame Crackers (Estee) | ½ oz | 40 | 0 |
| Sesame Pita Crisps (Tuscany) | 1 oz | 96 | 0 |
| Sesame Twins (Lance) | 2 crackers | 40 | 0 |
| Stoned Wheat (Health Valley) | 1 oz | 120 | 0 |
| Tam Tams (Manischewitz) | 10 | 147 | 0 |
| Tam Tams No Salt (Manischewitz) | 5 | 70 | 0 |
| Tams Garlic (Manischewitz) | 10 | 153 | 0 |
| Tams Onion (Manischewitz) | 10 | 150 | 0 |
| Tams Wheat (Manischewitz) | 10 | 150 | 0 |
| Thin Wheat Snacks (Lance) | 7 crackers | 80 | 0 |
| Toastchee (Lance) | 1⅜ oz | 190 | 5 |

| FOOD | PORTION | CALORIES | CHOLESTEROL |
|---|---|---|---|
| Toasted Sesame Rye Crisp Bread (Ryvita) | 1 | 31 | 0 |
| Toasty (Lance) | 1¼ oz | 180 | 0 |
| Tomato-Flavor Tuscany Toast (Tuscany) | 1 oz | 95 | 0 |
| Town House (Keebler) | 9 crackers | 157 | tr |
| Triscuit | 7 pieces | 143 | 0 |
| Tuscany Toast (Tuscany) | 1 oz | 95 | 0 |
| Unsalted (Estee) | 2 | 30 | tr |
| Waldorf Low Salt (Keebler) | 9 crackers | 130 | 0 |
| Wheat American Heritage (Sunshine) | 4 | 60 | 0 |
| Wheat Twins (Lance) | 2 crackers | 30 | 0 |
| Wheat Wafers (Sunshine) | 8 | 80 | 0 |
| Wheatswafer (Lance) | 4 crackers | 60 | 0 |
| Wheatswafer (Lance) | 2 crackers | 30 | 0 |
| melba toast | 1 | 20 | 0 |
| saltine | 10 pieces | 121 | 0 |
| SNACK Cheese Crackers w/ Peanut Butter (Little Debbie) | 1 pkg (1.4 oz) | 190 | tr |

| FOOD | PORTION | CALORIES | CHOLESTEROL |
|---|---|---|---|
| Peanut Butter Cheese Crackers (Little Debbie) | 1 pkg (.93 oz) | 130 | tr |

## CRANBERRY

| CANNED | | | |
|---|---|---|---|
| CranOrange (Ocean Spray) | 2 oz | 100 | 0 |
| CranRaspberry (Ocean Spray) | 2 oz | 90 | 0 |
| Cranberry Sauce Jellied Old Fashioned (S&W) | ¼ cup | 90 | 0 |
| Cranberry Sauce Whole Berry Old Fashioned (S&W) | ¼ cup | 90 | 0 |
| Jellied Cranberry Sauce (Ocean Spray) | 2 oz | 90 | 0 |
| Whole Berry Sauce (Ocean Spray) | 2 oz | 90 | 0 |
| cranberry sauce, sweetened | ½ cup | 209 | 0 |
| FRESH | | | |
| Fresh Cranberries (Ocean Spray) | ¼ cup | 25 | 0 |
| cranberries; chopped | 1 cup | 54 | 0 |
| JUICE | | | |
| Cranberry (Smucker's) | 8 oz | 130 | 0 |

## CRANBERRY BEANS

| CANNED | | | |
|---|---|---|---|
| cranberry beans | ½ cup | 108 | 0 |

| FOOD | PORTION | CALORIES | CHOLESTEROL |
|------|---------|----------|-------------|
| **DRIED** | | | |
| cooked | ½ cup | 120 | 0 |
| raw | ½ cup | 328 | 0 |

## CRAYFISH

| FOOD | PORTION | CALORIES | CHOLESTEROL |
|------|---------|----------|-------------|
| **FRESH** | | | |
| cooked | 3 oz | 97 | 151 |
| raw | 3 oz | 76 | 118 |
| raw | 8 | 24 | 37 |

## CREAM
(*see also* SOUR CREAM, SOUR CREAM SUBSTITUTE, WHIPPED TOPPINGS)

| FOOD | PORTION | CALORIES | CHOLESTEROL |
|------|---------|----------|-------------|
| **LIQUID** | | | |
| Half & Half (Land O'Lakes) | 1 Tbsp | 20 | 5 |
| Whipping Cream (Land O'Lakes) | 1 Tbsp | 45 | 15 |
| Whipping Cream, Gourmet Heavy (Land O'Lakes) | 1 Tbsp | 60 | 20 |
| half & half | 1 Tbsp | 20 | 6 |
| half & half | 1 cup | 315 | 89 |
| heavy whipping | 1 Tbsp | 52 | 21 |
| light whipping | 1 Tbsp | 44 | 17 |
| light, coffee | 1 Tbsp | 29 | 10 |
| medium, 25% fat | 1 Tbsp | 37 | 13 |
| **WHIPPED** | | | |
| heavy whipping | 1 cup | 411 | 163 |
| light whipping | 1 cup | 345 | 132 |

| FOOD | PORTION | CALORIES | CHOLESTEROL |
|---|---|---|---|

## CREAM CHEESE

**LIGHT (REDUCED FAT)**

| FOOD | PORTION | CALORIES | CHOLESTEROL |
|---|---|---|---|
| Formagg Cottage | 1 oz | 80 | 0 |
| Formagg Cream Cheese Style | 1 oz | 80 | 0 |
| Philadelphia Brand Light Cream Cheese Product | 1 oz | 60 | 15 |

**NEUFCHATEL**

| FOOD | PORTION | CALORIES | CHOLESTEROL |
|---|---|---|---|
| Neufchatel (Kraft) | 1 oz | 80 | 25 |
| neufchatel | 1 oz | 74 | 22 |

**REGULAR**

| FOOD | PORTION | CALORIES | CHOLESTEROL |
|---|---|---|---|
| Philadelphia Brand | 1 oz | 100 | 30 |
| Philadelphia Brand w/ Pimentos | 1 oz | 90 | 30 |
| Philadelphia Brand w/ Chives | 1 oz | 90 | 30 |
| cream cheese | 1 oz | 99 | 31 |

**SOFT**

| FOOD | PORTION | CALORIES | CHOLESTEROL |
|---|---|---|---|
| Friendship | 1 oz | 103 | 31 |
| Philadelphia Brand | 1 oz | 100 | 30 |
| Philadelphia Brand w/ Chives & Onion | 1 oz | 100 | 30 |
| Philadelphia Brand w/ Honey | 1 oz | 100 | 25 |
| Philadelphia Brand w/ Olives & Pimento | 1 oz | 90 | 30 |
| Philadelphia Brand w/ Pineapple | 1 oz | 90 | 25 |

| FOOD | PORTION | CALORIES | CHOLESTEROL |
|---|---|---|---|
| Philadelphia Brand w/ Smoked Salmon | 1 oz | 90 | 25 |
| Philadelphia Brand w/ Strawberries | 1 oz | 90 | 25 |
| WHIPPED | | | |
| Philadelphia Brand | 1 oz | 100 | 30 |
| Philadelphia Brand w/ Bacon & Horseradish | 1 oz | 90 | 20 |
| Philadelphia Brand w/ Blue Cheese | 1 oz | 100 | 25 |
| Philadelphia Brand w/ Chives | 1 oz | 90 | 25 |
| Philadelphia Brand w/ Onions | 1 oz | 90 | 20 |
| Philadelphia Brand w/ Pimentos | 1 oz | 90 | 20 |
| Philadelphia Brand w/ Smoked Salmon | 1 oz | 100 | 25 |

## CREPES

| | | | |
|---|---|---|---|
| basic crepe, unfilled (home recipe) | 1 | 75 | 55 |

## CRESS
(*see also* WATERCRESS)

| FRESH | | | |
|---|---|---|---|
| garden, raw | ½ cup | 8 | 0 |
| garden; cooked | ½ cup | 16 | 0 |

| FOOD | PORTION | CALORIES | CHOLESTEROL |
|------|---------|----------|-------------|

# CROAKER

### FRESH
| Atlantic, raw | 3 oz | 89 | 52 |
| Atlantic, raw | 1 fillet (2.8 oz) | 83 | 48 |

### HOME RECIPE
| Atlantic; breaded & fried | 1 fillet (3.1 oz) | 192 | 73 |
| Atlantic; breaded & fried | 3 oz | 188 | 71 |

# CROISSANT

| Colonial Wheat Croissants (Rainbo) | 1 | 300 | 5 |
| croissant | 1 | 235 | 13 |

# CROUTONS

| Croutettes (Kellogg) | 1 cup | 144 | 0 |

# CUCUMBER

### FRESH
| raw | 1 | 39 | 0 |
| raw; sliced | ½ cup | 7 | 0 |

# CURRANTS

### DRIED
| currants, Zante | 1 cup | 204 | 0 |

### FRESH
| currants | ½ cup | 36 | 0 |

| FOOD | PORTION | CALORIES | CHOLESTEROL |
|------|---------|----------|-------------|

## CUSK

FRESH
| | | | |
|------|---------|----------|-------------|
| raw | 3 oz | 74 | 35 |
| raw | 1 fillet (4.3 oz) | 106 | 50 |

## CUSTARD
(*see also* PUDDING)

| | | | |
|------|---------|----------|-------------|
| Custard; as prep w/ skim milk (Delmark) | ½ cup | 97 | 6 |
| baked (home recipe) | ½ cup | 152 | 139 |
| custard; as prep from mix | ½ cup | 161 | 80 |
| zabaione (home recipe) | ½ cup | 159 | 409 |

## CUTTLEFISH

FRESH
| | | | |
|------|---------|----------|-------------|
| raw | 3 oz | 67 | 95 |

## DANDELION GREENS

FRESH
| | | | |
|------|---------|----------|-------------|
| cooked | ½ cup | 17 | 0 |
| raw; chopped | ½ cup | 13 | 0 |

## DANISH PASTRY

| | | | |
|------|---------|----------|-------------|
| fruit | 1 (2.3 oz) | 235 | 56 |
| plain | 1 (2 oz) | 220 | 49 |
| plain ring | 1 (12 oz) | 1305 | 292 |

| FOOD | PORTION | CALORIES | CHOLESTEROL |
|------|---------|----------|-------------|

## DATES

DRIED

| | | | |
|------|---------|----------|-------------|
| Dates, California Deglet Noor | 10 | 240 | 0 |
| Dates; diced (Bordo) | 2 oz | 203 | 0 |
| chopped | 1 cup | 489 | 0 |

## DIETING AIDS
(*see* NUTRITIONAL SUPPLEMENTS)

## DINNER
(*see also* ITALIAN FOOD, MEXICAN FOOD, PASTA DINNERS, POT PIE, ORIENTAL FOOD)

FROZEN

| | | | |
|------|---------|----------|-------------|
| Armour Classics Lite Steak Diane | 10 oz | 290 | 90 |
| Banquet All White Meat Fried Chicken Platter | 9 oz | 430 | 105 |
| Banquet Beans & Frankfurters Dinner | 10 oz | 510 | 34 |
| Banquet Beans & Frankfurters Dinner | 10 oz | 510 | 34 |
| Banquet Beef Platter | 10 oz | 460 | 70 |
| Banquet Chicken Pattie Platter | 7.5 oz | 370 | |
| Banquet Chopped Beef Dinner | 11 oz | 420 | 76 |
| Banquet Extra Helping Beef Dinner | 16 oz | 865 | 120 |
| Banquet Extra Helping Lasagne Dinner | 16.5 oz | 645 | 38 |
| Banquet Extra Helping Salisbury Steak Dinner | 18 oz | 910 | 171 |

| FOOD | PORTION | CALORIES | CHOLESTEROL |
|---|---|---|---|
| Banquet Extra Helping Salisbury Steak Dinner w/ Mushroom Gravy | 18 oz | 890 | 169 |
| Banquet Extra Helping Turkey Dinner | 19 oz | 750 | 63 |
| Banquet Family Favorites Chicken & Dumplings Dinner | 10 oz | 420 | 43 |
| Banquet Family Favorites Macaroni & Cheese Dinner | 10 oz | 415 | 28 |
| Banquet Family Favorites Noodles & Chicken Dinner | 10 oz | 340 | 45 |
| Banquet Family Favorites Spaghetti & Meatballs Dinner | 10 oz | 290 | 28 |
| Banquet Fish Platter | 8.75 oz | 445 | 92 |
| Banquet Ham Platter | 10 oz | 400 | 49 |
| Banquet Meat Loaf Dinner | 11 oz | 440 | 82 |
| Banquet Pot Pies Beef, Chicken, Turkey | 7 oz | 520 | 82–37 |
| Banquet Salisbury Steak Dinner | 11 oz | 495 | 76 |
| Banquet Turkey Dinner | 10.5 oz | 385 | 37 |
| Banquet Western Dinner | 11 oz | 630 | 87 |
| Budget Gourmet Cheese Manicotti w/ Meat Sauce | 10 oz | 450 | 50 |
| Budget Gourmet Chicken Cacciatore | 11 oz | 300 | 60 |
| Budget Gourmet Chicken & Egg Noodle w/ Broccoli | 10 oz | 450 | 130 |
| Budget Gourmet Chicken w/ Fettucini | 10 oz | 400 | 100 |

| FOOD | PORTION | CALORIES | CHOLESTEROL |
|---|---|---|---|
| Budget Gourmet Italian Sausage Lasagna | 10 oz | 420 | 80 |
| Budget Gourmet Italian Syle Meatballs with Noodles & Peppers | 10 oz | 310 | 55 |
| Budget Gourmet Linguini w/ Shrimp | 10 oz | 330 | 75 |
| Budget Gourmet Pasta Shells and Beef | 10 oz | 340 | 35 |
| Budget Gourmet Pepper Steak w/ Rice | 10 oz | 300 | 25 |
| Budget Gourmet Scallops & Shrimp Mariner | 11.5 oz | 320 | 70 |
| Budget Gourmet Seafood Newburg | 10 oz | 350 | 70 |
| Budget Gourmet Sirloin Salisbury Steak | 11.5 oz | 410 | 105 |
| Budget Gourmet Sirloin Tips in Burgundy Sauce | 11 oz | 310 | 65 |
| Budget Gourmet Sirloin Tips w/ Country Style Vegetables | 10 oz | 310 | 40 |
| Budget Gourmet Sliced Turkey Breast | 11.1 oz | 290 | 45 |
| Budget Gourmet Slim Selects Beef Stroganoff | 8.75 oz | 280 | 60 |
| Budget Gourmet Slim Selects Cheese Ravioli | 10 oz | 260 | 45 |
| Budget Gourmet Slim Selects Chicken Enchilada Suiza | 9 oz | 270 | 50 |
| Budget Gourmet Slim Selects Chicken-Au-Gratin | 9.1 oz | 260 | 70 |
| Budget Gourmet Slim Selects Fettucini w/ Meat Sauce | 10 oz | 290 | 25 |

| FOOD | PORTION | CALORIES | CHOLESTEROL |
|------|---------|----------|-------------|
| Budget Gourmet Slim Selects French Recipe Chicken | 10 oz | 260 | 60 |
| Budget Gourmet Slim Selects Glazed Turkey | 9 oz | 270 | 50 |
| Budget Gourmet Slim Selects Ham & Asparagus-Au-Gratin | 9 oz | 280 | 40 |
| Budget Gourmet Slim Selects Lasagne w/ Meat Sauce | 10 oz | 290 | 25 |
| Budget Gourmet Slim Selects Linguini w/ Scallops & Clams | 9.5 oz | 280 | 60 |
| Budget Gourmet Slim Selects Mandarin Chicken | 10 oz | 290 | 25 |
| Budget Gourmet Slim Selects Oriental Beef | 10 oz | 290 | 25 |
| Budget Gourmet Slim Selects Sirloin Enchilada Ranchero | 9 oz | 290 | 35 |
| Budget Gourmet Slim Selects Sirloin Salisbury Steak | 9 oz | 280 | 75 |
| Budget Gourmet Slim Selects Sirloin of Beef in Herb Sauce | 10 oz | 290 | 25 |
| Budget Gourmet Swedish Meatballs w/ Noodles | 10 oz | 600 | 140 |
| Budget Gourmet Sweet & Sour Chicken w/ Rice | 10 oz | 350 | 40 |
| Budget Gourmet Teriyaki Chicken | 12 oz | 360 | 55 |
| Budget Gourmet Three Cheese Lasagne | 10 oz | 400 | 65 |
| Budget Gourmet Turkey A La King w/ Rice | 10 oz | 390 | 75 |
| Budget Gourmet Veal Parmigiana | 12 oz | 440 | 165 |

| FOOD | PORTION | CALORIES | CHOLESTEROL |
|---|---|---|---|
| Budget Gourmet Yankee Pot Roast | 11 oz | 380 | 70 |
| Lean Cuisine Baked Rigatoni w/ Meat Sauce & Cheese | 9¾ oz | 260 | 35 |
| Lean Cuisine Beef & Pork Cannelloni w/ Mornay Sauce | 9⅝ oz | 270 | 45 |
| Lean Cuisine Cheese Cannelloni w/ Tomato Sauce | 9⅛ oz | 270 | 30 |
| Lean Cuisine Chicken & Vegetables w/ Vermicelli | 12¾ oz | 270 | 45 |
| Lean Cuisine Chicken a l'Orange w/ Almond Rice | 8 oz | 270 | 50 |
| Lean Cuisine Filet of Fish Divan | 12⅜ oz | 270 | 90 |
| Lean Cuisine Filet of Fish Florentine | 9 oz | 240 | 100 |
| Lean Cuisine Filet of Fish Jardiniere w/ Souffleed Potatoes | 11¼ oz | 280 | 95 |
| Lean Cuisine Glazed Chicken w/ Vegetable Rice | 8½ oz | 270 | 60 |
| Lean Cuisine Herbed Lamb w/ Rice | 10⅜ oz | 270 | 60 |
| Lean Cuisine Meatball Stew | 10 oz | 250 | 80 |
| Lean Cuisine Oriental Beef w/ Vegetables & Rice | 8⅝ oz | 270 | 45 |
| Lean Cuisine Salisbury Steak w/ Italian Style Sauce & Vegetables | 9½ oz | 270 | 95 |
| Lean Cuisine Sliced Turkey Breast in Mushroom Sauce | 8 oz | 220 | 50 |

| FOOD | PORTION | CALORIES | CHOLESTEROL |
|---|---|---|---|
| Lean Cuisine Spaghetti w/ Beef & Mushroom Sauce | 11½ oz | 280 | 25 |
| Lean Cuisine Stuffed Cabbage w/ Meat in Tomato Sauce | 10¾ oz | 220 | 40 |
| Lean Cuisine Turkey Dijon | 9½ oz | 280 | 65 |
| Lean Cuisine Vegetable & Pasta w/ Ham | 9⅜ oz | 280 | 45 |
| Sensible Chef Beef Pepper Steak w/ Rice Casserole | 9 oz | 250 | 54 |
| Sensible Chef Beef Stroganoff w/ Gravy Casserole | 9 oz | 240 | 69 |
| Sensible Chef Beef Tips w/ Vegetable & Noodles Casserole | 9 oz | 250 | 51 |
| Sensible Chef Chicken & Dumplings | 9 oz | 330 | 59 |
| Sensible Chef Chicken Ala King w/ Rice | 9 oz | 250 | 49 |
| Swanson Fried Chicken | 1 pkg (10.8 oz) | 583 | 184 |
| chicken fricassee | ¾ cup | 290 | 72 |

# DIP

| READY-TO-USE | | | |
|---|---|---|---|
| Acapulco (Ortega) | 1 oz | 8 | 0 |
| Avocado Guacamole (Kraft) | 2 Tbsp | 50 | 0 |
| Bacon & Horseradish (Kraft) | 2 Tbsp | 60 | 0 |

| FOOD | PORTION | CALORIES | CHOLESTEROL |
|---|---|---|---|
| Bacon & Horseradish Premium (Kraft) | 2 Tbsp | 50 | 10 |
| Blue Cheese Premium (Kraft) | 2 Tbsp | 45 | 10 |
| Clam (Kraft) | 2 Tbsp | 60 | 10 |
| Clam Premium (Kraft) | 2 Tbsp | 45 | 20 |
| Creamy Cucumber Premium (Kraft) | 2 Tbsp | 50 | 10 |
| Creamy Onion Premium (Kraft) | 2 Tbsp | 45 | 10 |
| French Onion (Kraft) | 2 Tbsp | 60 | 0 |
| French Onion Premium (Kraft) | 2 Tbsp | 45 | 10 |
| Garlic (Kraft) | 2 Tbsp | 60 | 0 |
| Green Onion (Kraft) | 2 Tbsp | 60 | 0 |
| Jalapeno Pepper (Kraft) | 2 Tbsp | 50 | 0 |
| Jalapeno Pepper Premium (Kraft) | 2 Tbsp | 60 | 15 |
| Nacho Cheese Premium (Kraft) | 2 Tbsp | 50 | 10 |

## DOCK

| FRESH | | | |
|---|---|---|---|
| cooked | 3½ oz | 20 | 0 |
| raw; chopped | ½ cup | 15 | 0 |

| FOOD | PORTION | CALORIES | CHOLESTEROL |
|---|---|---|---|

## DOLPHINFISH

FRESH

| | | | |
|---|---|---|---|
| raw | 1 fillet (7.2 oz) | 174 | 149 |
| raw | 3 oz | 73 | 62 |

## DOUGH

| | | | |
|---|---|---|---|
| Fillo Dough (Athens) | 1 oz | 74 | 0 |

## DOUGHNUT
(*see also* DUNKIN' DONUTS)

| | | | |
|---|---|---|---|
| Cake (Hostess) | 1 | 115 | 7 |
| Chocolate Covered (Hostess) | 1 | 129 | 4 |
| Cinnamon (Hostess) | 1 | 109 | 6 |
| Cinnamon Apple (Earth Grains) | 1 | 310 | 25 |
| Devil's Food (Earth Grains) | 1 | 330 | 20 |
| Donut Sticks (Little Debbie) | 1 pkg (1.67 oz) | 230 | tr |
| Donut Sticks (Little Debbie) | 1 pkg (2.5 oz) | 330 | tr |
| Glazed Old Fashioned (Earth Grains) | 1 | 310 | 20 |
| Krunch (Hostess) | 1 | 101 | 4 |
| Old Fashioned (Hostess) | 1 | 172 | 10 |

| FOOD | PORTION | CALORIES | CHOLESTEROL |
|------|---------|----------|-------------|
| Powdered Old Fashioned (Earth Grains) | 1 | 290 | 20 |
| Powdered Sugar (Hostess) | 1 | 112 | 7 |
| cake type, plain | 1 (1.5 oz) | 164 | 19 |
| cake type, sugared | 1 (1.6 oz) | 184 | 20 |
| jelly filled | 1 (2.3 oz) | 226 | 21 |
| raised, plain | 1 (1.5 oz) | 174 | 17 |

## DRESSING
(*see* STUFFING/DRESSING)

## DRINK MIXER
(*see also* SODA)

| FOOD | PORTION | CALORIES | CHOLESTEROL |
|------|---------|----------|-------------|
| Bitter Lemon (Schweppes) | 6 oz | 78 | 0 |
| Collins Mixer (Schweppes) | 6 oz | 70 | 0 |
| Lemon Sour (Schweppes) | 6 oz | 75 | 0 |
| Tonic Water (Schweppes) | 6 oz | 64 | 0 |
| Tonic Water Diet (Schweppes) | 6 oz | tr | 0 |
| whiskey sour mix | 2 oz | 55 | 0 |

## DRUM

FRESH
| freshwater, raw | 3 oz | 101 | 54 |
|-----------------|------|-----|----|
| freshwater, raw | 1 fillet (6.9 oz) | 236 | 127 |

| FOOD | PORTION | CALORIES | CHOLESTEROL |
|------|---------|----------|-------------|

## DUCK

FRESH
| flesh & skin, raw | ½ duck (1.4 lbs) | 2561 | 481 |
| flesh & skin, raw | 10 oz | 1159 | 218 |
| flesh & skin; roasted | 6 oz | 583 | 145 |
| flesh & skin; roasted | ½ duck (13.4 oz) | 1287 | 320 |
| flesh, raw | ½ duck (10.6 oz) | 399 | 233 |
| flesh, raw | 4.8 oz | 180 | 105 |
| flesh; roasted | 3.5 oz | 201 | 89 |
| flesh; roasted | ½ duck (7.8 oz) | 445 | 198 |
| wild, flesh & skin, raw | 8.4 oz | 505 | 191 |
| wild, flesh & skin, raw | 9.5 oz | 571 | 216 |

## DUMPLING

HOME RECIPE
| apple | 1 (10.5 oz) | 566 | 19 |
| dumpling | 2 (1 oz) | 70 | 33 |
| pear | 1 (10.2 oz) | 540 | 41 |

## EEL

FRESH
| cooked | 3 oz | 200 | 137 |
| cooked | 1 fillet (5.6 oz) | 375 | 257 |

| FOOD | PORTION | CALORIES | CHOLESTEROL |
|---|---|---|---|
| raw | 1 fillet (7.2 oz) | 375 | 257 |
| raw | 3 oz | 156 | 107 |
| SMOKED American smoked eel | 1¾ oz | 165 | 35 |

# EGG
(*see also* EGG SUBSTITUTE)

**CHICKEN**

| FOOD | PORTION | CALORIES | CHOLESTEROL |
|---|---|---|---|
| fried w/ butter | 1 | 83 | 246 |
| hard cooked | 1 | 79 | 274 |
| poached | 1 | 79 | 273 |
| raw | 1 | 79 | 274 |
| scrambled w/ butter & milk | 1 | 95 | 248 |
| white only | 1 | 16 | 0 |
| white only | 1 cup | 118 | 0 |
| yolk only | 1 | 63 | 272 |
| yolks | 1 cup | 897 | 3894 |

**DISHES**

| FOOD | PORTION | CALORIES | CHOLESTEROL |
|---|---|---|---|
| Cheese Omelet Sandwich (Microwave Chefwich) | 1 (5 oz) | 410 | 130 |
| Ham & Cheese Omelet Sandwich (Microwave Chefwich) | 1 (5 oz) | 380 | 150 |
| Sausage & Cheese Omelet Sandwich (Microwave Chefwich) | 1 (5 oz) | 410 | 120 |
| Western Style Omelet Sandwich (Microwave Chefwich) | 1 (5 oz) | 360 | 84 |

| FOOD | PORTION | CALORIES | CHOLESTEROL |
|---|---|---|---|
| **HOME RECIPE** | | | |
| creamed | ½ cup | 231 | 310 |
| deviled | 2 halves | 145 | 280 |
| egg foo young | 1 (5.1 oz) | 150 | 250 |
| omelet; as prep from 2 eggs, butter, milk | 4.5 oz | 189 | 497 |
| salad | ½ cup | 307 | 562 |
| **OTHER POULTRY** | | | |
| duck, raw | 1 | 130 | 619 |
| quail, raw | 1 | 14 | 76 |
| turkey, raw | 1 | 135 | 737 |

# EGG SUBSTITUTE

| FOOD | PORTION | CALORIES | CHOLESTEROL |
|---|---|---|---|
| Egg Beaters (Fleischmann's) | ¼ cup | 25 | 0 |
| Egg Beaters w/ Cheez (Fleischmann's) | ¼ cup | 130 | 5 |
| Egg Watchers (Tofutti) | 2 oz | 50 | 0 |
| Eggstra (Tillie Lewis) | 2 oz | 433 | 58 |
| Scramblers, frzn (Morningstar Farms) | 3.5 oz | 105 | 3 |
| frozen | ¼ cup | 96 | 1 |
| liquid | 1½ oz | 40 | tr |
| liquid | 1 cup | 211 | 3 |
| powder | 0.35 oz | 44 | 57 |
| powder | 0.7 oz | 88 | 114 |

| FOOD | PORTION | CALORIES | CHOLESTEROL |
|------|---------|----------|-------------|

## EGGNOG

| FOOD | PORTION | CALORIES | CHOLESTEROL |
|------|---------|----------|-------------|
| Eggnog (Land O'Lakes) | 8 oz | 300 | 123 |
| eggnog | 1 cup | 342 | 149 |
| eggnog | 1 qt | 1368 | 596 |
| eggnog flavor mix; as prep w/ milk | 9 oz | 260 | 33 |

## EGGPLANT

| FOOD | PORTION | CALORIES | CHOLESTEROL |
|------|---------|----------|-------------|
| FRESH | | | |
| cubed, cooked | ½ cup | 13 | 0 |
| raw; cut up | ½ cup | 11 | 0 |
| HOME RECIPE | | | |
| Baba Ghannouj | ¼ cup | 55 | 0 |

## ELDERBERRIES

| FOOD | PORTION | CALORIES | CHOLESTEROL |
|------|---------|----------|-------------|
| FRESH | | | |
| raw | 1 cup | 105 | 0 |

## ENDIVE

| FOOD | PORTION | CALORIES | CHOLESTEROL |
|------|---------|----------|-------------|
| FRESH | | | |
| raw; chopped | ½ cup | 4 | 0 |

## ENGLISH MUFFIN

| FOOD | PORTION | CALORIES | CHOLESTEROL |
|------|---------|----------|-------------|
| Best Foods Regular, Placentia | 1 | 130 | 0 |
| Roman Meal | 1 | 146 | 0 |
| Shop 'n Save | 1 | 130 | 0 |
| Thomas' Sourdough | 1 | 130 | 0 |
| Thomas' Honey Wheat | 1 | 129 | 0 |

| FOOD | PORTION | CALORIES | CHOLESTEROL |
|---|---|---|---|
| Thomas' Raisin | 1 | 153 | 0 |
| Thomas' Regular | 1 | 130 | 0 |
| HOME RECIPE | | | |
| cinnamon raisin | 1 | 186 | 0 |
| honey bran | 1 | 153 | 0 |
| plain | 1 | 158 | 0 |
| whole wheat | 1 | 167 | 1 |

## FALAFEL

| | | | |
|---|---|---|---|
| HOME RECIPE | | | |
| falafel | 1 pattie (.5 oz) | 57 | 0 |
| falafel | 3 patties (1.8 oz) | 170 | 0 |

## FAST FOODS
(*see individual names*)

## FAT
(*see also* BUTTER, BUTTER BLENDS, BUTTER SUBSTITUTE, MARGARINE, OIL)

| | | | |
|---|---|---|---|
| Crisco | 1 Tbsp | 110 | 0 |
| Crisco Butter Flavor | 1 Tbsp | 110 | 0 |
| beef fat; cooked | 1 oz | 193 | 27 |
| beef suet, raw | 1 oz | 242 | 19 |
| chicken fat, raw | 1 oz | 201 | 19 |
| chicken fat, raw | from ½ chicken (1.8 oz) | 327 | 30 |

| FOOD | PORTION | CALORIES | CHOLESTEROL |
|---|---|---|---|
| duck fat | 1 Tbsp | 115 | 13 |
| goose fat | 1 Tbsp | 115 | 13 |
| lard | 1 cup | 1849 | 195 |
| lard | 1 stick | 831 | 57 |
| lard | 1 Tbsp | 115 | 12 |
| lard | 1 tsp | 35 | 2 |
| mutton tallow, raw | 1 Tbsp | 116 | 13 |
| pork backfat | 1 oz | 230 | 16 |
| pork fat | 1 oz | 200 | 26 |
| pork fat, cured; roasted | 1 oz | 167 | 24 |
| pork fat, cured; uncooked | 1 oz | 164 | 19 |
| shortening, soybean & cottonseed | 1 Tbsp | 113 | 0 |
| shortening, soybean & cottonseed | 1 cup | 1812 | 0 |
| shortening, soybean & palm | 1 cup | 1812 | 0 |
| shortening, soybean & palm | 1 Tbsp | 113 | 0 |
| tallow (beef) | 1 Tbsp | 115 | 14 |
| tallow (beef) | 1 cup | 1849 | 223 |
| turkey fat | 1 Tbsp | 115 | 13 |

## FIGS

| | | | |
|---|---|---|---|
| **CANNED** | | | |
| Kadota Figs Whole Fancy (S&W) | ½ cup | 100 | 0 |
| **DRIED** | | | |
| cooked | ½ cup | 140 | 0 |
| whole | 10 | 477 | 0 |

| FOOD | PORTION | CALORIES | CHOLESTEROL |
|------|---------|----------|-------------|
| **FRESH** | | | |
| fig | 1 med | 50 | 0 |
| | | | |
| **FILBERTS** | | | |
| dried, blanched | 1 oz | 191 | 0 |
| dried, unblanched | 1 oz | 179 | 0 |
| dry roasted, unblanched | 1 oz | 188 | 0 |
| oil roasted, unblanched | 1 oz | 187 | 0 |
| | | | |
| **FISH** | | | |
| (see also individual names, FISH SUBSTITUTE) | | | |
| | | | |
| FROZEN | | | |
| breaded fillet; as prep | 1 (2 oz) | 155 | 64 |
| sticks; as prep | 1 stick (1 oz) | 76 | 31 |
| | | | |
| HOME RECIPE | | | |
| fish loaf; cooked | 3½ oz | 124 | 99 |
| | | | |
| **FISH SUBSTITUTE** | | | |
| Fillets, frzn (Worthington) | 3.5 oz | 209 | tr |
| Ocean Fillet (Loma Linda) | 1 (1.7 oz) | 130 | 0 |
| Ocean Fillet (Loma Linda) | 1 (2 oz) | 160 | 0 |
| Ocean Platter; mix not prep (Loma Linda) | ¼ cup | 50 | 0 |
| Vege-Scallops (Loma Linda) | 6 pieces (2.75 oz) | 70 | 0 |

| FOOD | PORTION | CALORIES | CHOLESTEROL |
|---|---|---|---|
| **FLATFISH** | | | |
| FRESH | | | |
| cooked | 1 fillet (4.5 oz) | 148 | 86 |
| cooked | 3 oz | 99 | 58 |
| raw | 3 oz | 78 | 41 |
| raw | 1 fillet (5.7 oz) | 149 | 78 |
| **FLOUNDER** | | | |
| FROZEN | | | |
| Flounder Primavera (King & Prince) | 9 oz | 270 | 90 |
| Flounder Primavera (King & Prince) | 6 oz | 180 | 60 |
| Flounder Primavera (King & Prince) | 4.5 oz | 135 | 45 |
| Flounder Del Rey (King & Prince) | 9 oz | 327 | 105 |
| **FLOUR** | | | |
| All-Purpose (Gold Medal) | 1 cup | 400 | 0 |
| All-Purpose (Red Band) | 1 cup | 390 | 0 |
| All-Purpose (White Deer) | 1 cup | 400 | 0 |
| Drifted Snow (General Mills) | 1 cup | 400 | 0 |
| High Protein Better for Bread (Gold Medal) | 1 cup | 400 | 0 |

| FOOD | PORTION | CALORIES | CHOLESTEROL |
|---|---|---|---|
| La Pina (Gold Medal) | 1 cup | 390 | 0 |
| Self-Rising (Gold Medal) | 1 cup | 380 | 0 |
| Self-Rising (Red Band) | 1 cup | 380 | 0 |
| Softasilk (General Mills) | ¼ cup | 100 | 0 |
| Unbleached (Gold Medal) | 1 cup | 400 | 0 |
| White, Self-Rising (Aunt Jemima) | 1 cup | 479 | 0 |
| Whole Wheat (Gold Medal) | 1 cup | 390 | 0 |
| Whole Wheat (Red Band) | 1 cup | 400 | 0 |
| Whole Wheat Blend (Gold Medal) | 1 cup | 370 | 0 |
| Wondra | 1 cup | 400 | 0 |
| cottonseed, lowfat | 1 oz | 94 | 0 |
| cottonseed, partially defatted | 1 Tbsp | 18 | 0 |
| cottonseed, partially defatted | 1 cup | 337 | 0 |
| peanut, defatted | 1 Tbsp | 13 | 0 |
| peanut, defatted | 1 cup | 196 | 0 |
| peanut, defatted | 1 oz | 92 | 0 |
| peanut, lowfat | 1 oz | 120 | 0 |
| peanut, lowfat | 1 cup | 257 | 0 |
| potato | ½ cup | 316 | 0 |
| rice | 1 cup | 479 | 0 |
| sesame, lowfat | 1 oz | 95 | 0 |

| FOOD | PORTION | CALORIES | CHOLESTEROL |
|------|---------|----------|-------------|

## FRANKFURTER
(*see* HOT DOG)

## FRENCH BEANS

| | | | |
|------|---------|----------|-------------|
| DRIED | | | |
| cooked | 1 cup | 228 | 0 |
| raw | 1 cup | 631 | 0 |

## FRENCH FRIES
(*see* POTATOES)

## FRENCH TOAST

| | | | |
|------|---------|----------|-------------|
| French toast | 1 slice | 155 | 112 |

## FROG LEG

| | | | |
|------|---------|----------|-------------|
| frog leg; as prep w/ seasoned flour & fried (home recipe) | 1 (.8 oz) | 70 | 12 |
| frog legs, raw | 4 lg (3.5 oz) | 73 | 50 |

## FROSTING
(*see* CAKE)

## FRUCTOSE
(*see also* SUGAR, SUGAR SUBSTITUTE)

| | | | |
|------|---------|----------|-------------|
| Fructose (Estee) | 1 tsp | 12 | 0 |

| FOOD | PORTION | CALORIES | CHOLESTEROL |
|------|---------|----------|-------------|

# FRUIT DRINKS

**FROZEN**

| | | | |
|------|---------|----------|-------------|
| Cranberry Juice Cocktail; as prep (Seneca) | 6 oz | 110 | 0 |
| Cranberry-Apple Juice Cocktail; as prep (Seneca) | 6 oz | 110 | 0 |
| Grape-Cranberry Juice Cocktail; as prep (Seneca) | 6 oz | 110 | 0 |
| Raspberry Cranberry Juice Cocktail; as prep (Seneca) | 6 oz | 110 | 0 |
| White Grape Juice; as prep (Seneca) | 6 oz | 110 | 0 |
| cranberry juice cocktail; as prep | 6 oz glass | 102 | 0 |
| fruit punch; as prep w/ water | 1 cup | 113 | 0 |
| lemonade; as prep w/ water | 1 cup | 100 | 0 |
| limeade; as prep w/ water | 1 cup | 102 | 0 |

**MIX**

| | | | |
|------|---------|----------|-------------|
| Berry Blend; as prep (Crystal Light) | 8 oz | 3 | 0 |
| Black Cherry; as prep (Kool-Aid) | 8 oz | 98 | 0 |
| Cherry Sugar Free; as prep (Kool-Aid) | 8 oz | 3 | 0 |
| Citrus Blend; as prep (Crystal Light) | 8 oz | 3 | 0 |

| FOOD | PORTION | CALORIES | CHOLESTEROL |
|------|---------|----------|-------------|
| Grape; as prep (Crystal Light) | 8 oz | 3 | 0 |
| Grape; as prep (Kool-Aid) | 8 oz | 98 | 0 |
| Lemon-Lime Sugar; as prep (Country Time) | 8 oz | 5 | 0 |
| Lemon-Lime Sweetened; as prep (Country Time) | 8 oz | 82 | 0 |
| Lemon-Lime; as prep (Crystal Light) | 8 oz | 4 | 0 |
| Lemonade Sugar Free; as prep (Kool-Aid) | 8 oz | 4 | 0 |
| Lemonade Sugar Free; as prep (Country Time) | 8 oz | 5 | 0 |
| Lemonade Sugar Sweetened; as prep (Kool-Aid) | 8 oz | 78 | 0 |
| Lemonade Sweetened; as prep (Country Time) | 8 oz | 82 | 0 |
| Lemonade Flavor Crystals; as prep (Wyler's) | 8 oz | 92 | 0 |
| Lemonade; as prep (Crystal Light) | 8 oz | 5 | 0 |
| Lemonade; as prep (Kool-Aid) | 8 oz | 99 | 0 |
| Mountain Berry Punch Sugar Sweetened; as prep (Kool-Aid) | 8 oz | 78 | 0 |

| FOOD | PORTION | CALORIES | CHOLESTEROL |
|------|---------|----------|-------------|
| Orange; as prep (Crystal Light) | 8 oz | 4 | 0 |
| Orange; as prep (Kool-Aid) | 8 oz | 98 | 0 |
| Rainbow Punch; as prep (Kool-Aid) | 8 oz | 98 | 0 |
| Raspberry Sugar Sweetened; as prep (Kool-Aid) | 8 oz | 79 | 0 |
| Sunshine Punch; as prep (Kool-Aid) | 8 oz | 99 | 0 |
| Tang Orange Sugar Free; as prep (General Foods) | 8 oz | 5 | 0 |
| Tang Orange; as prep (General Foods) | 8 oz | 87 | 0 |
| Tropical Punch Sugar Free; as prep (Kool-Aid) | 8 oz | 3 | 0 |
| Tropical Punch Sugar Sweetened; as prep (Kool-Aid) | 8 oz | 84 | 0 |
| Wild Strawberry Artifical Flavor Crystals; as prep (Wyler's) | 8 oz | 80 | 0 |
| Wild Strawberry Artifical Flavor Crystals; as prep (Wyler's) | 8 oz | 80 | 0 |
| fruit punch; as prep w/ water | 9 oz | 97 | 0 |
| lemonade powder; as prep w/ water | 9 oz | 113 | 0 |

| FOOD | PORTION | CALORIES | CHOLESTEROL |
|---|---|---|---|
| **READY-TO-USE** | | | |
| Any Flavor (Land O'Lakes) | 8 oz | 120 | 0 |
| Apple (SIPPS) | 8.45 oz | 130 | 0 |
| Apple Cranberry (Mott's) | 10 oz | 176 | 0 |
| Apple Cranberry (Mott's) | 9.5 oz | 167 | 0 |
| Apple Raspberry (Mott's) | 9.5 oz | 150 | 0 |
| Apple Raspberry (Mott's) | 10 oz | 158 | 0 |
| Black Cherry Cooler (Health Valley) | 13 oz | 144 | 0 |
| Cran-Blueberry (Ocean Spray) | 6 oz | 120 | 0 |
| Cran-Grape (Ocean Spray) | 6 oz | 130 | 0 |
| Cran-Orange (Ocean Spray) | 6 oz | 100 | 0 |
| Cran-Raspberry (Ocean Spray) | 6 oz | 110 | 0 |
| Cran-Raspberry Low Calorie (Ocean Spray) | 6 oz | 40 | 0 |
| Cran-Tastic (Ocean Spray) | 6 oz | 110 | 0 |
| Cranapple (Ocean Spray) | 6 oz | 130 | 0 |
| Cranapple Low Calorie (Ocean Spray) | 6 oz | 40 | 0 |

| FOOD | PORTION | CALORIES | CHOLESTEROL |
|---|---|---|---|
| Cranberry Apple Cooler (Health Valley) | 13 oz | 144 | 0 |
| Cranberry Juice Cocktail (Ocean Spray) | 6 oz | 110 | 0 |
| Cranberry Juice Cocktail (Seneca) | 6 oz | 110 | 0 |
| Cranberry Juice Cocktail Low Calorie (Ocean Spray) | 6 oz | 40 | 0 |
| Cranberry-Apple Juice Cocktail (Seneca) | 6 oz | 110 | 0 |
| Cranicot (Ocean Spray) | 6 oz | 110 | 0 |
| Fruit Punch (Mott's) | 9.5 oz | 150 | 0 |
| Fruit Punch (Mott's) | 10 oz | 170 | 0 |
| Fruit Punch (SIPPS) | 8.45 oz | 130 | 0 |
| Grape (SIPPS) | 8.45 oz | 130 | 0 |
| Grape Apple (Mott's) | 10 oz | 167 | 0 |
| Grape Apple (Mott's) | 9.5 oz | 158 | 0 |
| Lemon-Lime Cooler (SIPPS) | 8.45 oz | 130 | 0 |
| Lemonade (SIPPS) | 8.45 oz | 85 | 0 |
| Lemonade (Shasta) | 12 oz | 146 | 0 |

| FOOD | PORTION | CALORIES | CHOLESTEROL |
|---|---|---|---|
| Mauna La'i Hawaiian Guava Fruit Drink (Ocean Spray) | 6 oz | 100 | 0 |
| Mauna La'i Hawaiian Guava Passion Fruit Drink (Ocean Spray) | 6 oz | 100 | 0 |
| Mixed Berry (SIPPS) | 8.45 oz | 130 | 0 |
| Orange (SIPPS) | 8.45 oz | 130 | 0 |
| Orange Fruit Juice Blend (Mott's) | 10 oz | 144 | 0 |
| Pineapple Grapefruit Juice Cocktail (Ocean Spray) | 6 oz | 110 | 0 |
| Pink Grapefruit Juice Cocktail (Ocean Spray) | 6 oz | 80 | 0 |
| Raspberry Cranberry Juice Cocktail (Seneca) | 6 oz | 110 | 0 |
| Sunny Delight Florida Citrus Punch (Sundor) | 6 oz | 90 | 0 |
| Sunshine Punch (SIPPS) | 8.45 oz | 130 | 0 |
| Wild Cherry (SIPPS) | 8.45 oz | 130 | 0 |
| Wild Cherry Cooler (Health Valley) | 13 oz | 144 | 0 |
| cranberry apricot | 6 oz | 118 | 0 |
| cranberry apple | 6 oz | 123 | 0 |
| cranberry grape | 6 oz | 103 | 0 |

| FOOD | PORTION | CALORIES | CHOLESTEROL |
|---|---|---|---|
| cranberry juice cocktail | 1 cup | 147 | 0 |
| cranberry juice cocktail | 6 oz | 108 | 0 |
| fruit punch | 6 oz | 87 | 0 |
| grape | 6 oz | 94 | 0 |
| orange | 6 oz | 94 | 0 |
| orange & apricot | 1 cup | 128 | 0 |
| pineapple & grapefruit | 1 cup | 117 | 0 |
| pineapple & orange | 1 cup | 125 | 0 |

## FRUIT, MIXED
   (see also individual names)

| | | | |
|---|---|---|---|
| CANNED | | | |
| Fruit Cocktail in Heavy Syrup (S&W) | ½ cup | 90 | 0 |
| Fruit Cocktail Natural Lite (S&W) | ½ cup | 60 | 0 |
| Fruit Cocktail Natural Style (S&W) | ½ cup | 90 | 0 |
| Fruit Salad, chilled (Kraft) | ½ cup | 50 | 0 |
| Mixed Fruit Chunky Natural Style (S&W) | ½ cup | 90 | 0 |
| fruit cocktail, in heavy syrup | ½ cup | 93 | 0 |
| fruit cocktail, in juice | ½ cup | 56 | 0 |
| fruit cocktail, in water | ½ cup | 40 | 0 |
| fruit salad, in heavy syrup | ½ cup | 94 | 0 |
| fruit salad, in juice | ½ cup | 62 | 0 |

| FOOD | PORTION | CALORIES | CHOLESTEROL |
|------|---------|----------|-------------|
| fruit salad, tropical, in heavy syrup | ½ cup | 110 | 0 |
| **DRIED** | | | |
| Fruit 'n Nut Mix (Planters) | 1 oz | 150 | 0 |
| mixed | 11 oz pkg | 712 | 0 |
| **FROZEN** | | | |
| Mixed Fruit in Syrup (Birds Eye) | ½ cup | 123 | 0 |
| **JUICE** | | | |
| Apple Citrus (Tree Top) | 6 oz | 90 | 0 |
| Apple Citrus, frzn; as prep (Tree Top) | 6 oz | 90 | 0 |
| Apple Cranberry (Mott's) | 6 oz | 83 | 0 |
| Apple Cranberry (Mott's) | 9.5 oz | 147 | 0 |
| Apple Cranberry (Mott's) | 8.45 oz | 136 | 0 |
| Apple Cranberry (Tree Top) | 6 oz | 100 | 0 |
| Apple Cranberry, frzn; as prep (Tree Top) | 6 oz | 100 | 0 |
| Apple Grape (Mott's) | 6 oz | 86 | 0 |
| Apple Grape (Mott's) | 8.45 oz | 128 | 0 |
| Apple Grape (Mott's) | 9.5 oz | 139 | 0 |

| FOOD | PORTION | CALORIES | CHOLESTEROL |
|------|---------|----------|-------------|
| Apple Grape<br>(Tree Top) | 6 oz | 100 | 0 |
| Apple Grape, frzn; as prep<br>(Tree Top) | 6 oz | 100 | 0 |
| Apple Pear<br>(Tree Top) | 6 oz | 90 | 0 |
| Apple Pear, frzn; as prep<br>(Tree Top) | 6 oz | 90 | 0 |
| Apple Raspberry<br>(Mott's) | 6 oz | 83 | 0 |
| Apple Raspberry<br>(Mott's) | 8.45 oz | 124 | 0 |
| Apple Raspberry<br>(Tree Top) | 6 oz | 80 | 0 |
| Apple Raspberry, frzn; as<br>prep<br>(Tree Top) | 6 oz | 80 | 0 |
| Apricot Pineapple Nectar<br>(S&W) | 6 oz | 120 | 0 |
| Orange Banana<br>(Chiquita) | 6 oz | 90 | 0 |
| Orange Banana<br>(Smucker's) | 8 oz | 120 | 0 |
| Orange Fruit Juice Blend<br>(Mott's) | 9.5 oz | 139 | 0 |
| Orange-Grapefruit Juice 100%<br>Pure Unsweetened<br>(Kraft) | 6 oz | 80 | 0 |
| Orange-Pineapple Juice 100%<br>Pure Unsweetened<br>(Kraft) | 6 oz | 80 | 0 |
| Pineapple-Grapefruit<br>(Dole) | 6 oz | 90 | 0 |

| FOOD | PORTION | CALORIES | CHOLESTEROL |
|------|---------|----------|-------------|
| Pineapple-Orange (Dole) | 6 oz | 100 | 0 |
| Pineapple-Orange Banana (Dole) | 6 oz | 90 | 0 |
| Pineapple–Pink Grapefruit (Dole) | 6 oz | 101 | 0 |
| orange-grapefruit | 1 cup | 107 | 0 |

## FRUIT SNACKS

| FOOD | PORTION | CALORIES | CHOLESTEROL |
|------|---------|----------|-------------|
| Flavor Tree Cherry Fruit People | 1 oz | 111 | 0 |
| Flavor Tree Fruit Bears | 1.05 oz | 117 | 0 |
| Flavor Tree Fruit Circus | 1.05 oz | 117 | 0 |
| Flavor Tree Fruit Nibbles | ½ pkg | 118 | 0 |
| Flavor Tree Fruit People | 1 oz | 111 | 0 |
| Flavor Tree Lemon Fruit People | 1 oz | 111 | 0 |
| Flavor Tree Orange Fruit People | 1 oz | 111 | 0 |
| Flavor Tree Strawberry Fruit Roll | 1 roll | 67 | 0 |
| Flavor Tree Strawberry Fruit People | 1 oz | 111 | 0 |
| Sunkist Fun Fruit Alphabets | .9 oz | 100 | 0 |
| Sunkist Fun Fruit Animals | .9 oz | 100 | 0 |
| Sunkist Fun Fruit Berry Bunch | .9 oz | 100 | 0 |
| Sunkist Fun Fruit Cherry | .9 oz | 100 | 0 |
| Sunkist Fun Fruit Dinosaurs Strawberry | .9 oz | 100 | 0 |

| FOOD | PORTION | CALORIES | CHOLESTEROL |
|------|---------|----------|-------------|
| Sunkist Fun Fruit Fantastic Fruit Punch | .9 oz | 100 | 0 |
| Sunkist Fun Fruit Grape | .9 oz | 100 | 0 |
| Sunkist Fun Fruit Numbers | .9 oz | 100 | 0 |
| Sunkist Fun Fruit Raspberry | .9 oz | 100 | 0 |
| Sunkist Fun Fruit Strawberry | .9 oz | 100 | 0 |
| Sunkist Fun Fruit Tropical Fruit | .9 oz | 100 | 0 |

# GARBANZO
(see CHICKPEAS)

# GARLIC
| | | | |
|------|---------|----------|-------------|
| powder | 1 tsp | 9 | 0 |
| raw | 1 clove | 4 | 0 |

# GEFILTEFISH
READY-TO-USE
| | | | |
|------|---------|----------|-------------|
| sweet recipe | 1 piece (1.5 oz) | 35 | 12 |

# GELATIN
DRINKS
| | | | |
|------|---------|----------|-------------|
| Orange Flavored Drinking Gelatin w/ NutraSweet (Knox) | 1 envelope | 39 | 0 |

| FOOD | PORTION | CALORIES | CHOLESTEROL |
|------|---------|----------|-------------|
| **MIX** | | | |
| Apricot; as prep (Jell-O) | ½ cup | 80 | 0 |
| Black Cherry; as prep (Jell-O) | ½ cup | 81 | 0 |
| Black Raspberry; as prep (Jell-O) | ½ cup | 81 | 0 |
| Blackberry; as prep (Jell-O) | ½ cup | 81 | 0 |
| Cherry Sugar Free (Diamond Crystal) | ½ cup | 8 | 0 |
| Cherry Sugar Free; as prep (Jell-O) | 1 pop | 9 | 0 |
| Cherry w/ NutraSweet; as prep (D-Zerta) | ½ cup | 8 | 0 |
| Cherry; as prep (Jell-O) | ½ cup | 81 | 0 |
| Concord Grape; as prep (Jell-O) | ½ cup | 81 | 0 |
| Gelatin Desserts; as prep (Estee) | ½ cup | 8 | 0 |
| Hawaiian Pineapple Sugar Free; as prep (Jell-O) | 1 pop | 8 | 0 |
| Lemon Sugar Free; as prep (Jell-O) | 1 pop | 8 | 0 |
| Lemon Sugar Free (Diamond Crystal) | ½ cup | 8 | 0 |
| Lemon w/ NutraSweet; as prep (D-Zerta) | ½ cup | 8 | 0 |

| FOOD | PORTION | CALORIES | CHOLESTEROL |
|------|---------|----------|-------------|
| Lemon; as prep (Jell-O) | ½ cup | 81 | 0 |
| Lime Sugar Free; as prep (Jell-O) | 1 pop | 8 | 0 |
| Lime Sugar Free (Diamond Crystal) | ½ cup | 8 | 0 |
| Lime w/ NutraSweet; as prep (D-Zerta) | ½ cup | 9 | 0 |
| Lime; as prep (Jell-O) | ½ cup | 81 | 0 |
| Mixed Fruit Sugar Free; as prep (Jell-O) | 1 pop | 8 | 0 |
| Mixed Fruit; as prep (Jell-O) | ½ cup | 81 | 0 |
| Orange Pineapple; as prep (Jell-O) | ½ cup | 81 | 0 |
| Orange Sugar Free; as prep (Jell-O) | 1 pop | 8 | 0 |
| Orange Sugar Free (Diamond Crystal) | ½ cup | 8 | 0 |
| Orange w/ NutraSweet; as prep (D-Zerta) | ½ cup | 8 | 0 |
| Orange; as prep (Jell-O) | ½ cup | 81 | 0 |
| Peach Sugar Free; as prep (Jell-O) | 1 pop | 8 | 0 |
| Peach; as prep (Jell-O) | ½ cup | 81 | 0 |

| FOOD | PORTION | CALORIES | CHOLESTEROL |
|------|---------|----------|-------------|
| Raspberry Sugar Free; as prep (Jell-O) | 1 pop | 8 | 0 |
| Raspberry Sugar Free (Diamond Crystal) | ½ cup | 8 | 0 |
| Raspberry w/ NutraSweet; as prep (D-Zerta) | ½ cup | 8 | 0 |
| Raspberry; as prep (Jell-O) | ½ cup | 81 | 0 |
| Strawberry Banana Sugar Free; as prep (Jell-O) | 1 pop | 8 | 0 |
| Strawberry Banana; as prep (Jell-O) | ½ cup | 81 | 0 |
| Strawberry Sugar Free; as prep (Jell-O) | 1 pop | 8 | 0 |
| Strawberry Sugar Free (Diamond Crystal) | ½ cup | 8 | 0 |
| Strawberry w/ NutraSweet; as prep (D-Zerta) | ½ cup | 8 | 0 |
| Strawberry; as prep (Jell-O) | ½ cup | 81 | 0 |
| Triple Berry Sugar Free; as prep (Jell-O) | 1 pop | 8 | 0 |
| Wild Strawberry; as prep (Jell-O) | ½ cup | 81 | 0 |
| dry, unsweetened | 1 Tbsp | 23 | 0 |

| FOOD | PORTION | CALORIES | CHOLESTEROL |
|------|---------|----------|-------------|

## GIBLETS

| FOOD | PORTION | CALORIES | CHOLESTEROL |
|------|---------|----------|-------------|
| capon, raw | 4 oz | 150 | 335 |
| capon; simmered | 1 cup | 238 | 629 |
| chicken; simmered | 1 cup | 228 | 570 |
| chicken; flour coated, fried | 1 cup | 402 | 647 |
| chicken, raw | 2.6 oz | 93 | 196 |
| duck; simmered | 1 cup | 238 | 629 |
| turkey, raw | 8.6 oz | 314 | 688 |
| turkey; simmered | 1 cup | 243 | 606 |

## GINKGO NUTS

| FOOD | PORTION | CALORIES | CHOLESTEROL |
|------|---------|----------|-------------|
| canned | 1 oz | 32 | 0 |
| dried | 1 oz | 99 | 0 |

## GIZZARD

| FOOD | PORTION | CALORIES | CHOLESTEROL |
|------|---------|----------|-------------|
| chicken, raw | 1.3 oz | 41 | 48 |
| chicken; simmered | 1 cup | 222 | 281 |
| turkey, raw | 4 oz | 133 | 178 |
| turkey; simmered | 1 cup | 236 | 336 |

## GOOSE

**FRESH**

| FOOD | PORTION | CALORIES | CHOLESTEROL |
|------|---------|----------|-------------|
| flesh & skin, raw | ½ goose (2.9 lb) | 4893 | 1055 |
| flesh & skin, raw | 11.2 oz | 1187 | 256 |
| flesh & skin; roasted | 6.6 oz | 574 | 172 |
| flesh & skin; roasted | ½ goose (1.7 lbs) | 2362 | 708 |

| FOOD | PORTION | CALORIES | CHOLESTEROL |
|------|---------|----------|-------------|
| flesh, raw | ½ goose (2.3 lbs) | 1237 | 640 |
| flesh, raw | 6.5 oz | 299 | 155 |
| flesh; roasted | 5 oz | 340 | 138 |
| flesh; roasted | ½ goose (1.3 lbs) | 1406 | 569 |

## GOOSEBERRIES

| | | | |
|------|---------|----------|-------------|
| canned, in light syrup | ½ cup | 93 | 0 |
| raw | 1 cup | 67 | 0 |

## GRANOLA
(see also CEREAL)

| BARS | | | |
|------|---------|----------|-------------|
| Kudos Chocolate Chip | 1.2 oz | 180 | 8 |
| Kudos Nutty Fudge | 1.3 oz | 190 | 7 |
| Kudos Peanut Butter | 1.3 oz | 190 | 6 |
| New Trail, Chocolate Covered Cocoa Creme | 1 | 200 | 5 |
| New Trail, Chocolate Covered Peanut Butter | 1 | 200 | 5 |
| Sunbelt Chewy Granola Chocolate Chip | 1 bar (1.25 oz) | 150 | tr |
| Sunbelt Chewy Granola Oats & Honey | 1 bar (1 oz) | 130 | tr |
| Sunbelt Chewy Granola w/ Almonds | 1 bar (1 oz) | 120 | tr |
| Sunbelt Chewy Granola w/ Chocolate Chip | 1 bar (1.75 oz) | 220 | tr |
| Sunbelt Chewy Granola w/ Raisins | 1 bar (1.25 oz) | 150 | tr |

| FOOD | PORTION | CALORIES | CHOLESTEROL |
|---|---|---|---|
| Sunbelt Fudge Dipped Chewy Granola Chocolate Chip | 1 bar (1.63 oz) | 220 | tr |
| Sunbelt Fudge Dipped Chewy Granola Oats & Honey | 1 bar (1.38 oz) | 190 | tr |
| Sunbelt Fudge Dipped Chewy Granola w/ Peanuts | 1 bar (1.5 oz) | 200 | tr |
| Sunbelt Fudge Dipped Chewy Granola w/ Peanuts | 1 bar (2.25 oz) | 300 | tr |
| Sunbelt Granola Cereal Fruit & Nut | 1 bar (1 oz) | 120 | tr |
| **CEREAL** | | | |
| Cinnamon & Raisin (Nature Valley) | ⅓ cup | 120 | 0 |
| Cinnamon & Raisin w/ skim milk (Nature Valley) | ⅓ cup + ½ cup milk | 160 | 3 |
| Coconut & Honey (Nature Valley) | ⅓ cup | 150 | 0 |
| Coconut & Honey w/ skim milk (Nature Valley) | ⅓ cup + ½ cup milk | 190 | 3 |
| Erewhon Date Nut | 1 oz | 130 | 0 |
| Erewhon Honey Almond | 1 oz | 130 | 0 |
| Erewhon Maple | 1 oz | 130 | 0 |
| Erewhon Spiced Apple | 1 oz | 130 | 0 |
| Erewhon Sunflower Crunch | 1 oz | 130 | 0 |
| Erewhon w/ Bran | 1 oz | 130 | 0 |
| Health Valley Real Granola | 1 oz | 120 | 0 |
| Nature Valley Fruit & Nut | ⅓ cup | 170 | 3 |

| FOOD | PORTION | CALORIES | CHOLESTEROL |
|------|---------|----------|-------------|
| Nature Valley Fruit & Nut w/ skim milk | ⅓ cup + ½ cup milk | 170 | 3 |
| Nature Valley Toasted Oat Mixture | ⅓ cup | 130 | 0 |
| Nature Valley Toasted Oat Mixture w/ skim milk | ⅓ cup + ½ cup milk | 170 | 3 |
| Post Hearty Granola | ¼ cup | 127 | 0 |
| Post Hearty Granola w/ Raisins | ¼ cup | 123 | 0 |
| Post Hearty Granola w/ whole milk | ¼ cup + ½ cup milk | 203 | 17 |

## GRAPEFRUIT

| FOOD | PORTION | CALORIES | CHOLESTEROL |
|------|---------|----------|-------------|
| Grapefruit (Tree Top) | 6 oz | 120 | 0 |
| Sections Chilled Unsweetened (Kraft) | ½ cup | 50 | 0 |
| Sections Natural Style (S&W) | ½ cup | 40 | 0 |
| Sections in Light Syrup (S&W) | ½ cup | 80 | 0 |
| in juice | ½ cup | 46 | 0 |
| in light syrup | ½ cup | 76 | 0 |
| in water | ½ cup | 44 | 0 |
| FRESH Pink (Ocean Spray) | ½ med | 50 | 0 |
| Ruby Red (Chiquita) | ½ fruit | 40 | 0 |

| FOOD | PORTION | CALORIES | CHOLESTEROL |
|------|---------|----------|-------------|
| White (Ocean Spray) | ½ med | 45 | 0 |
| grapefruit | ½ fruit | 38 | 0 |
| JUICE Grapefruit (Mott's) | 9.5 oz | 118 | 0 |
| Grapefruit (Mott's) | 10 oz | 124 | 0 |
| Grapefruit Juice (Ocean Spray) | 6 oz | 70 | 0 |
| Grapefruit Juice 100% Pure Unsweetened (Kraft) | 6 oz | 70 | 0 |
| Pink Premium Grapefruit Juice (Ocean Spray) | 6 oz | 60 | 0 |
| Unsweetened (S&W) | 6 oz | 80 | 0 |
| fresh | 1 cup | 96 | 0 |
| frzn, unsweetened | 1 cup | 93 | 0 |
| frzn; as prep | 1 cup | 102 | 0 |
| frzn; not prep | 6 oz container | 302 | 0 |

## GRAPES

| | | | |
|------|---------|----------|-------------|
| CANNED Thompson Seedless Premium (S&W) | ½ cup | 100 | 0 |
| grapes, in heavy syrup | ½ cup | 94 | 0 |
| FRESH grapes | 10 | 36 | 0 |

| FOOD | PORTION | CALORIES | CHOLESTEROL |
|------|---------|----------|-------------|
| **JUICE** | | | |
| Concord Unsweetened (S&W) | 6 oz | 100 | 0 |
| Grape (Seneca) | 6 oz | 115 | 0 |
| Grape, frzn; as prep (Seneca) | 6 oz | 100 | 0 |
| Natural Grape, frzn; as prep (Seneca) | 6 oz | 115 | 0 |
| frzn, sweetened; as prep | 1 cup | 128 | 0 |
| frzn, sweetened; not prep | 6 oz container | 386 | 0 |
| grape | 1 cup | 155 | 0 |

# GRAVY
(*see also* SAUCE)

| FOOD | PORTION | CALORIES | CHOLESTEROL |
|------|---------|----------|-------------|
| **CANNED** | | | |
| au jus | 1 cup | 38 | 1 |
| au jus | 1 can (10.5 oz) | 48 | 1 |
| beef | 1 can (10.2 oz) | 155 | 9 |
| beef | 1 cup | 124 | 7 |
| chicken | 1 cup | 189 | 5 |
| chicken | 1 can (10.5 oz) | 236 | 6 |
| mushroom | 1 can (10.5 oz) | 150 | 0 |
| mushroom | 1 cup | 120 | 0 |
| turkey | 1 cup | 122 | 5 |

| FOOD | PORTION | CALORIES | CHOLESTEROL |
|------|---------|----------|-------------|
| turkey | 1 can (10.5 oz) | 152 | 6 |
| **DRY** | | | |
| Brown Gravy Mix; as prep (Estee) | ¼ cup | 14 | 0 |
| Chicken (Diamond Crystal) | 2 oz | 30 | 2 |
| Chicken and Herb Gravy Mix; as prep (Estee) | ¼ cup | 20 | tr |
| au jus; as prep w/ water | 1 cup | 19 | 1 |
| au jus; not prep | 1 pkg (.8 oz) | 79 | 4 |
| brown; as prep w/ water | 1 cup | 9 | tr |
| brown; not prep | 1 pkg (.9 oz) | 85 | 2 |
| chicken; as prep w/ water | 1 cup | 83 | 3 |
| chicken; not prep | 1 pkg (.8 oz) | 83 | 2 |
| mushroom; as prep w/ water | 1 cup | 70 | 1 |
| mushroom; not prep | 1 pkg (.7 oz) | 70 | 1 |
| onion; as prep w/ water | 1 cup | 80 | 1 |
| onion; not prep | 1 pkg (.8 oz) | 77 | tr |
| pork; as prep w/ water | 1 cup | 76 | 3 |
| pork; not prep | 1 pkg (.7 oz) | 76 | 2 |
| turkey; as prep w/ water | 1 cup | 87 | 3 |
| turkey; not prep | 1 pkg (.9 oz) | 87 | 2 |

| FOOD | PORTION | CALORIES | CHOLESTEROL |
|------|---------|----------|-------------|

## GREAT NORTHERN BEANS

CANNED

| | | | |
|------|---------|----------|-------------|
| Great Northern Beans (Hanover) | ½ cup | 110 | 0 |
| great northern | 1 cup | 300 | 0 |

DRIED

| | | | |
|------|---------|----------|-------------|
| Great Northern (Hurst Brand) | 1 cup | 277 | 0 |
| cooked | 1 cup | 210 | 0 |
| raw | 1 cup | 621 | 0 |

## GREEN BEANS

CANNED

| | | | |
|------|---------|----------|-------------|
| Cut Green Beans (Owatonna) | ½ cup | 20 | 0 |
| Cut Premium Blue Lake (S&W) | ½ cup | 20 | 0 |
| Cuts (Libby) | ½ cup | 20 | 0 |
| Cuts (Seneca) | ½ cup | 20 | 0 |
| Cuts Natural Pack (Libby) | ½ cup | 20 | 0 |
| Cuts Natural Pack (Seneca) | ½ cup | 20 | 0 |
| Dilled (S&W) | ½ cup | 60 | 0 |
| French (Libby) | ½ cup | 20 | 0 |

| FOOD | PORTION | CALORIES | CHOLESTEROL |
|---|---|---|---|
| French (Seneca) | ½ cup | 20 | 0 |
| French Natural Pack (Libby) | ½ cup | 20 | 0 |
| French Natural Pack (Seneca) | ½ cup | 20 | 0 |
| French Style (Owatonna) | ½ cup | 20 | 0 |
| French Style Premium Blue Lake (S&W) | ½ cup | 20 | 0 |
| Whole (Libby) | ½ cup | 20 | 0 |
| Whole (Seneca) | ½ cup | 20 | 0 |
| Whole Fancy Stringless (S&W) | ½ cup | 20 | 0 |
| Whole Vertical Pack (S&W) | ½ cup | 20 | 0 |
| FROZEN Bavarian Style Beans & Spaetzle (Birds Eye) | ½ cup | 98 | 14 |
| Cut Beans (Southland) | 3 oz | 25 | 0 |
| Cut Green Beans (Hanover) | ½ cup | 20 | 0 |
| French (Southland) | 3 oz | 25 | 0 |
| French Green Beans w/ Toasted Almonds (Birds Eye) | ½ cup | 52 | 0 |

| FOOD | PORTION | CALORIES | CHOLESTEROL |
|------|---------|----------|-------------|
| French Style Blue Lake (Hanover) | ½ cup | 25 | 0 |
| French; cooked (Health Valley) | 4.7 oz | 36 | 0 |
| Green Beans Cut (Birds Eye) | ½ cup | 25 | 0 |
| Green Beans French (Birds Eye) | ½ cup | 26 | 0 |
| Green Beans Italian (Birds Eye) | ½ cup | 31 | 0 |
| Green Beans Whole (Birds Eye) | ½ cup | 30 | 0 |
| Italian Cut (Hanover) | ½ cup | 35 | 0 |
| Whole (Birds Eye) | ½ cup | 23 | 0 |
| Whole Blue Lake (Hanover) | ½ cup | 30 | 0 |

## GROUNDCHERRIES

| FOOD | PORTION | CALORIES | CHOLESTEROL |
|------|---------|----------|-------------|
| fresh | ½ cup | 37 | 0 |

## GROUPER

**FRESH**

| FOOD | PORTION | CALORIES | CHOLESTEROL |
|------|---------|----------|-------------|
| cooked | 1 fillet (7.1 oz) | 238 | 95 |
| cooked | 3 oz | 100 | 40 |
| raw | 3 oz | 78 | 31 |
| raw | 1 fillet (9.1 oz) | 238 | 95 |

| FOOD | PORTION | CALORIES | CHOLESTEROL |
|---|---|---|---|
| **GUAVA** | | | |
| FRESH | | | |
| guava | 1 | 45 | 0 |
| HOME RECIPE | | | |
| guava sauce | ½ cup | 43 | 0 |
| **GUINEA HEN** | | | |
| meat, w/o skin, raw | ½ bird (9.3 oz) | 290 | 166 |
| **HADDOCK** | | | |
| FRESH | | | |
| cooked | 1 fillet (5.3 oz) | 168 | 110 |
| cooked | 3 oz | 95 | 63 |
| raw | 3 oz | 74 | 49 |
| raw | 1 fillet (6.8 oz) | 168 | 111 |
| roe, raw | 3½ oz | 130 | 360 |
| SMOKED | | | |
| smoked | 3 oz | 99 | 65 |
| smoked | 1 oz | 33 | 21 |
| **HALIBUT** | | | |
| FRESH | | | |
| Altantic & Pacific, raw | ½ fillet (7.2 oz) | 223 | 65 |
| Atlantic & Pacific, raw | 3 oz | 93 | 27 |
| Atlantic & Pacific; cooked | 3 oz | 119 | 35 |

| FOOD | PORTION | CALORIES | CHOLESTEROL |
|------|---------|----------|-------------|
| Atlantic & Pacific; cooked | ½ fillet (5.6 oz) | 223 | 65 |
| Greenland, raw | ½ fillet (7.2 oz) | 380 | 94 |
| Greenland, raw | 3 oz | 158 | 39 |

## HAM

(*see also* HAM DISHES, LUNCHEON MEATS/COLD CUTS, PORK, TURKEY)

| FOOD | PORTION | CALORIES | CHOLESTEROL |
|------|---------|----------|-------------|
| Armour Golden Star Boneless | 1 oz | 33 | 13 |
| Armour Golden Star Canned | 1 oz | 32 | 11 |
| Armour Lower Salt Boneless | 1 oz | 34 | 13 |
| Armour Lower Salt, 93% Fat Free | 1 oz | 35 | 14 |
| Armour Star Boneless | 1 oz | 41 | 15 |
| Armour Star Canned | 1 oz | 34 | 11 |
| Armour Star Speedy Cut | 1 oz | 44 | 15 |
| Armour 1877 Boneless | 1 oz | 42 | 15 |
| Carl Buddig | 1 oz | 50 | 20 |
| Oscar Mayer Boiled w/ Natural Juices | 1 slice (21 g) | 23 | 12 |
| Oscar Mayer Breakfast Ham Water Added | 1 slice (43 g) | 52 | 21 |
| Oscar Mayer Chopped w/ Natural Juices | 1 slice (28 g) | 55 | 17 |
| Oscar Mayer Cracked Black Pepper | 1 slice (21 g) | 24 | 11 |
| Oscar Mayer Ham & Cheese Loaf | 1 slice (28 g) | 76 | 18 |
| Oscar Mayer Ham Salad Spread w/ Natural Juices | 1 oz | 59 | 10 |

| FOOD | PORTION | CALORIES | CHOLESTEROL |
|---|---|---|---|
| Oscar Mayer Ham and Cheese Spread | 1 oz | 67 | 15 |
| Oscar Mayer Honey w/ Natural Juices | 1 slice (21 g) | 26 | 11 |
| Oscar Mayer Jubilee Boneless | 1 oz | 46 | 15 |
| Oscar Mayer Jubilee Canned w/ Natural Juices | 1 oz | 31 | 13 |
| Oscar Mayer Jubilee Slice w/ Water Added | 1 oz | 29 | 14 |
| Oscar Mayer Jubilee Steak w/ Water Added | 1 slice (2 oz) | 59 | 28 |
| Oscar Mayer Smoked Cooked | 1 slice (21 g) | 23 | 12 |
| Oscar Mayer Baked Cooked | 1 slice (21 g) | 21 | 10 |
| The Spreadables, Ham Salad | ¼ can | 100 | 24 |
| canned; chopped | 1 slice (21 g) | 50 | 10 |
| canned; chopped | 1 oz | 68 | 14 |
| center slice, lean only, raw | 4 oz | 220 | |
| chopped | 1 slice (21 g) | 48 | 11 |
| chopped | 1 oz | 65 | 15 |
| ham (13% fat), canned; roasted | 3 oz | 192 | 52 |
| ham (13% fat), canned; unheated | 1 oz | 54 | 11 |
| ham patties; uncooked | 1 patty (2.3 oz) | 206 | 46 |
| ham salad spread | 1 Tbsp | 32 | 6 |

| FOOD | PORTION | CALORIES | CHOLESTEROL |
|---|---|---|---|
| ham salad spread | 1 oz | 61 | 10 |
| ham, boneless (11% fat); roasted | 3 oz | 151 | 50 |
| ham, boneless, extra lean; roasted | 3 oz | 140 | 48 |
| ham, boneless, extra lean; unheated | 1 slice (1 oz) | 46 | 15 |
| ham, center slice, lean & fat; unheated | 4 oz | 229 | 61 |
| ham, extra lean, canned; roasted | 3 oz | 142 | 34 |
| ham, extra lean, canned; unheated | 1 oz | 41 | 11 |
| minced | 1 slice (21 g) | 55 | 15 |
| minced | 1 oz | 75 | 20 |
| patties; grilled | 1 patty (2 oz) | 203 | 43 |
| sliced, extra lean (5% fat) | 1 slice (28 g) | 37 | 13 |
| sliced, regular (11 % fat) | 1 slice (28 g) | 52 | 16 |
| steak, boneless, extra lean; unheated | 1 oz | 35 | 13 |
| whole, lean & fat; roasted | 3 oz | 207 | 52 |
| whole, lean only; roasted | 3 oz | 133 | 47 |

## HAM DISHES

**HOME RECIPE**

| | | | |
|---|---|---|---|
| croquettes | 1 (3.1 oz) | 217 | 77 |
| salad | ½ cup | 287 | 237 |

| FOOD | PORTION | CALORIES | CHOLESTEROL |
|---|---|---|---|
| **HAZELNUTS** | | | |
| dried, blanched | 1 oz | 191 | 0 |
| dried, unblanched | 1 oz | 179 | 0 |
| dry roasted, unblanched | 1 oz | 188 | 0 |
| oil roasted, unblanched | 1 oz | 187 | 0 |
| **HEART** | | | |
| beef, raw | 4 oz | 132 | 158 |
| beef; simmered | 3 oz | 148 | 164 |
| chicken, raw | 6.1 g | 9 | 8 |
| chicken; simmered | 1 cup | 268 | 350 |
| pork, raw | 1 heart (7.9 oz) | 267 | 296 |
| pork; braised | 1 heart (4.3 oz) | 191 | 285 |
| turkey, raw | 1 oz | 41 | 33 |
| turkey; simmered | 1 cup | 257 | 327 |

**HERBAL TEA**
(*see* TEA/HERBAL TEA)

**HERBS/SPICES**

| FOOD | PORTION | CALORIES | CHOLESTEROL |
|---|---|---|---|
| DRIED | | | |
| Bar-B-Q Shaker (Diamond Crystal) | ½ tsp | 4 | 0 |
| Chef Seasoning (Diamond Crystal) | 1 pkg (.45 oz) | 2 | 0 |
| Chef Shaker (Diamond Crystal) | ½ tsp | 4 | 0 |

| FOOD | PORTION | CALORIES | CHOLESTEROL |
|---|---|---|---|
| French Shaker (Diamond Crystal) | ½ tsp | 4 | 0 |
| Italian Shaker (Diamond Crystal) | ½ tsp | 4 | 0 |
| Mexican Shaker (Diamond Crystal) | ½ tsp | 4 | 0 |
| allspice, ground | 1 tsp | 5 | 0 |
| anise seed | 1 tsp | 7 | 0 |
| basil, ground | 1 tsp | 4 | 0 |
| bay leaf, crumbled | 1 tsp | 2 | 0 |
| caraway seed | 1 tsp | 7 | 0 |
| cardamom, ground | 1 tsp | 6 | 0 |
| cayenne | 1 tsp | 6 | 0 |
| celery seed | 1 tsp | 8 | 0 |
| chervil | 1 tsp | 1 | 0 |
| chili powder | 1 tsp | 8 | 0 |
| chives, freeze-dried | 1 Tbsp | 1 | 0 |
| cinnamon, ground | 1 tsp | 6 | 0 |
| cloves, ground | 1 tsp | 7 | 0 |
| coriander leaf | 1 tsp | 2 | 0 |
| coriander leaf, dried | 1 tsp | 2 | 0 |
| coriander seed | 1 tsp | 5 | 0 |
| cumin seed | 1 tsp | 8 | 0 |
| curry powder | 1 tsp | 6 | 0 |
| dill seed | 1 tsp | 6 | 0 |
| dill weed, dried | 1 tsp | 3 | 0 |
| fennel seed | 1 tsp | 7 | 0 |
| fenugreek seed | 1 tsp | 12 | 0 |

| FOOD | PORTION | CALORIES | CHOLESTEROL |
|---|---|---|---|
| ginger, ground | 1 tsp | 6 | 0 |
| mace, ground | 1 tsp | 8 | 0 |
| marjoram, dried | 1 tsp | 2 | 0 |
| mustard seed, yellow | 1 tsp | 15 | 0 |
| nutmeg, ground | 1 tsp | 12 | 0 |
| onion powder | 1 tsp | 7 | 0 |
| oregano, ground | 1 tsp | 5 | 0 |
| paprika | 1 tsp | 6 | 0 |
| parsley | 1 Tbsp | 1 | 0 |
| parsley, dried | 1 tsp | 1 | 0 |
| parsley, freeze-dried | 1 Tbsp | 1 | 0 |
| pepper, black | 1 tsp | 5 | 0 |
| pepper, red | 1 tsp. | 6 | 0 |
| pepper, white | 1 tsp. | 7 | 0 |
| poppy seed | 1 tsp | 15 | 0 |
| poultry seasoning | 1 tsp | 5 | 0 |
| pumpkin pie spice | 1 tsp | 6 | 0 |
| rosemary, dried | 1 tsp | 4 | 0 |
| saffron | 1 tsp | 2 | 0 |
| sage, ground | 1 tsp | 2 | 0 |
| savory, ground | 1 tsp | 4 | 0 |
| tarragon, ground | 1 tsp | 5 | 0 |
| thyme, ground | 1 tsp | 4 | 0 |
| turmeric, ground | 1 tsp | 8 | 0 |
| FRESH | | | |
| coriander | ¼ cup | 4 | 0 |
| ginger root | 5 slices | 8 | 0 |

| FOOD | PORTION | CALORIES | CHOLESTEROL |
|---|---|---|---|
| ginger root | ½ oz | 7 | 0 |
| parsley, raw; chopped | ½ cup | 10 | 0 |

## HERRING

**CANNED**

| | | | |
|---|---|---|---|
| w/ tomato sauce | 1.9 oz | 97 | 53 |

**FRESH**

| | | | |
|---|---|---|---|
| Atlantic, raw | 3 oz | 134 | 51 |
| Atlantic, raw | 1 fillet (6.5 oz) | 291 | 110 |
| Atlantic; cooked | 1 fillet (5 oz) | 290 | 110 |
| Atlantic; cooked | 3 oz | 172 | 65 |
| Pacific, raw | 1 fillet (6.5 oz) | 359 | 141 |
| Pacific, raw | 3 oz | 166 | 65 |
| roe, raw | 3½ oz | 130 | 360 |

**READY-TO-USE**

| | | | |
|---|---|---|---|
| Atlantic, kippered | 1 fillet (1.4 oz) | 87 | 33 |
| Atlantic, pickled | ½ oz | 39 | 12 |
| kippered, fillet | 1 sm piece (.7 oz) | 42 | 17 |
| kippered, fillet | 1 med piece (.7 oz) | 84 | 34 |

| FOOD | PORTION | CALORIES | CHOLESTEROL |
|------|---------|----------|-------------|

## HICKORY NUTS

| | | | |
|------|---------|----------|-------------|
| dried | 1 oz | 187 | 0 |

## HONEYDEW

| | | | |
|------|---------|----------|-------------|
| FRESH | | | |
| Honey Dew (Chiquita) | 1 cup | 70 | 0 |
| honeydew; cubed | 1 cup | 60 | 0 |

## HORSERADISH

| | | | |
|------|---------|----------|-------------|
| Gold's Hot | 1 Tbsp | 4 | 0 |
| Gold's Red | 1 Tbsp | 4 | 0 |
| Gold's White | 1 Tbsp | 4 | 0 |
| Kraft Horseradish Mustard | 1 Tbsp | 4 | 0 |
| Kraft Horseradish Sauce | 1 Tbsp | 50 | 5 |
| Kraft Cream Style Prepared (Kraft) | 1 Tbsp | 8 | 0 |
| Kraft Prepared | 1 Tbsp | 4 | 0 |
| Sauceworks Horseradish Sauce | 1 Tbsp | 50 | 5 |

## HOT CAKES
(*see* PANCAKES)

## HOT DOG
(*see also* MEAT SUBSTITUTE, SAUSAGE, SAUSAGE SUBSTITUTE)

| | | | |
|------|---------|----------|-------------|
| CHICKEN | | | |
| Chicken Weiners (Health Valley) | 3.5 oz | 290 | 53 |
| Wampler Longacre | 1 (1.6 oz) | 115 | 54 |

| FOOD | PORTION | CALORIES | CHOLESTEROL |
|---|---|---|---|
| Wampler Longacre | 1 (2 oz) | 144 | 54 |
| Weaver | 1 (1.6 oz) | 115 | 39 |
| chicken | 1 (1.5 oz) | 116 | 45 |
| **MEAT** | | | |
| Beef Weiners (Health Valley) | 3.5 oz | 288 | 53 |
| Beef, Armour Lower Salt Jumbo | 1 | 170 | 30 |
| Beef, Armour Star Jumbo | 1 | 190 | 30 |
| Chili Dog Sandwich, frzn (Microwave Chefwich) | 1 (5 oz) | 400 | 20 |
| Frankfurters (Hebrew National) | 1 (1.6 oz) | 140 | 14 |
| Frankfurters (Hebrew National) | 1 (1.8 oz) | 160 | 16 |
| Frankfurters Deli (Hebrew National) | 1 (2.3 oz) | 200 | 20 |
| Meat, Armour Lower Salt Jumbo | 1 | 170 | 30 |
| Meat, Armour Star Jumbo | 1 | 190 | 30 |
| Oscar Mayer Bacon & Cheddar Cheese | 1 (1.6 oz) | 143 | 30 |
| Oscar Mayer Beef Franks | 1 (1.6 oz) | 144 | 29 |
| Oscar Mayer Beef w/ Cheddar Franks | 1 (1.6 oz) | 130 | 29 |
| Oscar Mayer Bun-Length Franks | 1 (2 oz) | 186 | 32 |
| Oscar Mayer Bun-Length Wieners | 1 (2 oz) | 181 | 27 |

| FOOD | PORTION | CALORIES | CHOLESTEROL |
|------|---------|----------|-------------|
| Oscar Mayer Cheese Hot Dogs | 1 (1.6 oz) | 145 | 31 |
| Oscar Mayer German Brand Frankfurters | 1 (2.7 oz) | 230 | 30 |
| Oscar Mayer Wieners | 1 (1.6 oz) | 144 | 27 |
| Oscar Mayer Wieners Little | 1 (.3 oz) | 28 | 5 |
| beef | 1 (1¾ oz) | 184 | 27 |
| beef | 1 (1.5 oz) | 142 | 27 |
| beef | 1 (1.9 oz) | 180 | 35 |
| beef & pork | 1 (1¾ oz) | 183 | 29 |
| pork, cheesefurter, smokie | 1 (1.5 oz) | 141 | 29 |
| TURKEY Cheese Franks (Bil Mar Foods) | 1 (1.6 oz) | 109 | 29 |
| Mr. Turkey Franks | 1 (1.6 oz) | 106 | 31 |
| Mr. Turkey Franks | 1 (½ oz) | 79 | 23 |
| Mr. Turkey Franks | 1 (2 oz) | 132 | 39 |
| Turkey Cheese Franks (Louis Rich) | 1 (1.6 oz) | 108 | 38 |
| Turkey Franks (Louis Rich) | 1 (1.6 oz) | 103 | 42 |
| Turkey Weiners (Health Valley) | 3.5 oz | 238 | 53 |
| Wampler Longacre | 1 (1.6 oz) | 102 | 37 |
| turkey | 1 (1.5 oz) | 102 | 48 |

## HUMMUS

| HOME RECIPE hummus | ⅓ cup | 140 | 0 |

| FOOD | PORTION | CALORIES | CHOLESTEROL |
|------|---------|----------|-------------|
| hummus | 1 cup | 420 | 0 |

## HYACINTH BEANS

DRIED
| | | | |
|------|---------|----------|-------------|
| cooked | 1 cup | 228 | 0 |
| raw | 1 cup | 723 | 0 |

## ICE CREAM AND FROZEN DESSERTS
(*see also* ICE CREAM, NON-DAIRY)

| | | | |
|------|---------|----------|-------------|
| Berry Blend Pops (Crystal Light) | 1 bar | 14 | 0 |
| Berry Punch (Jell-O) | 1 pop | 31 | 0 |
| Blueberry Fruit 'N Juice Bars (Dole) | 1 bar | 90 | 5 |
| Cherry (Jell-O) | 1 pop | 32 | 0 |
| Cherry Fresh Lites (Dole) | 1 bar | 25 | 0 |
| Cherry Fruit & Juice Bars (Chiquita) | 1 bar (2 oz) | 50 | 0 |
| Cherry Fruit Bars (Jell-O) | 1 bar (1.8 oz) | 39 | 0 |
| Cherry Italian Ice (Good Humor) | 6 oz | 138 | 0 |
| Cherry Vanilla, Coffee, Peach, or Strawberry Ice Cream (Breyers) | ½ cup | 135 | 15–20 |
| Cherry/Orange Ice Stripes (Good Humor) | 1.5 oz | 35 | 0 |
| Chocolate (Ben & Jerry's) | 4 oz | 290 | 49 |

| FOOD | PORTION | CALORIES | CHOLESTEROL |
|------|---------|----------|-------------|
| Chocolate Creamy Lites Bar (Carnation) | 1 bar | 50 | 8 |
| Chocolate Fudge Heaven Sundae Bar (Carnation) | 1 bar | 150 | 7 |
| Chocolate Malted Bars (Carnation) | 1 bar | 70 | 19 |
| Chocolate/Vanilla Cool 'N Creamy Bars (Crystal Light) | 1 bar | 55 | 1 |
| Double Chocolate Fudge Cool 'N Creamy Bars (Crystal Light) | 1 bar | 55 | 1 |
| Dutch Chocolate (American Glace) | 4 oz | 48 | 0 |
| French Vanilla (Ben & Jerry's) | 4 oz | 267 | 66 |
| Fruit Flavored Sherbet (Land O'Lakes) | 4 oz | 130 | 5 |
| Fruit Punch Fruit Slush (Wyler's) | 4 oz | 140 | 0 |
| Fruit Punch SunTops (Dole) | 1 bar | 40 | 0 |
| Fruit Punch Pops (Crystal Light) | 1 bar | 14 | 0 |
| Grape (Jell-O) | 1 pop | 31 | 0 |
| Grape SunTops (Dole) | 1 bar | 40 | 0 |
| Grape/Lemon Italian Ice (Good Humor) | 6 oz | 138 | 0 |

| FOOD | PORTION | CALORIES | CHOLESTEROL |
|---|---|---|---|
| Grape/Lemon Ice Stripes (Good Humor) | 1.5 oz | 35 | 0 |
| Lemon Fresh Lites (Dole) | 1 bar | 25 | 0 |
| Lemon White Italian Ice (Good Humor) | 6 oz | 138 | 0 |
| Lemon/Cherry w/ Gummy Dinosaur Colossal Fossil (Good Humor) | 3 oz | 75 | 0 |
| Lemon/Grape w/ Gummy Dinosaur Colossal Fossil (Good Humor) | 3 oz | 75 | 0 |
| Lemon/Lime Swirl (Jell-O) | 1 pop | 33 | 0 |
| Lemonade SunTops (Dole) | 1 bar | 40 | 0 |
| Mandarin Orange Sorbet (Dole) | 4 oz | 110 | 0 |
| Mixed Berry (Jell-O) | 1 pop | 31 | 0 |
| Mixed Berry Bars (Jell-O) | 1 bar (1.8 oz) | 42 | 0 |
| Orange (Jell-O) | 1 pop | 31 | 0 |
| Orange Bars (Jell-O) | 1 bar (1.8 oz) | 42 | 0 |
| Orange Pops (Crystal Light) | 1 bar | 13 | tr |
| Orange Sherbet Push-Up (Good Humor) | 3 oz | 56 | 0 |
| Orange/Pineapple Swirl (Jell-O) | 1 pop | 31 | 0 |

| FOOD | PORTION | CALORIES | CHOLESTEROL |
|---|---|---|---|
| Orange/Raspberry Italian Ice (Good Humor) | 6 oz | 138 | 0 |
| Orange/Vanilla Cool 'N Creamy Bars (Crystal Light) | 1 bar | 31 | tr |
| Original Cheesecake Bar (Carnation) | 1 bar | 120 | 12 |
| Passion-fruit (Vitari) | 4 oz | 80 | 0 |
| Peach (Vitari) | 4 oz | 80 | 0 |
| Peach Fruit 'N Juice Bars (Dole) | 1 bar | 90 | 5 |
| Peach Sorbet (Dole) | 4 oz | 120 | 0 |
| Pina Colada Fruit 'N Juice Bars (Dole) | 1 bar | 90 | 0 |
| Pineapple Fruit 'N Juice Bars (Dole) | 1 bar | 70 | 0 |
| Pineapple Sorbet (Dole) | 4 oz | 120 | 0 |
| Pineapple Orange Fresh Lites (Dole) | 1 bar | 25 | 0 |
| Pineapple Pops (Crystal Light) | 1 bar | 13 | 0 |
| Pink Lemonade Pops (Crystal Light) | 1 bar | 14 | 0 |
| Raspberry (Jell-O) | 1 pop | 29 | 0 |
| Raspberry Banana Fruit & Juice Bars (Chiquita) | 1 bar (2 oz) | 50 | 0 |

| FOOD | PORTION | CALORIES | CHOLESTEROL |
|------|---------|----------|-------------|
| Raspberry Bars (Jell-O) | 1 bar (1.8 oz) | 41 | 0 |
| Raspberry Fruit 'N Juice Bars (Dole) | 1 bar | 70 | 0 |
| Raspberry Pops (Crystal Light) | 1 bar | 14 | 0 |
| Raspberry Sorbet (Dole) | 4 oz | 110 | 0 |
| Raspberry Berry Swirl Bars (Carnation) | 1 bar | 70 | 10 |
| Raspberry Fresh Lites (Dole) | 1 bar | 25 | 0 |
| Raspberry Fruit & Juice Bars (Chiquita) | 1 bar (2 oz) | 50 | 0 |
| Raspberry Peach Bars (Jell-O) | 1 bar (1.8 oz) | 40 | 0 |
| Raspberry/Peach Swirl (Jell-O) | 1 pop | 29 | 0 |
| Skinny Dip | 4 oz | 36 | 0 |
| Strawberries and Cream (Good Humor) | 3 oz | 96 | 0 |
| Strawberry (Jell-O) | 1 pop | 31 | 0 |
| Strawberry Banana (Jell-O) | 1 pop | 31 | 0 |
| Strawberry Banana Bars (Jell-O) | 1 bar (1.8 oz) | 39 | 0 |
| Strawberry Banana Fruit & Juice Bars (Chiquita) | 1 bar (2 oz) | 50 | 0 |
| Strawberry Banana Swirl (Jell-O) | 1 pop | 31 | 0 |

| FOOD | PORTION | CALORIES | CHOLESTEROL |
|---|---|---|---|
| Strawberry Bars (Jell-O) | 1 bar (1.8 oz) | 41 | 0 |
| Strawberry Cheesecake Bars (Carnation) | 1 bar | 125 | 10 |
| Strawberry Creamy Lites Bar (Carnation) | 1 bar | 50 | 7 |
| Strawberry Finger Bar (Good Humor) | 2.5 oz | 49 | 0 |
| Strawberry Fruit 'N Juice Bars (Dole) | 1 bar | 70 | 0 |
| Strawberry Pops (Crystal Light) | 1 bar | 13 | 0 |
| Strawberry Sorbet (Dole) | 4 oz | 110 | 0 |
| Strawberry Tropical Mix (Jell-O) | 1 bar (1.8 oz) | 40 | 0 |
| Strawberry Berry Swirl Bar (Carnation) | 1 bar | 70 | 9 |
| Strawberry Fruit & Juice Bars (Chiquita) | 1 bar (2 oz) | 50 | 0 |
| Tahitian Vanilla (American Glace) | 4 oz | 48 | 0 |
| Tasti D-Lite | 4 oz | 40 | 5 |
| Tropical Orange SunTops (Dole) | 1 bar | 40 | 0 |
| Vanilla Caramel Nut, Heaven Bars (Carnation) | 1 bar | 225 | 9 |
| Vanilla Fudge Heaven Sundae Bars (Carnation) | 1 bar | 150 | 7 |
| Vanilla Fudge Nut (Carnation) | 1 bar | 222 | 9 |

| FOOD | PORTION | CALORIES | CHOLESTEROL |
|------|---------|----------|-------------|
| Vanilla Ice Cream (Land O'Lakes) | 4 oz | 140 | 30 |
| Vanilla Ice Milk (Land O'Lakes) | 4 oz | 90 | 10 |
| Watermelon Italian Ice (Good Humor) | 6 oz | 138 | 0 |
| Wild Cherry Pops (Crystal Light) | 1 bar | 13 | 0 |
| orange sherbet | ⅔ cup | 181 | 9 |
| orange sherbet (home recipe) | ½ cup | 120 | 9 |
| orange sherbet | 1 cup | 270 | 14 |
| vanilla ice milk | 1 cup | 184 | 18 |
| vanilla ice milk, soft serve | 1 cup | 223 | 13 |
| vanilla, 10% fat | 1 cup | 269 | 59 |
| vanilla, 16% fat | 1 cup | 349 | 88 |
| vanilla, French, soft serve | 1 cup | 377 | 153 |

## ICE CREAM, NON-DAIRY

| FOOD | PORTION | CALORIES | CHOLESTEROL |
|------|---------|----------|-------------|
| Mocha Mix Chocolate Chip | ½ cup | 160 | 0 |
| Mocha Mix Dutch Chocolate | ½ cup | 135 | 0 |
| Mocha Mix Mocha Almond Fudge | ½ cup | 150 | 0 |
| Mocha Mix Neapolitan | ½ cup | 130 | 0 |
| Mocha Mix Strawberry Swirl | ½ cup | 140 | 0 |
| Mocha Mix Toasted Almond | ½ cup | 150 | 0 |
| Mocha Mix Vanilla | ½ cup | 138 | 0 |
| Mocha Mix Vanilla Chocolate Almond | ½ cup | 150 | 0 |

| FOOD | PORTION | CALORIES | CHOLESTEROL |
|---|---|---|---|
| Tofulite | 4 oz | 150 | 0 |
| Tofutti Cappuccino Love Drops | 4 oz | 230 | 0 |
| Tofutti Chocolate Supreme | 4 oz | 210 | 0 |
| Tofutti Chocolate Cuties | 4 oz | 140 | 0 |
| Tofutti Chocolate Love Drops | 4 oz | 220 | 0 |
| Tofutti Lite lite Applejack Vanilla Twirl | 4 oz | 90 | 0 |
| Tofutti Lite lite Cappuccino Vanilla Twirl | 4 oz | 90 | 0 |
| Tofutti Lite lite Chocolate Vanilla Twirl | 4 oz | 90 | 0 |
| Tofutti Lite lite Chocolate Strawberry Twirl | 4 oz | 90 | 0 |
| Tofutti Lite lite Strawberry Vanilla Twirl | 4 oz | 90 | 0 |
| Tofutti Lite lite Vanilla Chocolate Strawberry Twirl | 4 oz | 90 | 0 |
| Tofutti Soft Serve Hi-Lite Chocolate | 4 oz | 100 | 0 |
| Tofutti Soft Serve Hi-Lite Vanilla | 4 oz | 90 | 0 |
| Tofutti Soft Serve Regular | 4 oz | 158 | 0 |
| Tofutti Vanilla | 4 oz | 200 | 0 |
| Tofutti Vanilla Almond Bark | 4 oz | 230 | 0 |
| Tofutti Vanilla Cuties | 4 oz | 130 | 0 |
| Tofutti Vanilla Love Drops | 4 oz | 220 | 0 |
| Tofutti Wildberry | 4 oz | 210 | 0 |

| FOOD | PORTION | CALORIES | CHOLESTEROL |
|---|---|---|---|

# ICE CREAM TOPPINGS
(*see also* SYRUP)

| FOOD | PORTION | CALORIES | CHOLESTEROL |
|---|---|---|---|
| Butterscotch Artifically Flavored Topping (Kraft) | 1 Tbsp | 60 | 0 |
| Butterscotch Flavored Topping (Smucker's) | 2 Tbsp | 140 | 0 |
| Caramel Topping (Kraft) | 1 Tbsp | 60 | 0 |
| Carmel Flavored Topping (Smucker's) | 2 Tbsp | 140 | 0 |
| Cherry (Smucker's) | 1 Tbsp | 53 | 0 |
| Chocolate Caramel Topping (Kraft) | 1 Tbsp | 60 | 0 |
| Chocolate Flavored Syrup Topping (Smucker's) | 2 Tbsp | 130 | 0 |
| Chocolate Fudge Magic Shell (Smucker's) | 2 Tbsp | 190 | 0 |
| Chocolate Fudge Topping (Smucker's) | 2 Tbsp | 130 | 0 |
| Chocolate Magic Shell (Smucker's) | 2 Tbsp | 190 | 0 |
| Chocolate Nut Magic Shell (Smucker's) | 2 Tbsp | 200 | 0 |
| Chocolate Topping (Kraft) | 1 Tbsp | 60 | 0 |
| Hot Caramel Topping (Smucker's) | 2 Tbsp | 150 | 0 |
| Hot Fudge Topping (Kraft) | 1 Tbsp | 70 | 0 |

| FOOD | PORTION | CALORIES | CHOLESTEROL |
|---|---|---|---|
| Hot Fudge Topping (Smucker's) | 2 Tbsp | 110 | 0 |
| Marshmallow (Smucker's) | 1 Tbsp | 68 | 0 |
| Marshmallow Creme (Kraft) | 1 Tbsp | 90 | 0 |
| Peanut Butter Magic Caramel (Smucker's) | 2 Tbsp | 150 | 0 |
| Pecans in Syrup (Smucker's) | 2 Tbsp | 130 | 0 |
| Pineapple (Smucker's) | 2 Tbsp | 130 | 0 |
| Pineapple (Smucker's) | 1 Tbsp | 54 | 0 |
| Pineapple Topping (Kraft) | 1 Tbsp | 50 | 0 |
| Red Raspberry Topping (Kraft) | 1 Tbsp | 50 | 0 |
| Strawberry (Smucker's) | 2 Tbsp | 120 | 0 |
| Strawberry (Smucker's) | 1 Tbsp | 44 | 0 |
| Strawberry Topping (Kraft) | 1 Tbsp | 50 | 0 |
| Walnut Topping (Kraft) | 1 Tbsp | 90 | 0 |
| Walnuts in Syrup (Smucker's) | 2 Tbsp | 130 | 0 |
| butterscotch sauce (home recipe) | 2 Tbsp | 151 | 40 |
| chocolate sauce (home recipe) | 2 Tbsp | 108 | 2 |
| hard sauce (home recipe) | 2 Tbsp | 142 | 15 |

| FOOD | PORTION | CALORIES | CHOLESTEROL |
|------|---------|----------|-------------|

## ICING
(*see* CAKE)

## INSTANT BREAKFAST
(*see* BREAKFAST DRINKS)

## ITALIAN FOOD
(*see also* DINNER, PASTA, PASTA DINNERS, PASTA SALAD)

FROZEN

| | | | |
|------|---------|----------|-------------|
| Italian Style International Recipe (Birds Eye) | ½ cup | 101 | 0 |
| Italian Style International Rice (Birds Eye) | ½ cup | 119 | 0 |

## JAM/JELLY/PRESERVE

ALL FRUIT

| | | | |
|------|---------|----------|-------------|
| All Flavors Simply Fruit Spread (Smucker's) | 1 tsp | 16 | 0 |
| Blueberry Fruit Spread (Pritikin Foods) | 1 tsp | 14 | 0 |
| Peach Fruit Spread (Pritikin Foods) | 1 tsp | 14 | 0 |
| Red Raspberry Fruit Spread (Pritikin Foods) | 1 tsp | 14 | 0 |
| Strawberry Fruit Spread (Pritikin Foods) | 1 tsp | 14 | 0 |

REDUCED CALORIE

| | | | |
|------|---------|----------|-------------|
| All Flavors Slenderella Low Calorie Imitation Jam (Smucker's) | 1 tsp | 8 | 0 |

| FOOD | PORTION | CALORIES | CHOLESTEROL |
|---|---|---|---|
| All Flavors Slenderella Low Calorie Imitation Jelly (Smucker's) | 1 tsp | 8 | 0 |
| All Flavors, Imitation Jelly, Single Service (Smucker's) | ⅜ oz pkg | 2 | 0 |
| All Flavors, Jellies, Single Service (Smucker's) | ½ oz pkg | 38 | 0 |
| All Flavors, Preserves, Single Service (Smucker's) | ½ oz pkg | 38 | 0 |
| All Flavors, Low Sugar Spreads (Smucker's) | 1 tsp | 8 | 0 |
| Grape Jelly Reduced Calorie (Kraft) | 1 tsp | 5 | 0 |
| Grape Imitation Jelly (Smucker's) | 1 tsp | 2 | 0 |
| Jellies, All Flavors (Estee) | 1 tsp | 2 | 0 |
| Preserves, All Flavors (Estee) | 1 tsp | 2 | 0 |
| Preserves, All Flavors (Louis Sherry) | 1 tsp | 2 | 0 |
| Strawberry Imitation Jelly (Smucker's) | 1 tsp | 2 | 0 |
| Strawberry Preserves Reduced Calorie (Kraft) | 1 tsp | 8 | 0 |
| REGULAR All Flavors Jelly (Home Brands) | 2 tsp | 35 | 0 |

| FOOD | PORTION | CALORIES | CHOLESTEROL |
|---|---|---|---|
| All Flavors Preserves (Smucker's) | 1 tsp | 18 | 0 |
| All Flavors Jam (Smucker's) | 1 tsp | 18 | 0 |
| Apple Butter (BAMA) | 2 tsp | 25 | 0 |
| Apple Butter (White House) | 1 oz | 50 | 0 |
| Apple Butter Natural (Smucker's) | 1 tsp | 12 | 0 |
| Apple Jelly (BAMA) | 2 tsp | 30 | 0 |
| Cider Apple Butter (Smucker's) | 1 tsp | 12 | 0 |
| Grape Jelly (BAMA) | 2 tsp | 30 | 0 |
| Jam, All Varieties (Kraft) | 1 tsp | 18 | 0 |
| Jelly, All Varieties (Kraft) | 1 tsp | 16 | 0 |
| Orange Marmalade (Smucker's) | 1 tsp | 18 | 0 |
| Peach Butter (Smucker's) | 1 tsp | 15 | 0 |
| Peach Preserves (BAMA) | 2 tsp | 30 | 0 |
| Preserves, All Varieties (Kraft) | 1 tsp | 16 | 0 |
| Preserves, All Flavors (Home Brands) | 2 tsp | 35 | 0 |
| Red Plum Jam (BAMA) | 2 tsp | 30 | 0 |

| FOOD | PORTION | CALORIES | CHOLESTEROL |
|------|---------|----------|-------------|
| Strawberry Preserves (BAMA) | 2 tsp | 30 | 0 |

## JAPANESE FOOD
(*see* ORIENTAL FOOD)

## JELLY
(*see* JAM/JELLY/PRESERVE)

## KALE

| FOOD | PORTION | CALORIES | CHOLESTEROL |
|------|---------|----------|-------------|
| FRESH | | | |
| cooked; chopped | ½ cup | 21 | 0 |
| raw; chopped | ½ cup | 21 | 0 |
| FROZEN | | | |
| chopped; cooked | ½ cup | 20 | 0 |
| frzn; not prep | 10 oz pkg | 79 | 0 |

## KETCHUP
(*see* CATSUP)

## KIDNEY

| FOOD | PORTION | CALORIES | CHOLESTEROL |
|------|---------|----------|-------------|
| beef, raw | 4 oz | 212 | 322 |
| beef; simmered | 3 oz | 122 | 329 |
| pork, raw | 3 oz | 84 | 270 |
| pork; braised | 3 oz | 128 | 408 |

## KIDNEY BEANS

| FOOD | PORTION | CALORIES | CHOLESTEROL |
|------|---------|----------|-------------|
| CANNED | | | |
| Dark Red Kidney Beans (Hanover) | ½ cup | 110 | 0 |

| FOOD | PORTION | CALORIES | CHOLESTEROL |
|------|---------|----------|-------------|
| Dark Red Lite 50% Less Salt (S&W) | ½ cup | 120 | 0 |
| Dark Red Premium (S&W) | ½ cup | 120 | 0 |
| Kidney, Dark Red (Trappey's) | ½ cup | 90 | 0 |
| Kidney, Jalapeno Light Red (Trappey's) | ½ cup | 90 | 0 |
| Kidney, Light Red (Trappey's) | ½ cup | 90 | 0 |
| Kidney, Red w/ Chili Gravy (Trappey's) | ½ cup | 100 | 0 |
| Light Red Kidney Beans in Sauce (Hanover) | ½ cup | 120 | 0 |
| kidney | 1 cup | 208 | 0 |
| red | 1 cup | 216 | 0 |
| **DRIED** California red, raw | 1 cup | 609 | 0 |
| California red; cooked | 1 cup | 219 | 0 |
| Kidney (Hurst Brand) | 1 cup | 254 | 0 |
| cooked | 1 cup | 225 | 0 |
| raw | 1 cup | 613 | 0 |
| red, raw | 1 cup | 619 | 0 |
| red; cooked | 1 cup | 225 | 0 |
| red, royal, raw | 1 cup | 605 | 0 |
| red, royal; cooked | 1 cup | 218 | 0 |

| FOOD | PORTION | CALORIES | CHOLESTEROL |
|---|---|---|---|
| SPROUTS | | | |
| cooked | 1 lb | 152 | 0 |
| raw | ½ cup | 27 | 0 |

## KIWIFRUIT

| | | | |
|---|---|---|---|
| FRESH | | | |
| Kiwifruit (California Kiwifruit Commission) | 2 | 90 | 0 |
| kiwifruit | 1 med | 46 | 0 |

## KOHLRABI

| | | | |
|---|---|---|---|
| FRESH | | | |
| raw; sliced | ½ cup | 19 | 0 |
| sliced, cooked | ½ cup | 24 | 0 |

## KUMQUATS

| | | | |
|---|---|---|---|
| FRESH | | | |
| kumquats | 1 | 12 | 0 |

## LAMB
(*see also* LAMB DISHES)

| | | | |
|---|---|---|---|
| FRESH | | | |
| chopped, lean & fat; cooked | ½ cup | 195 | 69 |
| ground, lean & fat; cooked | ½ cup | 153 | 54 |
| leg, w/o bone, lean & fat; roasted | 3 oz | 237 | 83 |
| leg, w/o bone, lean only; roasted | 3 oz | 158 | 85 |
| loin chop, w/ bone, lean & fat; broiled | 1 (2.5 oz) | 255 | 70 |

| FOOD | PORTION | CALORIES | CHOLESTEROL |
|---|---|---|---|
| loin chop, w/ bone, lean only; broiled | 1 (1.7 oz) | 92 | 49 |
| patty, lean & fat; cooked | 3 oz | 229 | 80 |
| rib chop, w/ bone, lean & fat; cooked | 1 (2.4 oz) | 273 | 66 |
| rib chop, w/ bone, lean only; cooked | 1 (1.5 oz) | 91 | 43 |
| shoulder shank, lean & fat; cooked | 3.2 oz | 306 | 89 |
| shoulder, lean & fat; roasted | 3 oz | 287 | 83 |
| shoulder, w/o bone, lean only; roasted | 3 oz | 174 | 85 |
| shoulder, w/o bone, lean & fat; roasted | 3 oz | 287 | 83 |

## LAMB DISHES

| | | | |
|---|---|---|---|
| curry | ¾ cup | 345 | 89 |
| lamb & potato casserole | ¾ cup | 277 | 89 |
| stew | ¾ cup | 124 | 29 |

## LAMB'S-QUARTERS

| FRESH | | | |
|---|---|---|---|
| chopped; cooked | ½ cup | 29 | 0 |

## LECITHIN
(*see* SOY)

## LEEKS

| DRIED | | | |
|---|---|---|---|
| freeze-dried | 1 Tbsp | 1 | 0 |

| FOOD | PORTION | CALORIES | CHOLESTEROL |
|---|---|---|---|
| **FRESH** | | | |
| chopped; cooked | ¼ cup | 8 | 0 |
| raw | 1 (4.4 oz) | 76 | 0 |
| raw; chopped | ¼ cup | 16 | 0 |

## LEMON

| FOOD | PORTION | CALORIES | CHOLESTEROL |
|---|---|---|---|
| **CANDIED** | | | |
| lemon peel | 1 oz | 90 | 0 |
| **FRESH** | | | |
| peel | 1 Tbsp | 0 | 0 |
| **HOME RECIPE** | | | |
| lemon sauce | 2 Tbsp | 57 | 48 |
| **JUICE** | | | |
| Lemon (Seneca) | 1 Tbsp | 6 | 0 |
| fresh | 1 Tbsp | 4 | 0 |
| frzn | 1 Tbsp | 3 | 0 |
| lemon | 1 Tbsp | 3 | 0 |

## LEMON EXTRACT

| FOOD | PORTION | CALORIES | CHOLESTEROL |
|---|---|---|---|
| Virginia Dare | 1 tsp | 22 | 0 |

## LEMONADE
(*see* FRUIT DRINKS)

## LENTILS

| FOOD | PORTION | CALORIES | CHOLESTEROL |
|---|---|---|---|
| Lentils; cooked (Hurst Brand) | 1 cup | 258 | 0 |
| Zesty Lentil Pilaf (Health Valley) | 4 oz | 110 | 0 |

| FOOD | PORTION | CALORIES | CHOLESTEROL |
|------|---------|----------|-------------|
| DRIED | | | |
| cooked | 1 cup | 231 | 0 |
| raw | 1 cup | 649 | 0 |
| SPROUTS | | | |
| sprouts | ½ cup | 40 | 0 |

## LETTUCE

| | | | |
|------|---------|----------|-------------|
| FRESH | | | |
| butterhead | 2 leaves | 2 | 0 |
| iceberg | 1 leaf | 3 | 0 |
| looseleaf; shredded | ½ cup | 5 | 0 |
| romaine; shredded | ½ cup | 4 | 0 |

## LIMA BEANS

| | | | |
|------|---------|----------|-------------|
| CANNED | | | |
| Lima Beans (Libby) | ½ cup | 80 | 0 |
| Lima Beans (Seneca) | ½ cup | 80 | 0 |
| Small Fancy (S&W) | ½ cup | 80 | 0 |
| large | 1 cup | 191 | 0 |
| lima beans | ½ cup | 93 | 0 |
| DRIED | | | |
| Baby Lima (Hurst Brand) | 1 cup | 262 | 0 |
| baby, raw | 1 cup | 677 | 0 |
| baby; cooked | 1 cup | 229 | 0 |
| cooked | ½ cup | 104 | 0 |

| FOOD | PORTION | CALORIES | CHOLESTEROL |
|---|---|---|---|
| large, raw | 1 cup | 602 | 0 |
| large; cooked | 1 cup | 217 | 0 |
| FROZEN Baby (Birds Eye) | ½ cup | 127 | 0 |
| Baby Lima Beans (Hanover) | ½ cup | 110 | 0 |
| Fordhook (Birds Eye) | ½ cup | 100 | 0 |
| Fordhook Lima Beans (Hanover) | ½ cup | 100 | 0 |
| Fordhook, raw | 10 oz | 301 | 0 |
| Thin; cooked (Health Valley) | 6.3 oz | 188 | 0 |
| lima beans, raw | ½ cup | 94 | 0 |
| lima beans; cooked | ½ cup | 85 | 0 |

## LIME

| | | | |
|---|---|---|---|
| JUICE fresh | 1 Tbsp | 4 | 0 |
| lime juice | 1 Tbsp | 3 | 0 |

## LINGCOD

| | | | |
|---|---|---|---|
| FRESH raw | ½ fillet (6.8 oz) | 164 | 100 |
| raw | 3 oz | 72 | 44 |

| FOOD | PORTION | CALORIES | CHOLESTEROL |
|------|---------|----------|-------------|

# LIQUOR/LIQUEUR

(*see also* BEER AND ALE, DRINK MIXER, WINE, WINE COOLERS)

| FOOD | PORTION | CALORIES | CHOLESTEROL |
|------|---------|----------|-------------|
| annisette | ⅔ oz | 74 | 0 |
| apricot brandy | ⅔ oz | 64 | 0 |
| benedictine | ⅔ oz | 69 | 0 |
| bloody mary | 1 cocktail (5 oz) | 116 | 0 |
| bourbon & soda | 1 cocktail (4 oz) | 105 | 0 |
| coffee liqueur | 1.5 oz | 174 | 0 |
| coffee w/ cream liqueur | 1.5 oz | 154 | 0 |
| creme de menthe | 1.5 oz | 186 | 0 |
| creme de menthe | ⅔ oz | 67 | 0 |
| curacao liqueur | ⅔ oz | 54 | 0 |
| daiquiri | 2½ oz | 87 | 0 |
| gin | 1.5 oz | 110 | 0 |
| gin & tonic | 1 cocktail (7.5 oz) | 171 | 0 |
| gin ricky | 4 oz | 150 | 0 |
| highball | 8 oz | 166 | 0 |
| manhattan | 2½ oz | 116 | 0 |
| martini | 1 cocktail (2.5 oz) | 156 | 0 |
| mint julep | 10 oz | 210 | 0 |
| old-fashioned | 2½ oz | 127 | 0 |
| piña colada | 1 cocktail (4.5 oz) | 262 | 0 |
| planter's punch | 3½ oz | 175 | 0 |

| FOOD | PORTION | CALORIES | CHOLESTEROL |
|------|---------|----------|-------------|
| rum | 1.5 oz | 97 | 0 |
| screwdriver | 1 cocktail (7 oz) | 174 | 0 |
| sherry | 2 oz | 84 | 0 |
| sloe gin fizz | 2½ oz | 132 | 0 |
| tequila sunrise | 1 cocktail (5.5 oz) | 189 | 0 |
| tom collins | 1 cocktail (7.5 oz) | 121 | 0 |
| vermouth, dry | 3½ oz | 105 | 0 |
| vermouth, sweet | 3½ oz | 167 | 0 |
| vodka | 1.5 oz | 97 | 0 |
| whiskey | 1.5 oz | 105 | 0 |
| whiskey sour | 1 cocktail (3 oz) | 123 | 0 |
| whiskey sour mix; as prep | 1 oz | 48 | 0 |

## LIVER
(see also PÂTÉ)

| FOOD | PORTION | CALORIES | CHOLESTEROL |
|------|---------|----------|-------------|
| beef, raw | 4 oz | 161 | 400 |
| beef; braised | 3 oz | 137 | 331 |
| beef; pan-fried | 3 oz | 184 | 410 |
| chicken, raw | 1.1 oz | 40 | 140 |
| duck, raw | 1.5 oz | 60 | 227 |
| pork, raw | 3 oz | 151 | 341 |
| pork; braised | 3 oz | 141 | 302 |
| turkey, raw | 3.6 oz | 140 | 475 |
| turkey; simmered | 1 cup | 237 | 876 |

| FOOD | PORTION | CALORIES | CHOLESTEROL |
|---|---|---|---|

# LOBSTER

**FRESH**

| FOOD | PORTION | CALORIES | CHOLESTEROL |
|---|---|---|---|
| northern, raw | 1 lobster (5.3 oz) | 136 | 143 |
| northern, raw | 3 oz | 77 | 81 |
| northern; cooked | 1 cup | 142 | 104 |
| northern; cooked | 3 oz | 83 | 61 |
| spiny, raw | 3 oz | 95 | 60 |
| spiny, raw | 1 lobster (7.3 oz) | 233 | 146 |

**FROZEN**

| FOOD | PORTION | CALORIES | CHOLESTEROL |
|---|---|---|---|
| Gulfstream Tails (King & Prince) | 6 oz | 170 | 171 |
| Gulfstream Tails (King & Prince) | 7 oz | 199 | 200 |
| Gulfstream Tails (King & Prince) | 8 oz | 227 | 227 |

**HOME RECIPE**

| FOOD | PORTION | CALORIES | CHOLESTEROL |
|---|---|---|---|
| newburg | 1 cup | 485 | 455 |

# LOGANBERRIES

**FROZEN**

| FOOD | PORTION | CALORIES | CHOLESTEROL |
|---|---|---|---|
| loganberries | 1 cup | 80 | 0 |

# LOQUATS

**FRESH**

| FOOD | PORTION | CALORIES | CHOLESTEROL |
|---|---|---|---|
| loquats | 1 | 5 | 0 |

| FOOD | PORTION | CALORIES | CHOLESTEROL |
|------|---------|----------|-------------|

# LOTUS ROOT

| FOOD | PORTION | CALORIES | CHOLESTEROL |
|------|---------|----------|-------------|
| FRESH cooked; sliced | 10 slices | 59 | 0 |
| raw; sliced | 10 slices | 45 | 0 |

# LOTUS SEEDS

| FOOD | PORTION | CALORIES | CHOLESTEROL |
|------|---------|----------|-------------|
| dried | 1 oz | 94 | 0 |

# LOX
(*see* SALMON)

# LUNCHEON MEATS/COLD CUTS
(*see also* CHICKEN, HAM, MEAT SUBSTITUTE, TURKEY)

| FOOD | PORTION | CALORIES | CHOLESTEROL |
|------|---------|----------|-------------|
| Beef (Carl Buddig) | 1 oz | 40 | 16 |
| Bologna Beef (Health Valley) | 3.5 oz | 310 | 49 |
| Bologna Midget (Hebrew National) | 1 oz | 60 | 14 |
| Corned Beef (Carl Buddig) | 1 oz | 40 | 16 |
| Oscar Mayer Bar-B-Q Loaf | 1 slice (28 g) | 48 | 13 |
| Oscar Mayer Bologna Beef Lebanon | 1 link (23 g) | 49 | 16 |
| Oscar Mayer Bologna | 1 slice (28 g) | 90 | 19 |
| Oscar Mayer Bologna Beef | 1 slice (28 g) | 90 | 18 |
| Oscar Mayer Bologna Beef Garlic Flavored | 1 slice (28 g) | 89 | 19 |

| FOOD | PORTION | CALORIES | CHOLESTEROL |
|---|---|---|---|
| Oscar Mayer Bologna w/ Cheese | 1 slice (23 g) | 74 | 16 |
| Oscar Mayer Braunschweiger German Brand | 1 oz | 94 | 46 |
| Oscar Mayer Braunschweiger Sliced | 1 slice (28 g) | 96 | 50 |
| Oscar Mayer Braunschweiger Tube | 1 oz | 96 | 43 |
| Oscar Mayer Cotto Salami | 1 slice (23 g) | 54 | 18 |
| Oscar Mayer Cotto Salami Beef | 1 slice (23 g) | 46 | 18 |
| Oscar Mayer Genoa Salami Beef | 1 slice (9 g) | 34 | 9 |
| Oscar Mayer Hard Salami | 1 slice (9 g) | 34 | 8 |
| Oscar Mayer Head Cheese | 1 slice (28 g) | 55 | 26 |
| Oscar Mayer Honey Loaf | 1 slice (28 g) | 35 | 14 |
| Oscar Mayer Jalapeno | 1 slice (28 g) | 72 | 10 |
| Oscar Mayer Liver Cheese Pork Fat Wrap | 1 slice (38 g) | 116 | 76 |
| Oscar Mayer Luncheon Meat | 1 slice (28 g) | 98 | 20 |
| Oscar Mayer Luxury Loaf | 1 slice (28 g) | 38 | 13 |
| Oscar Mayer New England Brand Sausage | 1 slice (23 g) | 31 | 14 |
| Oscar Mayer Old Fashioned Loaf | 1 slice (28 g) | 64 | 15 |

| FOOD | PORTION | CALORIES | CHOLESTEROL |
|---|---|---|---|
| Oscar Mayer Olive Loaf | 1 slice (28 g) | 62 | 13 |
| Oscar Mayer Pastrami | 1 slice (17 g) | 16 | 7 |
| Oscar Mayer Peppered Loaf | 1 slice (28 g) | 43 | 13 |
| Oscar Mayer Pickle & Pimiento Loaf | 1 slice (28 g) | 63 | 13 |
| Oscar Mayer Picnic Loaf | 1 slice (28 g) | 62 | 13 |
| Oscar Mayer Salami for Beer | 1 slice (23 g) | 55 | 16 |
| Oscar Mayer Salami for Beer Beef | 1 slice (23 g) | 66 | 17 |
| Oscar Mayer Sandwich Spread | 1 oz | 67 | 10 |
| Oscar Mayer Smoked Beef | 1 slice (14 g) | 14 | 7 |
| Oscar Mayer Summer Sausage Thuringer Cervelat | 1 slice (23 g) | 73 | 19 |
| Oscar Mayer Summer Sausage Thuringer Cervelat Beef | 1 slice (23 g) | 72 | 18 |
| Oscar Mayer Corned Beef | 1 slice (17 g) | 16 | 5 |
| Pastrami (Carl Buddig) | 1 oz | 40 | 16 |
| Pork Breakfast Sliced (Health Valley) | 3.5 oz | 560 | 77 |
| Salami (Health Valley) | 3.5 oz | 400 | 49 |

| FOOD | PORTION | CALORIES | CHOLESTEROL |
|---|---|---|---|
| Salami Midget (Hebrew National) | 1 oz | 57 | 11 |
| barbecue loaf, beef | 1 slice (23 g) | 40 | 9 |
| beerwurst | 1 slice (23 g) | 75 | 13 |
| beerwurst, beef | 1 slice (6 g) | 19 | 3 |
| beerwurst, pork | 1 slice (6 g) | 14 | 4 |
| beerwurst, pork | 1 slice (23 g) | 55 | 13 |
| berliner, pork & beef | 1 slice (23 g) | 53 | 11 |
| blood sausage | 1 slice (25 g) | 95 | 30 |
| bologna, beef | 1 slice (23 g) | 72 | 13 |
| bologna, beef & pork | 1 slice (23 g) | 73 | 13 |
| bologna, Lebanon beef | 1 slice (23 g) | 52 | 15 |
| bologna, pork | 1 slice (23 g) | 57 | 14 |
| braunschweiger | 1 oz | 102 | 44 |
| braunschweiger, pork | 1 slice (18 g) | 65 | 28 |
| corned beef loaf | 1 slice (28 g) | 46 | 12 |
| Dutch brand loaf, pork & beef | 1 slice (28 g) | 68 | 13 |

| FOOD | PORTION | CALORIES | CHOLESTEROL |
|---|---|---|---|
| ham & cheese loaf | 1 slice (28 g) | 147 | 33 |
| headcheese, pork | 1 slice (28 oz) | 60 | 23 |
| honey loaf, pork & beef | 1 slice (28 g) | 36 | 10 |
| honey roll sausage | 1 slice (23 g) | 42 | 12 |
| liver cheese, pork | 1 slice (38 g) | 115 | 66 |
| liver cheese, pork | 1 oz | 86 | 49 |
| liverwurst | 1 oz | 93 | 45 |
| liverwurst, pork | 1 slice (18 g) | 59 | 28 |
| luncheon meat, beef | 1 slice (28 g) | 87 | 18 |
| luncheon meat, beef | 1 slice (1 oz) | 87 | 18 |
| luncheon meat, beef, thin sliced | 5 slices (21 g) | 26 | 9 |
| luncheon meat, pork & beef | 1 slice (28 g) | 200 | 31 |
| luncheon meat, pork, canned | 1 slice (21 g) | 70 | 13 |
| luncheon meat, pork, canned | 1 oz | 95 | 18 |
| luncheon sausage, pork & beef | 1 slice (23 g) | 60 | 15 |
| luxury loaf, pork | 1 slice (28 g) | 40 | 10 |
| mortadella, beef & pork | 1 slice (15 g) | 47 | 8 |

| FOOD | PORTION | CALORIES | CHOLESTEROL |
|------|---------|----------|-------------|
| mother's loaf, pork | 1 slice (21 g) | 59 | 9 |
| New England brand sausage, pork & beef | 1 slice (23 g) | 37 | 11 |
| olive loaf, pork | 1 slice (28 g) | 67 | 11 |
| pastrami, beef | 1 slice (1 oz) | 99 | 26 |
| peppered loaf, pork & beef | 1 slice (28 g) | 42 | 13 |
| pickle & pimiento loaf, pork | 1 slice (28 g) | 74 | 10 |
| picnic loaf, pork & beef | 1 slice (28 g) | 66 | 11 |
| salami, cooked, beef | 1 slice (23 g) | 58 | 14 |
| salami, cooked, beef & pork | 1 slice (23 g) | 57 | 15 |
| salami, hard, pork & beef | 1 slice (10 g) | 42 | 8 |
| salami, hard, pork & beef | 1 pkg (4 oz) | 472 | 89 |
| sandwich spread, pork & beef | 1 Tbsp | 35 | 6 |
| sandwich spread, pork & beef | 1 oz | 67 | 11 |
| smoked chopped beef | 1 slice (1 oz) | 38 | 13 |
| summer sausage, Thuringer, cervelat | 1 slice (23 g) | 80 | 16 |

| FOOD | PORTION | CALORIES | CHOLESTEROL |
|------|---------|----------|-------------|

## LUPINS

DRIED
| | | | |
|------|---------|----------|-------------|
| cooked | 1 cup | 197 | 0 |
| raw | 1 cup | 668 | 0 |

## LYCHEES

FRESH
| | | | |
|------|---------|----------|-------------|
| lychees | 1 | 6 | 0 |

## MACADAMIA NUTS

| | | | |
|------|---------|----------|-------------|
| dried | 1 oz | 199 | 0 |
| oil roasted | 1 oz | 204 | 0 |

## MACARONI
(see PASTA)

## MACKEREL

CANNED
| | | | |
|------|---------|----------|-------------|
| jack | 1 can (12.7 oz) | 563 | 285 |
| jack | 1 cup | 296 | 150 |

FRESH
| | | | |
|------|---------|----------|-------------|
| Atlantic, raw | 3 oz | 174 | 60 |
| Atlantic, raw | 1 fillet (3.9 oz) | 229 | 78 |
| Atlantic; cooked | 1 fillet (3.1 oz) | 231 | 66 |
| Atlantic; cooked | 3 oz | 223 | 64 |
| king, raw | ½ fillet (6.9 oz) | 207 | 106 |

| FOOD | PORTION | CALORIES | CHOLESTEROL |
|------|---------|----------|-------------|
| king, raw | 3 oz | 89 | 45 |
| Spanish, raw | 3 oz | 118 | 65 |
| Spanish, raw | 1 fillet (6.6 oz) | 260 | 142 |
| Spanish; cooked | 1 fillet (5.1 oz) | 230 | 107 |
| Spanish; cooked | 3 oz | 134 | 62 |

## MALTED MILK

| | | | |
|------|---------|----------|-------------|
| **LIQUID** | | | |
| chocolate | 1 cup | 233 | 34 |
| natural flavor | 1 cup | 236 | 37 |
| **POWDER** | | | |
| Carnation Chocolate | 3 heaping tsp (21 g) | 79 | 1 |
| Carnation Original | 3 heaping tsp (21 g) | 90 | 4 |
| Malted Milk Chocolate Instant; as prep w/ whole milk (Kraft) | 3 tsp + 1 cup milk | 240 | 25 |
| Malted Milk Natural Instant; as prep w/ whole milk (Kraft) | 3 tsp + 1 cup milk | 240 | 25 |
| chocolate | ¾ oz | 83 | 1 |
| natural flavor | ¾ oz | 86 | 4 |

## MANGO

| | | | |
|------|---------|----------|-------------|
| **FRESH** | | | |
| mango | 1 | 135 | 0 |

| FOOD | PORTION | CALORIES | CHOLESTEROL |
|------|---------|----------|-------------|

# MARGARINE
(*see also* BUTTER BLENDS, BUTTER SUBSTITUTE)

REDUCED CALORIE

| FOOD | PORTION | CALORIES | CHOLESTEROL |
|------|---------|----------|-------------|
| Blue Bonnet Diet | 1 Tbsp | 50 | 0 |
| Fleischmann's Diet | 1 Tbsp | 50 | 0 |
| Fleischmann's Diet w/ Lite Salt | 1 Tbsp | 50 | 0 |
| Kraft Spread | 1 Tbsp | 50 | 0 |
| Kraft Spread (stick) | 1 Tbsp | 60 | 0 |
| Mazola Light Corn Oil Spread | 1 Tbsp | 50 | 0 |
| Mazola Light Corn Oil Spread | 1 cup | 835 | 0 |
| Mazola, Diet | 1 Tbsp | 50 | 0 |
| Mazola, Diet | 1 cup | 815 | 0 |
| Parkay Diet Soft | 1 Tbsp | 50 | 0 |
| Parkay Light Corn Oil Spread | 1 Tbsp | 70 | 0 |
| Parkay Spread | 1 Tbsp | 60 | 0 |
| Weight Watchers | 1 Tbsp | 50 | 0 |
| corn | 1 tsp | 17 | 0 |
| corn | 1 cup | 801 | 0 |
| soybean | 1 cup | 801 | 0 |
| soybean | 1 tsp | 17 | 0 |
| soybean & cottonseed | 1 tsp | 17 | 0 |
| soybean & cottonseed | 1 cup | 801 | 0 |
| soybean & palm | 1 cup | 801 | 0 |
| soybean & palm | 1 tsp | 17 | 0 |
| REGULAR | | | |
| Blue Bonnet | 1 Tbsp | 100 | 0 |

| FOOD | PORTION | CALORIES | CHOLESTEROL |
|---|---|---|---|
| Fleischmann's | 1 Tbsp | 100 | 0 |
| Fleischmann's Light Corn Oil Stick | 1 Tbsp | 80 | 0 |
| Fleischmann's Sweet, Unsalted | 1 Tbsp | 100 | 0 |
| Krona (Lever) | 1 Tbsp | 100 | 15 |
| Land O'Lakes, Premium Corn Oil Stick | 1 Tbsp | 100 | 0 |
| Land O'Lakes, Regular Stick | 1 Tbsp | 100 | 0 |
| Mazola | 1 Tbsp | 100 | 0 |
| Mazola | 1 cup | 1650 | 0 |
| Mazola, Unsalted | 1 Tbsp | 100 | 0 |
| Mazola, Unsalted | 1 cup | 1635 | 0 |
| Mother's | 1 Tbsp | 100 | 0 |
| Mother's, Unsalted | 1 Tbsp | 100 | 0 |
| Nucoa | 1 Tbsp | 100 | 0 |
| Nucoa | 1 cup | 1630 | 0 |
| Parkay | 1 Tbsp | 100 | 0 |
| Shedd's Spread Country Crock Classic Quarters | 1 Tbsp | 80 | 0 |
| coconut, safflower, palm | 1 tsp | 34 | 0 |
| coconut, safflower, palm | 1 stick | 815 | 0 |
| corn | 1 stick | 815 | 0 |
| corn | 1 tsp | 34 | 0 |
| corn, soybean & cottonseed | 1 stick | 815 | 0 |
| corn, soybean & cottonseed | 1 tsp | 34 | 0 |
| corn, soybean & cottonseed, unsalted | 1 tsp | 34 | 0 |

| FOOD | PORTION | CALORIES | CHOLESTEROL |
|---|---|---|---|
| corn, soybean & cottonseed, unsalted | 1 stick | 809 | 0 |
| soybean & palm | 1 tsp | 34 | 0 |
| soybean & palm | 1 stick | 815 | 0 |
| soybean, hydrogenated | 1 stick | 815 | 0 |
| soybean, hydrogenated | 1 tsp | 34 | 0 |
| sunflower, soybean & cottonseed | 1 stick | 815 | 0 |
| sunflower, soybean & cottonseed | 1 tsp | 34 | 0 |
| **SOFT** | | | |
| Blue Bonnet Light Tasty Spread | 1 Tbsp | 60 | 0 |
| Blue Bonnet Spread | 1 Tbsp | 80 | 0 |
| Blue Bonnet Spread Stick (70% fat) | 1 Tbsp | 90 | 0 |
| Blue Bonnet Spread Stick (75% fat) | 1 Tbsp | 90 | 0 |
| Blue Bonnet Soft | 1 Tbsp | 100 | 0 |
| Fleischmann's | 1 Tbsp | 100 | 0 |
| Fleischmann's Light Corn Oil Spread | 1 Tbsp | 80 | 0 |
| Fleischmann's Sweet, Unsalted | 1 Tbsp | 100 | 0 |
| I Can't Believe It's Not Butter! (Lever) | 1 Tbsp | 90 | 0 |
| Land O'Lakes Regular Soft Tub | 1 Tbsp | 100 | 0 |
| Mother's, Unsalted | 1 Tbsp | 100 | 0 |
| Mother's, Salted | 1 Tbsp | 100 | 0 |

| FOOD | PORTION | CALORIES | CHOLESTEROL |
|---|---|---|---|
| Nucoa | 1 Tbsp | 90 | 0 |
| Nucoa | 1 cup | 1415 | 0 |
| Parkay Corn Oil Soft | 1 Tbsp | 100 | 0 |
| Parkay Soft | 1 Tbsp | 100 | 0 |
| Promise | 1 Tbsp | 90 | 0 |
| Shedd's Spread Country Crock | 1 Tbsp | 80 | 0 |
| corn | 1 tsp | 34 | 0 |
| corn | 1 cup | 1626 | 0 |
| safflower | 1 tsp | 34 | 0 |
| safflower | 1 cup | 1626 | 0 |
| safflower, cottonseed & peanut | 1 cup | 1626 | 0 |
| safflower, cottonseed & peanut | 1 tsp | 34 | 0 |
| soybean, salted | 1 tsp | 34 | 0 |
| soybean, salted | 1 cup | 1626 | 0 |
| soybean, unsalted | 1 cup | 1626 | 0 |
| soybean, unsalted | 1 tsp | 34 | 0 |
| soybean & cottonseed | 1 cup | 1626 | 0 |
| soybean & cottonseed | 1 tsp | 34 | 0 |
| soybean & cottonseed, unsalted | 1 tsp | 34 | 0 |
| soybean & cottonseed, unsalted | 1 cup | 1626 | 0 |
| soybean & palm | 1 cup | 1626 | 0 |
| soybean & palm | 1 tsp | 34 | 0 |
| soybean & safflower | 1 tsp | 34 | 0 |

| FOOD | PORTION | CALORIES | CHOLESTEROL |
|---|---|---|---|
| soybean & safflower | 1 cup | 1626 | 0 |
| sunflower & peanut | 1 cup | 1626 | 0 |
| sunflower & peanut | 1 tsp | 34 | 0 |
| **SQUEEZE** | | | |
| Fleischmann's | 1 Tbsp | 100 | 0 |
| Parkay Squeeze | 1 Tbsp | 100 | 0 |
| soybean & cottonseed | 1 tsp | 34 | 0 |
| **WHIPPED** | | | |
| Blue Bonnet Soft Whipped | 1 Tbsp | 70 | 0 |
| Blue Bonnet Whipped Stick | 1 Tbsp | 70 | 0 |
| Fleischmann's Lightly Salted | 1 Tbsp | 70 | 0 |
| Fleischmann's Unsalted | 1 Tbsp | 70 | 0 |
| Miracle Brand | 1 Tbsp | 60 | 0 |
| Miracle Brand (stick) | 1 Tbsp | 70 | 0 |
| Parkay | 1 Tbsp | 60 | 0 |
| Parkay (stick) | 1 Tbsp | 60 | 0 |

# MARSHMALLOW

| FOOD | PORTION | CALORIES | CHOLESTEROL |
|---|---|---|---|
| Funmallows (Kraft) | 1 | 25 | 0 |
| Funmallows Miniature (Kraft) | 10 | 18 | 0 |
| Jet-Puffed (Kraft) | 1 | 25 | 0 |
| Miniature (Kraft) | 10 | 18 | 0 |
| miniature | 1 | 2 | 0 |

| FOOD | PORTION | CALORIES | CHOLESTEROL |
|------|---------|----------|-------------|

## MATZO

| FOOD | PORTION | CALORIES | CHOLESTEROL |
|------|---------|----------|-------------|
| Daily Thin Tea (Manischewitz) | 1 | 103 | 0 |
| Dietetic Thins (Manischewitz) | 1 | 91 | 0 |
| Egg n' Onion (Manischewitz) | 1 | 112 | 15 |
| Matzo Cracker Miniatures (Manischewitz) | 10–20 | 90 | 0 |
| Matzo Farfel (Manischewitz) | 1 cup | 280 | 0 |
| Matzo Meal (Manischewitz) | 1 cup | 514 | 0 |
| Passover (Manischewitz) | 1 | 129 | 0 |
| Passover Egg (Manischewitz) | 1 | 132 | 25 |
| Passover Egg Matzo Crackers (Manischewitz) | 10 | 108 | 20 |
| Unsalted (Manischewitz) | 1 | 110 | 0 |
| Wheat Matzo Crackers (Manischewitz) | 10 | 90 | 0 |
| Whole Wheat w/ Bran (Manischewitz) | 1 | 110 | 0 |

## MAYONNAISE
   (*see also* MAYONNAISE TYPE SALAD DRESSING, RELISH)

REDUCED CALORIE

| Best Foods Light | 1 Tbsp | 50 | 5 |
| Best Foods Light | 1 cup | 760 | 90 |

| FOOD | PORTION | CALORIES | CHOLESTEROL |
|------|---------|----------|-------------|
| Diamond Crystal | 1 Tbsp | 50 | 5 |
| Hellman's Light | 1 Tbsp | 50 | 5 |
| Hellman's Light | 1 cup | 760 | 90 |
| Kraft Light Reduced Calorie Mayonnaise | 1 Tbsp | 45 | 5 |
| imitation | 1 cup | 232 | 103 |
| imitation | 1 Tbsp | 15 | 6 |
| soybean | 1 Tbsp | 34 | 4 |
| soybean | 1 cup | 556 | 58 |
| REGULAR Best Foods Real | 1 Tbsp | 100 | 5 |
| Best Foods Real | 1 cup | 1570 | 95 |
| Hellman's Real | 1 Tbsp | 100 | 5 |
| Kraft Real Mayonnaise | 1 Tbsp | 100 | 5 |
| Kraft Sandwich Spread | 1 Tbsp | 50 | 5 |
| Mother's | 1 Tbsp | 100 | 10 |
| mayonnaise | 2 Tbsp | 196 | 16 |
| sandwich spread | 1 Tbsp | 60 | 12 |
| soybean | 1 Tbsp | 99 | 8 |
| soybean | 1 cup | 1577 | 130 |

## MAYONNAISE TYPE SALAD DRESSING
(*see also* MAYONNAISE, RELISH)

| FOOD | PORTION | CALORIES | CHOLESTEROL |
|------|---------|----------|-------------|
| Bright Day Dressing | 1 Tbsp | 60 | 0 |
| Miracle Whip Salad Dressing | 1 Tbsp | 70 | 5 |
| Weight Watchers Reduced Calorie Dressing | 1 Tbsp | 40 | 5 |

| FOOD | PORTION | CALORIES | CHOLESTEROL |
|---|---|---|---|
| mayonnaise type salad dressing | 1 cup | 916 | 60 |
| mayonnaise type salad dressing | 2 Tbsp | 114 | 8 |
| REDUCED CALORIE | | | |
| soybean w/o cholesterol | 1 cup | 1084 | 0 |
| soybean w/o cholesterol | 1 Tbsp | 68 | 0 |

## MEAT SUBSTITUTE
(see also CHICKEN SUBSTITUTE, SAUSAGE SUBSTITUTE, TURKEY SUBSTITUTE)

| | | | |
|---|---|---|---|
| Bolono, frzn (Worthington) | 3.5 oz | 138 | 1 |
| Corn Dogs (Loma Linda) | 1 (2.5 oz) | 250 | 0 |
| Dinner Cuts (Loma Linda) | 2 (3.5 oz) | 110 | 0 |
| Dinner Cuts No Salt Added (Loma Linda) | 2 (3.5 oz) | 110 | 0 |
| Fripats, frzn (Worthington) | 3.5 oz | 294 | 1 |
| Griddle Steaks (Loma Linda) | 1 (1.7 oz) | 160 | 0 |
| Griddle Steaks (Loma Linda) | 1 (2 oz) | 190 | 0 |
| Leanies, frzn (Worthington) | 3.5 oz | 252 | 2 |
| Meatless Big Franks (Loma Linda) | 1 (1.8 oz) | 100 | 0 |
| Meatless Bologna (Loma Linda) | 2 slices (2 oz) | 150 | 0 |

| FOOD | PORTION | CALORIES | CHOLESTEROL |
|---|---|---|---|
| Meatless Redi-Burger (Loma Linda) | ½" slice (2.4 oz) | 130 | 0 |
| Meatless Roast Beef (Loma Linda) | 2 slices (2 oz) | 107 | 0 |
| Meatless Salami (Loma Linda) | 2 slices (2 oz) | 98 | 0 |
| Meatless Salami, frzn (Worthington) | 3.5 oz | 198 | 1 |
| Meatless Savory Meatballs (Loma Linda) | 7 (2.5 oz) | 190 | 0 |
| Meatless Sizzle Burger (Loma Linda) | 1 (2.5 oz) | 210 | 0 |
| Meatless Sizzle Franks (Loma Linda) | 2 (2.4 oz) | 170 | 0 |
| Meatless Swiss Steak w/ Gravy (Loma Linda) | 1 steak (2.6 oz) | 140 | 0 |
| Meatless Vita-Burger Chunks (Loma Linda) | ¼ cup | 70 | 0 |
| Meatless Vita-Burger Granules (Loma Linda) | 3 Tbsp | 70 | 0 |
| Nuteena (Loma Linda) | ½" slice (2.4 oz) | 160 | 0 |
| Okara Pattie, frzn (Natural Touch) | 3.5 oz | 208 | tr |
| Olive Loaf (Loma Linda) | 2 slices (2 oz) | 119 | 0 |
| Patties, frzn (Morningstar Farms) | 3.5 oz | 240 | 2 |
| Patty Mix (Loma Linda) | ¼ cup | 50 | 0 |

| FOOD | PORTION | CALORIES | CHOLESTEROL |
|---|---|---|---|
| Prime Stakes, canned (Worthington) | 3.5 oz | 182 | 2 |
| Prosage Chub, frzn (Worthington) | 3.5 oz | 245 | 1 |
| Prosage Links, frzn (Worthington) | 3.5 oz | 280 | 2 |
| Prosage Patties, frzn (Worthington) | 3.5 oz | 279 | 2 |
| Proteena (Loma Linda) | ½" slice (2.5 oz) | 140 | 0 |
| Saucettes, canned (Worthington) | 3.5 oz | 210 | 2 |
| Savory Dinner Loaf; mix not prep (Loma Linda) | ¼ cup | 50 | 0 |
| Stakelets, frzn (Worthington) | 3.5 oz | 178 | 1 |
| Stew Pac (Loma Linda) | 2 oz | 70 | 0 |
| Tastee Cuts (Loma Linda) | 2 pieces (2.5 oz) | 70 | 0 |
| Tender Bits (Loma Linda) | 4 pieces (2 oz) | 80 | 0 |
| Tender Rounds w/ Gravy (Loma Linda) | 6 pieces (2.6 oz) | 120 | 0 |
| Tofu Pups (Lightlife) | 1 (1.5 oz) | 92 | 0 |
| Vege-Burger (Loma Linda) | ½ cup | 110 | 0 |
| Vege-Burger NSA (Loma Linda) | ½ cup | 140 | 0 |
| Vegelona (Loma Linda) | ½ slice | 100 | 0 |

| FOOD | PORTION | CALORIES | CHOLESTEROL |
|---|---|---|---|
| Wham, frzn (Worthington) | 3.5 oz | 184 | 2 |
| simulated sausage | 1 link (25 g) | 64 | 0 |
| simulated sausage | 1 patty (38 g) | 97 | 0 |

# MELON
(*see also individual names*)

FRESH
| Cantalene (Chiquita) | 1 cup | 60 | 0 |
|---|---|---|---|
| Honey Mist (Chiquita) | 1 cup | 80 | 0 |

FROZEN
| melon balls | 1 cup | 55 | 0 |
|---|---|---|---|

# MEXICAN FOOD
(*see also* CHIPS, DINNER, SNACKS)

CANNED
| Jalapeno Sliced (Trappey's) | 1 oz | 6 | 0 |
|---|---|---|---|
| Jalapeno Whole (Trappey's) | 2 med peppers | 8 | 0 |
| Mexican Sauce (Pritikin Foods) | 4 oz | 50 | 0 |
| Mexican Style Stewed Tomatoes (S&W) | ½ cup | 40 | 0 |
| Picante Sauce (Estee) | 2 Tbsp | 8 | 0 |

| FOOD | PORTION | CALORIES | CHOLESTEROL |
|---|---|---|---|
| Taco Sauce (Estee) | 2 Tbsp | 14 | 0 |
| tomatoes w/ green chilies | ½ cup | 18 | 0 |
| **FRESH** | | | |
| chili peppers, hot, raw | 1 pepper | 18 | 0 |
| chili peppers, hot, raw; chopped | ½ cup | 30 | 0 |
| tamale | 1 (3.9 oz) | 155 | 10 |
| tortilla; baked | 1 (.7 oz) | 43 | 0 |
| tortilla; steamed | 1 (.7 oz) | 43 | 0 |
| **FROZEN** | | | |
| 3 Beef Enchiladas (El Charrito) | 1 pkg (11 oz) | 560 | 55 |
| 3 Cheese Enchiladas (El Charrito) | 1 pkg (11 oz) | 470 | 30 |
| 3 Chicken Enchiladas (El Charrito) | 1 pkg (11 oz) | 440 | 60 |
| 4 Grande Beef Enchiladas (El Charrito) | 1 pkg (16.5 oz) | 890 | 65 |
| 6 Beef Enchiladas (El Charrito) | 1 pkg (16.25 oz) | 880 | 75 |
| 6 Beef & Cheese Enchiladas (El Charrito) | 1 pkg (16.25 oz) | 880 | 70 |
| 6 Cheese Enchiladas (El Charrito) | 1 pkg (16.25 oz) | 780 | 45 |
| Beef Enchilada Dinner (El Charrito) | 1 pkg (13.75 oz) | 620 | 45 |
| Beef & Bean Burritos (Patio) | 5 oz | 361 | 24 |
| Beef & Bean Green Chili (Patio) | 5 oz | 330 | 26 |

| FOOD | PORTION | CALORIES | CHOLESTEROL |
|---|---|---|---|
| Beef & Red Bean Chili Burritos (Patio) | 5 oz | 333 | 20 |
| Beef Enchilada Dinner (Patio) | 13.25 oz | 514 | 28 |
| Burrito Dinner (Patio) | 12 oz | 517 | 24 |
| Burrito Grande B&B (El Charrito) | 1 pkg (6 oz) | 430 | 25 |
| Burrito Grande Green Chili B&B (El Charrito) | 1 pkg (6 oz) | 410 | 20 |
| Burrito Grande Jalapeno (El Charrito) | 1 pkg (6 oz) | 410 | 25 |
| Burrito Grande Red Chili B&B (El Charrito) | 1 pkg (6 oz) | 410 | 25 |
| Burrito Green Chili B&B (El Charrito) | 1 pkg (5 oz) | 370 | 20 |
| Burrito Red Chili B&B (El Charrito) | 1 pkg (5 oz) | 380 | 20 |
| Burrito Red Hot B&B (El Charrito) | 1 pkg (5 oz) | 540 | 20 |
| Burrito Red Hot Beef (El Charrito) | 1 pkg (5 oz) | 340 | 20 |
| Cheese Enchilada Dinner (El Charrito) | 1 pkg (13.75 oz) | 570 | 30 |
| Cheese Enchilada Dinner (Patio) | 12.25 oz | 378 | 17 |
| Chicken Enchilada Dinner (El Charrito) | 1 pkg (13.75 oz) | 510 | 50 |
| Fiesta Dinner (Patio) | 12.25 oz | 461 | 28 |

| FOOD | PORTION | CALORIES | CHOLESTEROL |
|---|---|---|---|
| Grande Beef Enchilada Dinner (El Charrito) | 1 pkg (21 oz) | 950 | 70 |
| Grande Mexican Style Dinner (El Charrito) | 1 pkg (20 oz) | 850 | 65 |
| Grande Satillo Dinner (El Charrito) | 1 pkg (20.75 oz) | 820 | 45 |
| Mexican Dinner (Patio) | 13.25 | 533 | 41 |
| Mexican Style Dinner (El Charrito) | 1 pkg (14.25 oz) | 690 | 45 |
| Queso Dinner (El Charrito) | 1 pkg (13.25 oz) | 490 | 15 |
| Ranchera Dinner (Patio) | 13 oz | 468 | 33 |
| Red Hot Burritos (Patio) | 5 oz | 352 | 21 |
| Satillo Dinner (El Charrito) | 1 pkg (13.5 oz) | 570 | 30 |
| Tortillas, Corn (El Charrito) | 2 | 95 | 0 |
| Tortillas, Flour (El Charrito) | 2 | 170 | 0 |
| **HOME RECIPE** | | | |
| burrito | 1 (8 oz) | 332 | 34 |
| enchiladas, eggplant | 1 | 142 | 7 |
| taco salad | 1 cup | 292 | 71 |
| tacos verde blanco y rojo | 1 (5.6 oz) | 296 | 38 |
| **MIX** | | | |
| Taco Meat Seasoning, Mild (Ortega) | 1 oz | 90 | 0 |

| FOOD | PORTION | CALORIES | CHOLESTEROL |
|---|---|---|---|
| Taco Meat Seasoning, Mild; as prep w/ ground beef (Ortega) | 3 oz | 180 | 60 |
| Tortilla, Corn Masa Harina; not prep (Quaker) | 1 cup | 421 | 0 |
| Tortilla, Wheat Masa Trigo; not prep (Quaker) | 1 cup | 458 | 0 |

## MILK
(*see also* CHOCOLATE, COCOA, MILK DRINKS)

| FOOD | PORTION | CALORIES | CHOLESTEROL |
|---|---|---|---|
| **CANNED** | | | |
| Carnation Evaporated | ½ cup | 170 | 37 |
| Carnation Evaporated Lowfat | ½ cup | 110 | 18 |
| Carnation Evaporated Skimmed | ½ cup | 100 | 5 |
| Pet 99 Evaporated Skimmed | ½ cup | 100 | 1 |
| Pet Evaporated | ½ cup | 170 | 36 |
| condensed, sweetened | 1 oz | 123 | 13 |
| evaporated | 1 oz | 42 | 9 |
| evaporated, skim | 1 oz | 25 | 1 |
| **DRIED** | | | |
| Carnation Nonfat Dry; as prep w/ water | 8 oz | 80 | 4 |
| Carnation Nonfat Dry; as prep w/ water | 1 qt | 320 | 16 |
| Flash Instant Nonfat; as prep | 8 oz | 80 | 5 |
| buttermilk, sweet cream | 1 Tbsp | 25 | 5 |
| instantized | 1 cup | 244 | 12 |

| FOOD | PORTION | CALORIES | CHOLESTEROL |
|---|---|---|---|
| nonfat | ¼ cup | 109 | 6 |
| whey, sweet | 1 cup | 512 | 9 |
| whole | ¼ cup | 159 | 31 |
| **LIQUID, LOWFAT** Lowfat Buttermilk (Land O'Lakes) | 8 oz | 100 | 10 |
| Lowfat Friendship Buttermilk | 8 oz | 120 | 14 |
| Lowfat Lactaid | 8 oz | 102 | 10 |
| Lowfat Land O'Lakes, 1% | 8 oz | 100 | 10 |
| Lowfat Land O'Lakes, 2% | 8 oz | 120 | 20 |
| lowfat, 1%, nonfat milk solids added | 1 cup | 104 | 10 |
| lowfat, 1%, protein fortified | 1 cup | 119 | 10 |
| lowfat, 1% | 1 cup | 102 | 10 |
| lowfat, 2%, protein fortified | 1 cup | 137 | 19 |
| lowfat, 2% | 1 cup | 121 | 18 |
| lowfat buttermilk | 1 cup | 99 | 9 |
| lowfat whey, sweet | 1 cup | 66 | 5 |
| **LIQUID, REGULAR** Regular Land O'Lakes | 8 oz | 150 | 35 |
| regular filled milk | 1 cup | 154 | 4 |
| regular goat milk | 1 cup | 168 | 28 |
| regular human milk | 1 fl oz | 21 | 4 |
| regular imitation milk | 1 cup | 150 | tr |
| regular Indian buffalo | 1 cup | 236 | 46 |
| regular sheep | 1 cup | 26 | 4 |
| regular whole, 3.3% fat | 1 cup | 150 | 33 |

| FOOD | PORTION | CALORIES | CHOLESTEROL |
|---|---|---|---|
| regular whole, low sodium | 1 cup | 149 | 33 |
| **LIQUID, SKIM** | | | |
| Skim Land O'Lakes | 8 oz | 90 | 5 |
| skim | 1 cup | 86 | 4 |
| skim, nonfat milk solids added | 1 cup | 90 | 5 |
| skim, protein fortified | 1 cup | 100 | 5 |

## MILK DRINKS
(see also BREAKFAST DRINKS, CHOCOLATE, COCOA)

| | | | |
|---|---|---|---|
| Chocolate Milk (Land O'Lakes) | 8 oz | 210 | 30 |
| Chocolate Milk, 1% (Land O'Lakes) | 8 oz | 160 | 5 |
| Chocolate Skim Milk (Land O'Lakes) | 8 oz | 140 | 5 |
| chocolate, lowfat, 1% | 1 cup | 158 | 7 |
| chocolate, lowfat, 2% | 1 cup | 179 | 17 |
| chocolate, whole | 1 cup | 208 | 30 |
| strawberry flavor mix; as prep w/ whole milk | 9 oz | 234 | 33 |

## MILK SUBSTITUTE
(see also COFFEE WHITENERS)

| | | | |
|---|---|---|---|
| Vitamite (Deihl) | 8 oz | 100 | 0 |

## MILKFISH

| **FRESH** | | | |
|---|---|---|---|
| raw | 3 oz | 126 | 44 |

| FOOD | PORTION | CALORIES | CHOLESTEROL |
|------|---------|----------|-------------|
| **MILKSHAKE** | | | |
| Chocolate (Micro Magic) | 1 shake (11.5 oz) | 440 | 50 |
| Strawberry (Micro Magic) | 1 shake (11.5 oz) | 440 | 49 |
| Vanilla (Micro Magic) | 1 shake (11.5 oz) | 490 | 56 |
| chocolate thick shake | 10.6 oz | 356 | 32 |
| chocolate, fast food | 10 oz | 360 | 37 |
| strawberry, fast food | 10 oz | 319 | 31 |
| vanilla, fast food | 10 oz | 314 | 32 |
| vanilla thick shake | 11 oz | 350 | 37 |
| **MINERAL WATER/BOTTLED WATER** | | | |
| Artesia | 7 oz | 0 | 0 |
| Artesia Almund | 7 oz | 0 | 0 |
| Artesia Cranberi | 7 oz | 0 | 0 |
| Artesia Lemin | 7 oz | 0 | 0 |
| Artesia Orange | 7 oz | 0 | 0 |
| Crystal Geyser Sparkling Mineral Water | 6 oz | 0 | 0 |
| Crystal Geyser Sparkling Mineral Water Cherry Chocolate | 6 oz | 0 | 0 |
| Crystal Geyser Sparkling Mineral Water Lemon | 6 oz | 0 | 0 |
| Crystal Geyser Sparkling Mineral Water Lime | 6 oz | 0 | 0 |
| Crystal Geyser Sparkling Mineral Water Natural Wild Cherry w/ Vitafort | 6 oz | 0 | 0 |

| FOOD | PORTION | CALORIES | CHOLESTEROL |
|---|---|---|---|
| Crystal Geyser Sparkling Mineral Water Orange | 6 oz | 0 | 0 |
| Diamond Spring Water | 1 qt (liter) | 0 | 0 |
| Mountain Valley Water | 1 qt (liter) | 0 | 0 |
| Perrier | 6.5 oz | 0 | 0 |
| Poland Springs | 8 oz | 0 | 0 |
| Vichy (Schweppes) | 6 oz | 0 | 0 |

## MISO

| | | | |
|---|---|---|---|
| miso | ½ cup | 284 | 0 |

## MOCHA

| | | | |
|---|---|---|---|
| Bavarian Mint Mocha Sugar Free; as prep (Hills Bros.) | 6 oz | 35 | 0 |
| Bavarian Mint Mocha; as prep (Hills Bros.) | 6 oz | 50 | 0 |
| Cafe Mocha; as prep (Hills Bros.) | 6 oz | 50 | 0 |
| Cafe Mocha; as prep (MJB Co.) | 6 oz | 50 | 0 |
| Cherry Mocha; as prep (MJB Co.) | 6 oz | 50 | 0 |
| Fudge Mocha Sugar Free; as prep (MJB Co.) | 6 oz | 40 | 0 |
| Mint Mocha Sugar Free; as prep (MJB Co.) | 6 oz | 35 | 0 |
| Mint Mocha; as prep (MJB Co.) | 6 oz | 50 | 0 |

| FOOD | PORTION | CALORIES | CHOLESTEROL |
|------|---------|----------|-------------|
| Swiss Mocha; as prep (Hills Bros.) | 6 oz | 40 | 0 |
| Vanilla Mocha Sugar Free; as prep (MJB Co.) | 6 oz | 40 | 0 |

## MOLASSES

| | | | |
|------|---------|----------|-------------|
| Grandma's Gold Label | 1 Tbsp | 70 | 0 |
| Grandma's Green Label | 1 Tbsp | 70 | 0 |
| blackstrap | 1 Tbsp | 43 | 0 |
| molasses | 1 Tbsp | 46 | 0 |

## MONKFISH

| | | | |
|------|---------|----------|-------------|
| FRESH | | | |
| raw | 3 oz | 64 | 21 |

## MOTHBEANS

| | | | |
|------|---------|----------|-------------|
| DRIED | | | |
| cooked | 1 cup | 207 | 0 |
| raw | 1 cup | 673 | 0 |

## MOUSSE

| | | | |
|------|---------|----------|-------------|
| Chocolate Mousse No Bake Dessert (Jell-O) | 1 pkg (3.5 oz) | 415 | 4 |
| Chocolate Mousse No Bake Dessert; as prep (Jell-O) | ½ cup | 141 | 9 |
| Chocolate Fudge Mousse No Bake Dessert (Jell-O) | 1 pkg (3.5 oz) | 406 | 4 |

| FOOD | PORTION | CALORIES | CHOLESTEROL |
|------|---------|----------|-------------|
| Chocolate Fudge Mousse No Bake Dessert; as prep (Jell-O) | ½ cup | 138 | 9 |
| HOME RECIPE | | | |
| crab | ¼ cup | 364 | 136 |
| orange | ½ cup | 87 | 1 |

## MUFFIN

| FOOD | PORTION | CALORIES | CHOLESTEROL |
|------|---------|----------|-------------|
| FROZEN | | | |
| Apple Cinnamon Spice Hearty Fruit Muffins (Sara Lee) | 1 | 220 | 0 |
| Banana Nut Bran Hearty Fruit Muffins (Sara Lee) | 1 | 230 | 0 |
| Blueberry Hearty Fruit Muffins (Sara Lee) | 1 | 200 | 0 |
| Golden Corn Hearty Fruit Muffins (Sara Lee) | 1 | 250 | 0 |
| Oatmeal 'N Fruit Hearty Fruit Muffins (Sara Lee) | 1 | 230 | 0 |
| Raisin Bran Hearty Fruit Muffins (Sara Lee) | 1 | 220 | 0 |
| HOME RECIPE | | | |
| apple | 1 (1.6 oz) | 137 | 21 |
| blueberry | 1 (1.9 oz) | 147 | 22 |
| bran | 1 (1.9 oz) | 104 | 21 |
| corn | 1 (1.6 oz) | 169 | 40 |

| FOOD | PORTION | CALORIES | CHOLESTEROL |
|------|---------|----------|-------------|
| orange | 1 (1.6 oz) | 137 | 33 |
| plain | 1 (1.6 oz) | 158 | 25 |
| whole wheat | 1 (1.6 oz) | 123 | 31 |
| MIX | | | |
| Blueberry Muffin Mix Bakery Style; as prep (Duncan Hines) | 1 | 190 | 10 |
| Bran & Honey Nut Muffin Mix Bakery Style; as prep (Duncan Hines) | 1 | 200 | 10 |
| Bran Date Muffin; as prep (Jiffy) | 1 | 110 | 10 |
| Cinnamon Swirl Muffin Mix Bakery Style; as prep (Duncan Hines) | 1 | 200 | 10 |
| Corn Muffin; as prep (Jiffy) | 1 | 115 | 10 |
| READY-TO-EAT | | | |
| Oat Bran Blueberry (Health Valley) | 2 oz | 140 | 0 |
| Oat Bran Almond/Date (Health Valley) | 2 oz | 170 | 0 |
| Oat Bran Raisin (Health Valley) | 2 oz | 140 | 0 |

## MULLET

| FOOD | PORTION | CALORIES | CHOLESTEROL |
|------|---------|----------|-------------|
| FRESH | | | |
| striped, raw | 3 oz | 99 | 42 |
| striped, raw | 1 fillet (4.2 oz) | 139 | 59 |

| FOOD | PORTION | CALORIES | CHOLESTEROL |
|------|---------|----------|-------------|
| striped; cooked | 1 fillet (3.3 oz) | 139 | 59 |
| striped; cooked | 3 oz | 127 | 54 |

## MUNG BEANS

DRIED
| | | | |
|------|---------|----------|-------------|
| cooked | 1 cup | 213 | 0 |
| mung beans long rice | 1 cup | 492 | 0 |
| raw | 1 cup | 719 | 0 |

SPROUTS
| | | | |
|------|---------|----------|-------------|
| cooked | ½ cup | 13 | 0 |
| raw | ½ cup | 16 | 0 |
| stir-fried | ½ cup | 31 | 0 |

## MUSHROOM

CANNED
| | | | |
|------|---------|----------|-------------|
| Mushrooms (Libby) | ¼ cup | 35 | 0 |
| Mushrooms (Seneca) | ¼ cup | 35 | 0 |
| mushrooms | ½ cup | 19 | 0 |

DRIED
| | | | |
|------|---------|----------|-------------|
| shitake | 4 | 44 | 0 |

FRESH
| | | | |
|------|---------|----------|-------------|
| raw | 1 | 5 | 0 |
| raw; sliced | ½ cup | 9 | 0 |
| shitake; cooked | 4 | 40 | 0 |
| sliced; cooked | ½ cup | 21 | 0 |

| FOOD | PORTION | CALORIES | CHOLESTEROL |
|---|---|---|---|
| **FROZEN**<br>Mushroom Vegetable Crisp<br>(Ore Ida) | 2⅔ oz | 130 | 5 |

## MUSSEL

| | | | |
|---|---|---|---|
| **FRESH** | | | |
| blue, raw | 3 oz | 73 | 24 |
| blue, raw | 1 cup | 129 | 42 |
| blue; cooked | 3 oz | 147 | 48 |

## MUSTARD

| | | | |
|---|---|---|---|
| **READY-TO-USE** | | | |
| Kosciuszko | 1 tbsp | 11 | 0 |
| Kraft Horseradish Mustard | 1 Tbsp | 4 | 0 |
| Kraft Pure Prepared | 1 Tbsp | 4 | 0 |
| Plochman's Yellow Mustard | 1 Tbsp | 11 | 0 |
| Plochman's Dijon Mustard | 1 Tbsp | 11 | 0 |
| Plochman's Spicy Brown Mustard | 1 Tbsp | 11 | 0 |
| Plochman's Stone Ground Mustard | 1 Tbsp | 11 | 0 |
| Sauceworks Hot Mustard Sauce | 1 Tbsp | 35 | 5 |

## MUSTARD GREENS

| | | | |
|---|---|---|---|
| **FRESH** | | | |
| cooked; chopped | ½ cup | 11 | 0 |
| raw; chopped | ½ cup | 7 | 0 |

| FOOD | PORTION | CALORIES | CHOLESTEROL |
|------|---------|----------|-------------|
| **FROZEN** | | | |
| frzn; chopped, cooked | ½ cup | 14 | 0 |
| frzn; not prep | ½ cup | 15 | 0 |

## NATTO

| | | | |
|------|---------|----------|-------------|
| natto | ½ cup | 187 | 0 |

## NAVY BEANS

| FOOD | PORTION | CALORIES | CHOLESTEROL |
|------|---------|----------|-------------|
| **CANNED** | | | |
| Navy Beans (Hanover) | ½ cup | 100 | 0 |
| navy | 1 cup | 296 | 0 |
| **DRIED** | | | |
| Navy (Hurst Brand) | 1 cup | 277 | 0 |
| cooked | 1 cup | 259 | 0 |
| raw | 1 cup | 697 | 0 |
| **SPROUTS** | | | |
| cooked | 3½ oz | 78 | 0 |
| raw | ½ cup | 35 | 0 |

## NECTARINE

| | | | |
|------|---------|----------|-------------|
| **FRESH** | | | |
| nectarine | 1 | 67 | 0 |

## NEUFCHATEL CHEESE
(*see* CREAM CHEESE)

## NON-DAIRY CREAMERS
(*see* COFFEE WHITENERS)

| FOOD | PORTION | CALORIES | CHOLESTEROL |
|------|---------|----------|-------------|

## NON-DAIRY WHIPPED TOPPINGS
(*see* WHIPPED TOPPINGS)

## NOODLES
(*see also* PASTA DINNERS)

| FOOD | PORTION | CALORIES | CHOLESTEROL |
|------|---------|----------|-------------|
| noodle pudding (home recipe) | ½ cup | 132 | 27 |
| CANNED chow mein noodles | ½ cup | 228 | 3 |
| DRY Egg Noodles (Creamette) | 2 oz | 221 | 70 |
| Egg Noodles (Skinner) | 2 oz | 220 | 55 |
| Egg Noodles Enriched (Ronzoni) | 2 oz | 211 | 61 |
| Egg Noodles, uncooked (Mueller's) | 2 oz | 220 | 55 |
| Fine, Medium, Wide & Extra Wide (P&R) | 2 oz | 220 | 55 |
| Spinach Egg Noodles (Ronzoni) | 2 oz | 209 | 61 |
| Spinach Egg Noodles Light 'N Fluffy (Skinner) | 2 oz | 220 | 55 |
| egg noodles | ½ cup | 100 | 25 |

## NUTRITIONAL SUPPLEMENTS
(*see also* BREAKFAST BAR, BREAKFAST DRINKS)

| FOOD | PORTION | CALORIES | CHOLESTEROL |
|------|---------|----------|-------------|
| DIET Slender Chocolate (Carnation) | 10 oz | 220 | 4 |

| FOOD | PORTION | CALORIES | CHOLESTEROL |
|------|---------|----------|-------------|
| Slender Chocolate Fudge (Carnation) | 10 oz | 220 | 4 |
| Slender Chocolate Malt (Carnation) | 10 oz | 220 | 4 |
| Slender Milk Chocolate (Carnation) | 10 oz | 220 | 4 |
| Slender Vanilla (Carnation) | 10 oz | 220 | 5 |
| Slender Bars Chocolate (Carnation) | 2 bars | 270 | tr |
| Slender Bars Chocolate Chip (Carnation) | 2 bars | 270 | tr |
| Slender Bars Chocolate Peanut Butter (Carnation) | 2 bars | 270 | tr |
| Slender Bars Vanilla (Carnation) | 2 bars | 270 | tr |
| Slender Instant Chocolate (Carnation) | 1 pkg (1.06 oz) | 110 | 3 |
| Slender Instant Chocolate; as prep w/ 2% milk (Carnation) | 1 pkg + 6 oz milk | 200 | 15 |
| Slender Instant Dutch Chocolate (Carnation) | 1 pkg (1.06 oz) | 110 | 2 |
| Slender Instant Dutch Chocolate; as prep w/ 2% milk (Carnation) | 1 pkg + 6 oz milk | 200 | 14 |
| Slender Instant French Vanilla (Carnation) | 1 pkg (1.04 oz) | 110 | 3 |
| Slender Instant French Vanilla; as prep w/ 2% milk (Carnation) | 1 pkg + 6 oz milk | 200 | 15 |

| FOOD | PORTION | CALORIES | CHOLESTEROL |
|------|---------|----------|-------------|
| REGULAR | | | |
| Ensure Black Walnut (Ross) | 8 oz | 254 | 3 |
| Ensure Coffee (Ross) | 8 oz | 254 | 3 |
| Ensure Eggnog (Ross) | 8 oz | 254 | 3 |
| Ensure Strawberry (Ross) | 8 oz | 254 | 3 |
| Ensure Vanilla (Ross) | 8 oz | 254 | 3 |
| Ensure Plus, Coffee (Ross) | 8 oz | 355 | 4 |
| Ensure Plus, Eggnog (Ross) | 8 oz | 355 | 4 |
| Ensure Plus, Strawberry (Ross) | 8 oz | 355 | 4 |
| Ensure Plus, Vanilla (Ross) | 8 oz | 355 | 4 |
| Isocal (Mead Johnson) | 8 oz | 250 | 3 |
| Isocal HCN (Mead Johnson) | 8 oz | 473 | 7 |
| Lonalac (Mead Johnson) | 1 oz | 20 | tr |
| Malsovit Mealwafers | 2 | 152 | 0 |
| Meal-on-the-Go Food Bar | 1 (3 oz) | 340 | tr |
| Nutri-Care Strawberry | 1 pkg (1.13 oz) | 120 | 5 |
| Nutri-Care, Strawberry; as prep w/ 1 cup whole milk | 1 pkg (1.13 oz) | 280 | 45 |

| FOOD | PORTION | CALORIES | CHOLESTEROL |
|------|---------|----------|-------------|
| Nutri-Care, Strawberry; as prep w/ 1 cup 2% milk | 1 pkg (1.13 oz) | 260 | 25 |
| Sustacal (Mead Johnson) | 8 oz | 240 | 2 |
| Sustacal HC (Mead Johnson) | 8 oz | 360 | 4 |
| Sustacal Pudding (Mead Johnson) | 5 oz | 240 | tr |

## NUTS, MIXED
(*see also individual names*)

| FOOD | PORTION | CALORIES | CHOLESTEROL |
|------|---------|----------|-------------|
| Cashews & Peanuts, Honey Roasted (Planters) | 1 oz | 170 | 0 |
| Mixed Nuts Deluxe, Oil Roasted (Planters) | 1 oz | 180 | 0 |
| Mixed Nuts, Dry Roasted (Planters) | 1 oz | 170 | 0 |
| Mixed Nuts, Dry Roasted, Unsalted (Planters) | 1 oz | 170 | 0 |
| Mixed Nuts, Oil Roasted (Planters) | 1 oz | 180 | 0 |
| Mixed Nuts, Oil Roasted, Unsalted (Planters) | 1 oz | 180 | 0 |
| Mixed Nuts w/ Peanuts (Guy's) | 1 oz | 180 | 0 |
| Nut Topping (Planters) | 1 oz | 180 | 0 |
| Tasty Mix (Guy's) | 1 oz | 130 | 0 |

| FOOD | PORTION | CALORIES | CHOLESTEROL |
|---|---|---|---|
| Tavern Nuts (Planters) | 1 oz | 170 | 0 |
| mixed, dry roasted, w/ peanuts | 1 oz | 169 | 0 |
| mixed, oil roasted, w/ peanuts | 1 oz | 175 | 0 |
| mixed, oil roasted, w/o peanuts | 1 oz | 175 | 0 |

## OCTOPUS

| FRESH | | | |
|---|---|---|---|
| raw | 3 oz | 70 | 41 |

## OIL
(see also FAT)

| Bertolli Classico | 1 Tbsp | 120 | 0 |
|---|---|---|---|
| Bertolli Extra Light | 1 Tbsp | 120 | 0 |
| Bertolli Extra Virgin | 1 Tbsp | 120 | 0 |
| Crisco | 1 Tbsp | 120 | 0 |
| Italica | 1 Tbsp | 120 | 0 |
| Mazola | 1 Tbsp | 120 | 0 |
| Mazola | 1 cup | 1955 | 0 |
| Mazola No-Stick | 2.5 second spray | 6 | 0 |
| Peanut (Planters) | 1 Tbsp | 120 | 0 |
| Pompeian | 1 Tbsp | 130 | 0 |
| Popcorn (Planters) | 1 Tbsp | 120 | 0 |
| Puritan | 1 Tbsp | 120 | 0 |

| FOOD | PORTION | CALORIES | CHOLESTEROL |
|------|---------|----------|-------------|
| almond | 1 cup | 1927 | 0 |
| almond | 1 Tbsp | 120 | 0 |
| apricot kernel | 1 cup | 1927 | 0 |
| apricot kernel | 1 Tbsp | 120 | 0 |
| cocoa butter | 1 Tbsp | 120 | 0 |
| coconut | 1 Tbsp | 120 | 0 |
| corn | 1 cup | 1927 | 0 |
| corn | 1 Tbsp | 120 | 0 |
| cottonseed | 1 cup | 1927 | 0 |
| cottonseed | 1 Tbsp | 120 | 0 |
| grapeseed | 1 Tbsp | 120 | 0 |
| hazelnut | 1 cup | 1927 | 0 |
| hazelnut | 1 Tbsp | 120 | 0 |
| olive | 1 Tbsp | 119 | 0 |
| olive | 1 cup | 1909 | 0 |
| palm | 1 cup | 1927 | 0 |
| palm | 1 Tbsp | 120 | 0 |
| palm kernel | 1 Tbsp | 120 | 0 |
| palm kernel | 1 cup | 1927 | 0 |
| palm, Babassu | 1 Tbsp | 120 | 0 |
| peanut | 1 cup | 1909 | 0 |
| peanut | 1 Tbsp | 119 | 0 |
| poppyseed | 1 Tbsp | 120 | 0 |
| rapeseed | 1 Tbsp | 120 | 0 |
| rapeseed | 1 cup | 1927 | 0 |
| rice bran | 1 Tbsp | 120 | 0 |
| safflower | 1 Tbsp | 120 | 0 |

| FOOD | PORTION | CALORIES | CHOLESTEROL |
|------|---------|----------|-------------|
| safflower | 1 cup | 1927 | 0 |
| sesame | 1 Tbsp | 120 | 0 |
| soybean | 1 Tbsp | 120 | 0 |
| soybean | 1 cup | 1927 | 0 |
| soybean & cottonseed | 1 Tbsp | 120 | 0 |
| soybean & cottonseed | 1 cup | 1927 | 0 |
| soybean, hydrogenated | 1 cup | 1927 | 0 |
| soybean, hydrogenated | 1 Tbsp | 120 | 0 |
| sunflower | 1 Tbsp | 120 | 0 |
| sunflower | 1 cup | 1927 | 0 |
| walnut | 1 cup | 1927 | 0 |
| walnut | 1 Tbsp | 120 | 0 |
| wheat germ | 1 Tbsp | 120 | 0 |

## OKRA

| FOOD | PORTION | CALORIES | CHOLESTEROL |
|------|---------|----------|-------------|
| Okra Cut (Trappey's) | ½ cup | 25 | 0 |
| **FRESH** | | | |
| raw | 8 pods | 36 | 0 |
| raw; sliced | ½ cup | 19 | 0 |
| sliced; cooked | ½ cup | 25 | 0 |
| **FROZEN** | | | |
| Cut Okra (Hanover) | ½ cup | 25 | 0 |
| Okra Vegetable Crisp (Ore Ida) | 3 oz | 160 | 5 |
| Whole Okra (Hanover) | ½ cup | 35 | 0 |

| FOOD | PORTION | CALORIES | CHOLESTEROL |
|------|---------|----------|-------------|
| frzn; not prep | 10 oz pkg | 85 | 0 |
| okra; sliced, cooked | ½ cup | 34 | 0 |
| okra; cooked | 10 oz pkg | 94 | 0 |

## OLIVES

| FOOD | PORTION | CALORIES | CHOLESTEROL |
|------|---------|----------|-------------|
| Ripe Extra Large (S&W) | 1 oz | 47 | 0 |
| Ripe Large (S&W) | 1 oz | 47 | 0 |
| Ripe Pitted Extra Large (S&W) | 1 oz | 47 | 0 |
| Ripe Pitted Jumbo (S&W) | 1 oz | 47 | 0 |
| Ripe Pitted Large (S&W) | 1 oz | 47 | 0 |
| Spanish Green (Tee Pee) | 2 oz | 98 | 0 |

## ONION

| FOOD | PORTION | CALORIES | CHOLESTEROL |
|------|---------|----------|-------------|
| CANNED Whole Small (S&W) | ½ cup | 35 | 0 |
| onions; chopped | ½ cup | 21 | 0 |
| DRIED onions | 1 Tbsp | 16 | 0 |
| FRESH onions; chopped, cooked | ½ cup | 29 | 0 |
| raw; chopped | 1 Tbsp | 3 | 0 |
| FROZEN Chopped (Ore Ida) | 2 oz | 20 | 0 |

| FOOD | PORTION | CALORIES | CHOLESTEROL |
|------|---------|----------|-------------|
| Chopped (Southland) | 2 oz | 15 | 0 |
| Onions Small Whole (Birds Eye) | ½ cup | 40 | 0 |
| Onions Small w/ Cream Sauce (Birds Eye) | ½ cup | 100 | tr |
| Rings (Ore Ida) | 2 oz | 140 | 0 |
| chopped; cooked | 1 Tbsp | 4 | 0 |
| chopped; cooked | ½ cup | 30 | 0 |
| chopped; not prep | 1 pkg (10 oz) | 83 | 0 |
| onion rings | 9 oz pkg | 658 | 0 |
| onion rings | 16 oz pkg | 1170 | 0 |
| onion rings; cooked | 2 rings | 81 | 0 |
| whole; not prep | 10 oz pkg | 101 | 0 |

# ORANGE

| FOOD | PORTION | CALORIES | CHOLESTEROL |
|------|---------|----------|-------------|
| CANDIED orange peel | 1 oz | 90 | 0 |
| CANNED Mandarin Natural Style (S&W) | ½ cup | 60 | 0 |
| Mandarin Oranges in Light Syrup (Dole) | ½ cup | 76 | 0 |
| Mandarin Selected Sections in Heavy Syrup (S&W) | ½ cup | 76 | 0 |

| FOOD | PORTION | CALORIES | CHOLESTEROL |
|------|---------|----------|-------------|
| **FRESH** | | | |
| orange | 1 | 62 | 0 |
| peel | 1 Tbsp | 0 | 0 |
| peel; grated | 1 tsp | 0 | 0 |
| **JUICE** | | | |
| Orange (Tree Top) | 6 oz | 90 | 0 |
| Orange Juice (Ocean Spray) | 6 oz | 90 | 0 |
| Orange Juice 100% Pure Unsweetened (Kraft) | 6 oz | 90 | 0 |
| Unsweetened 100% Juice (S&W) | 6 oz | 83 | 0 |
| chilled | 1 cup | 110 | 0 |
| fresh | 1 cup | 111 | 0 |
| frzn; as prep | 1 cup | 112 | 0 |
| frzn; not prep | 6 oz container | 339 | 0 |
| orange juice | 1 cup | 104 | 0 |

## ORANGE EXTRACT

| Virginia Dare | 1 tsp | 22 | 0 |
|---|---|---|---|

## ORGAN MEATS
(*see* BRAINS, GIBLETS, GIZZARD, HEART, KIDNEY, LIVER)

## ORIENTAL FOOD
(*see also* DINNER, RICE)

| CANNED | | | |
|---|---|---|---|
| Chun King Divider Pak Beef Chow Mein | 7 oz | 100 | 15 |

| FOOD | PORTION | CALORIES | CHOLESTEROL |
|---|---|---|---|
| Chun King Divider Pak Beef Chow Mein | 8 oz | 110 | 20 |
| Chun King Divider Pak Beef Pepper Oriental | 7 oz | 110 | 15 |
| Chun King Divider Pak Chicken Chow Mein | 7 oz | 110 | 15 |
| Chun King Divider Pak Chicken Chow Mein | 8 oz | 120 | 10 |
| Chun King Divider Pak Pork Chow Mein Mein | 7 oz | 120 | 25 |
| Chun King Divider Pak Shrimp Chow Mein | 7 oz | 100 | 30 |
| Chun King Stir-Fry Entree Chow Mein w/ Chicken | 6 oz | 220 | 45 |
| Chun King Stir-Fry Entree Chow Mein w/Beef | 6 oz | 290 | 50 |
| Chun King Stir-Fry Entree Pepper Steak | 6 oz | 250 | 50 |
| Chun King Stir-Fry Entree Sukiyaki | 6 oz | 290 | 50 |
| Chun King Stir-Fry Entree Egg Foo Young | 5 oz | 140 | 140 |
| chop suey w/ meat | 1 cup | 144 | 5 |
| chow mein chicken | 1 cup | 95 | 8 |
| chow mein noodles | ½ cup | 228 | 3 |
| **FROZEN** Birds Eye Chinese Style International Recipe | ½ cup | 68 | tr |
| Birds Eye Chinese Style Stir-Fry Vegetable | ½ cup | 36 | 0 |

| FOOD | PORTION | CALORIES | CHOLESTEROL |
|---|---|---|---|
| Birds Eye Chow Mein Style International Recipe | ½ cup | 89 | tr |
| Birds Eye Japanese Style International Recipe | ½ cup | 88 | tr |
| Birds Eye Japanese Style Stir-Fry Vegetalbe | ½ cup | 29 | 0 |
| Birds Eye Mandarin Style International Recipe | ½ cup | 86 | tr |
| Budget Gourmet Slim Select Mandarin Chicken | 10 oz | 290 | 25 |
| Budget Gourmet Slim Select Oriental Beef | 10 oz | 290 | 25 |
| Budget Gourmet Teriyaki Chicken | 12 oz | 360 | 55 |
| La Choy Fresh & Lite Almond Chicken | 9.75 oz | 290 | 33 |
| La Choy Fresh & Lite Beef Teriyaki | 10 oz | 280 | 48 |
| La Choy Fresh & Lite Beef & Broccoli | 11 oz | 290 | 54 |
| La Choy Fresh & Lite Imperial Chicken Chow Mein | 11 oz | 270 | 45 |
| La Choy Fresh & Lite Pepper Steak | 10 oz | 290 | 54 |
| La Choy Fresh & Lite Shrimp w/ Lobster Sauce | 10 oz | 220 | 99 |
| La Choy Fresh & Lite Spicy Chicken Oriental | 9.75 oz | 290 | 27 |
| La Choy Fresh & Lite Sweet & Sour Chicken | 10 oz | 280 | 33 |
| Lean Cuisine Chicken Chow Mein w/ Rice | 11¼ oz | 250 | 30 |

| FOOD | PORTION | CALORIES | CHOLESTEROL |
|---|---|---|---|
| Lean Cuisine Shrimp & Chicken Cantonese w/ Noodles | 10⅛ oz | 260 | 105 |
| Lean Cuisine Szechwan Beef w/ Noodles & Vegetables | 9¼ oz | 280 | 90 |
| **HOME RECIPE** | | | |
| chicken teriyaki | ¾ cup | 399 | 92 |
| chop suey w/ pork | 1 cup | 375 | 62 |
| chow mein chicken | 1 cup | 255 | 78 |
| chow mein pork | 1 cup | 425 | 89 |
| chow mein shrimp | 1 cup | 221 | 55 |
| egg foo yung | 1 (5.1 oz) | 150 | 250 |
| wonton; fried | ½ cup | 111 | 31 |
| **MIX** | | | |
| Kikkoman Chow Mein Seasoning | 1⅛ oz pkg | 98 | tr |
| Kikkoman Teriyaki Baste & Glaze | 1 Tbsp | 27 | 0 |

# OYSTER

| FOOD | PORTION | CALORIES | CHOLESTEROL |
|---|---|---|---|
| **CANNED** | | | |
| Whole (Bumble Bee) | ½ cup (3.5 oz) | 100 | 55 |
| eastern | 1 cup | 170 | 136 |
| eastern | 3 oz | 58 | 46 |
| **FRESH** | | | |
| eastern, raw | 6 med | 58 | 46 |
| eastern, raw | 1 cup | 170 | 136 |
| eastern; cooked | 6 med | 58 | 46 |

| FOOD | PORTION | CALORIES | CHOLESTEROL |
|---|---|---|---|
| eastern; cooked | 3 oz | 117 | 93 |
| FROZEN<br>Carnation Jumbo or Extra Select Breaded Oysters (King & Prince) | 3.5 oz | 130 | 26 |
| HOME RECIPE<br>eastern; breaded & fried | 3 oz | 167 | 69 |
| eastern; breaded & fried | 6 med | 173 | 72 |
| oysters Rockefeller | 3 oysters | 66 | 38 |
| stew | 1 cup | 278 | 100 |

## PANCAKE/WAFFLE SYRUP
(*see also* SYRUP)

| FOOD | PORTION | CALORIES | CHOLESTEROL |
|---|---|---|---|
| Alaga Breakfast | 2 Tbsp | 108 | 0 |
| Alaga Butter Lite | 2 Tbsp | 54 | 0 |
| Alaga Honey Flavor | 2 Tbsp | 124 | 0 |
| Alaga Lite | 2 Tbsp | 54 | 0 |
| Estee | 1 Tbsp | 4 | 0 |
| Golden Griddle (Best Foods) | 1 Tbsp | 55 | 0 |
| Golden Griddle (Best Foods) | 1 cup | 885 | 0 |
| Karo Pancake Syrup | 1 Tbsp | 60 | 0 |
| Light Magic (Whitfield) | 2 Tbsp | 121 | 0 |
| Log Cabin Syrup Buttered | 1 oz | 106 | 2 |
| Log Cabin Syrup Country Kitchen | 1 oz | 101 | 0 |
| Log Cabin Syrup Lite | 1 oz | 61 | 0 |
| Log Cabin Syrup Maple Honey | 1 oz | 106 | 0 |

| FOOD | PORTION | CALORIES | CHOLESTEROL |
|------|---------|----------|-------------|
| Log Cabin Syrup Regular | 1 oz | 99 | 0 |
| Tastee | 2 Tbsp | 121 | 0 |
| Tastee Maple | 2 Tbsp | 113 | 0 |
| Yellow Label (Whitfield) | 2 Tbsp | 125 | 0 |
| Yellow Label Butter Flavor (Whitfield) | 2 Tbsp | 117 | 0 |
| Yellow Label Maple Flavor (Whitfield) | 2 Tbsp | 117 | 0 |

## PANCAKES

| | | | |
|------|---------|----------|-------------|
| FROZEN, READY-TO-USE Pancake (Morningstar Farms) | 3.5 oz | 232 | 4 |
| HOME RECIPE buckwheat | 1 (6" diam) | 137 | 0 |
| buckwheat | 1 (4" diam) | 68 | 0 |
| buttermilk | 1 (6" diam) | 164 | 54 |
| buttermilk | 1 (4" diam) | 61 | 20 |
| plain | 1 (6" diam) | 164 | 54 |
| plain | 1 (4" diam) | 61 | 20 |
| potato | 1 (4" diam) | 78 | 60 |
| zucchini | 1 (4" diam) | 69 | 31 |

| FOOD | PORTION | CALORIES | CHOLESTEROL |
|------|---------|----------|-------------|
| **MIX** | | | |
| Hungry Jack Extra Lights; as prep (Pillsbury) | 3 (4" diam) | 210 | 150 |
| Original Mix; as prep (Aunt Jemima) | 3 (4" diam) | 200 | 146 |
| Pancake Mix; as prep (Estee) | 3 (3" diam) | 100 | 0 |
| Pancake Mix; not prep (Health Valley) | 1 oz | 100 | 0 |

## PAPAYA

| | | | |
|------|---------|----------|-------------|
| **FRESH** | | | |
| Papayas (Produce Marketing Assoc) | ½ | 80 | 0 |
| papaya | 1 | 117 | 0 |
| **JUICE** | | | |
| nectar | 1 cup | 142 | 0 |

## PARSNIP

| | | | |
|------|---------|----------|-------------|
| **FRESH** | | | |
| cooked; sliced | ½ cup | 63 | 0 |
| raw; sliced | ½ cup | 50 | 0 |

## PASSION FRUIT

| | | | |
|------|---------|----------|-------------|
| **FRESH** | | | |
| passion fruit | 1 | 18 | 0 |

| FOOD | PORTION | CALORIES | CHOLESTEROL |
|------|---------|----------|-------------|

# PASTA
(*see also* NOODLES, PASTA DINNERS, PASTA SALAD)

DRY

| FOOD | PORTION | CALORIES | CHOLESTEROL |
|------|---------|----------|-------------|
| Acini de Pepe (San Giorgio) | 2 oz | 210 | 0 |
| All Shapes (Mueller's) | 2 oz | 210 | 0 |
| Alphabets (P&R) | 2 oz | 210 | 0 |
| Alphabets (San Giorgio) | 2 oz | 210 | 0 |
| Alphabets (Skinner) | 2 oz | 210 | 0 |
| Baby Pastina (San Giorgio) | 2 oz | 210 | 0 |
| Bows, Medium & Small (P&R) | 2 oz | 220 | 55 |
| Capellini (Delmonico) | 2 oz | 210 | 0 |
| Capellini (P&R) | 2 oz | 210 | 0 |
| Capellini (San Giorgio) | 2 oz | 210 | 0 |
| Ditalini (San Giorgio) | 2 oz | 210 | 0 |
| Elbow Macaroni (Delmonico) | 2 oz | 210 | 0 |
| Elbow Macaroni (San Giorgio) | 2 oz | 210 | 0 |
| Elbow Macaroni (Skinner) | 2 oz | 210 | 0 |

| FOOD | PORTION | CALORIES | CHOLESTEROL |
|---|---|---|---|
| Elbow Macaroni, Regular & Large (P&R) | 2 oz | 210 | 0 |
| Elbow Spaghetti (Delmonico) | 2 oz | 210 | 0 |
| Elbows Whole Wheat (Health Valley) | 2 oz | 170 | 0 |
| Elbows w/ 4 Vegetables Whole Wheat (Health Valley) | 2 oz | 170 | 0 |
| Fettuccini (P&R) | 2 oz | 210 | 0 |
| Fettucini (Skinner) | 2 oz | 210 | 0 |
| Fetuccini, Egg (P&R) | 2 oz | 220 | 55 |
| Fideo Enrollacio (Skinner) | 2 oz | 210 | 0 |
| Flakes (San Giorgio) | 2 oz | 210 | 0 |
| Fusilli Cut (San Giorgio) | 2 oz | 210 | 0 |
| Fusilli Cut (P&R) | 2 oz | 210 | 0 |
| Kluski (San Giorgio) | 2 oz | 220 | 55 |
| Lasagna (Delmonico) | 2 oz | 210 | 0 |
| Lasagna (Skinner) | 2 oz | 210 | 0 |
| Lasagna, Jumbo (P&R) | 2 oz | 210 | 0 |

| FOOD | PORTION | CALORIES | CHOLESTEROL |
|---|---|---|---|
| Lasagna Spinach Whole Wheat (Health Valley) | 2 oz | 170 | 0 |
| Lasagna Whole Wheat (Health Valley) | 2 oz | 170 | 0 |
| Lasagne (Mueller's) | 2 oz | 210 | 0 |
| Linguini (P&R) | 2 oz | 210 | 0 |
| Linguini (San Giorgio) | 2 oz | 210 | 0 |
| Linguini (Skinner) | 2 oz | 210 | 0 |
| Linguini (Skinner) | 2 oz | 210 | 0 |
| Linguini, Egg (Creamette) | 2 oz | 221 | 70 |
| Macaroni (Ronzoni) | 2 oz | 209 | 0 |
| Manicotti (P&R) | 2 oz | 210 | 0 |
| Manicotti (San Giorgio) | 2 oz | 210 | 0 |
| Manicotti (Skinner) | 2 oz | 210 | 0 |
| Mostaccioli (Delmonico) | 2 oz | 210 | 0 |
| Mostaccioli (Skinner) | 2 oz | 210 | 0 |
| Mostaccioli Rigati (San Giorgio) | 2 oz | 210 | 0 |
| Orzo (San Giorgio) | 2 oz | 210 | 0 |

| FOOD | PORTION | CALORIES | CHOLESTEROL |
|---|---|---|---|
| Perciatelli (P&R) | 2 oz | 210 | 0 |
| Perciatelli (San Giorgio) | 2 oz | 210 | 0 |
| Pot Pie Bows (San Giorgio) | 2 oz | 220 | 55 |
| Pot Pie Squares (San Giorgio) | 2 oz | 220 | 55 |
| Racing Wheels (San Giorgio) | 2 oz | 210 | 0 |
| Ribbon Pasta Whole Wheat (Pritikin Foods) | 2 oz | 220 | 0 |
| Rigatoni (Delmonico) | 2 oz | 210 | 0 |
| Rigatoni (San Giorgio) | 2 oz | 210 | 0 |
| Rigatoni (Skinner) | 2 oz | 210 | 0 |
| Rings (P&R) | 2 oz | 210 | 0 |
| Rippled Lasagne (San Giorgio) | 2 oz | 210 | 0 |
| Ripplets (Skinner) | 2 oz | 210 | 0 |
| Rotelle (Creamette) | 2 oz | 210 | 0 |
| Rotini (Delmonico) | 2 oz | 210 | 0 |
| Rotini (San Giorgio) | 2 oz | 210 | 0 |
| Rotini, Rainbow (Creamette) | 2 oz | 210 | 0 |

| FOOD | PORTION | CALORIES | CHOLESTEROL |
|---|---|---|---|
| Shell Macaroni (Skinner) | 2 oz | 210 | 0 |
| Shells, Large, Medium, Small & Jumbo (P&R) | 2 oz | 210 | 0 |
| Shells, Large, Medium, Small & Jumbo (San Giorgio) | 2 oz | 210 | 0 |
| Shells, Regular & Jumbo (Delmonico) | 2 oz | 210 | 0 |
| Spaghetti (Delmonico) | 2 oz | 210 | 0 |
| Spaghetti (San Giorgio) | 2 oz | 210 | 0 |
| Spaghetti (Skinner) | 2 oz | 210 | 0 |
| Spaghetti, Regular & Thin (P&R) | 2 oz | 210 | 0 |
| Spaghetti Wheels (Hanover) | ½ cup | 90 | 0 |
| Spaghetti Whole Wheat (Health Valley) | 2 oz | 170 | 0 |
| Spaghetti Whole Wheat (Pritikin Foods) | 2 oz | 220 | 0 |
| Spaghetti w/ Amaranth Whole Wheat (Health Valley) | 2 oz | 170 | 0 |
| Spaghetti w/ Spinach Whole Wheat (Health Valley) | 2 oz | 170 | 0 |
| Spaghetti, Egg (Creamette) | 2 oz | 221 | 70 |

| FOOD | PORTION | CALORIES | CHOLESTEROL |
|------|---------|----------|-------------|
| Spaghetti, Thin (Creamette) | 2 oz | 210 | 0 |
| Spaghetti; uncooked (Mueller's) | 2 oz | 210 | 0 |
| Spaghettini (Delmonico) | 2 oz | 210 | 0 |
| Spaghettini (San Giorgio) | 2 oz | 210 | 0 |
| Spinach Macaroni (Ronzoni) | 2 oz | 203 | 0 |
| Spinach Macaroni (Ronzoni) | 2 oz | 206 | 0 |
| Tubettini (San Giorgio) | 2 oz | 210 | 0 |
| Twirls (Skinner) | 2 oz | 210 | 0 |
| Twists, Tri Color (Mueller's) | 2 oz | 210 | 0 |
| Vermicelli (Delmonico) | 2 oz | 210 | 0 |
| Vermicelli (P&R) | 2 oz | 210 | 0 |
| Vermicelli (San Giorgio) | 2 oz | 210 | 0 |
| Vermicelli (Skinner) | 2 oz | 210 | 0 |
| Ziti (Creamette) | 2 oz | 210 | 0 |
| Ziti Cut (Delmonico) | 2 oz | 210 | 0 |
| Ziti Cut (San Giorgio) | 2 oz | 210 | 0 |

| FOOD | PORTION | CALORIES | CHOLESTEROL |
|---|---|---|---|

# PASTA DINNERS
(*see also* DINNER, PASTA SALAD)

| FOOD | PORTION | CALORIES | CHOLESTEROL |
|---|---|---|---|
| **CANNED** | | | |
| spaghetti w/ meatballs & tomato sauce | 1 cup | 258 | 23 |
| spaghetti w/ tomato sauce & cheese | 1 cup | 190 | 15 |
| | | | |
| **DRY MIX** | | | |
| Kraft American Style Spaghetti Dinner; as prep | 1 cup | 310 | 0 |
| Kraft Egg Noodle & Cheese Dinner; as prep | ¾ cup | 340 | 50 |
| Kraft Macaroni & Cheese Dinner Family Size; as prep | ¾ cup | 290 | 5 |
| Kraft Macaroni & Cheese Dinner; as prep | ¾ cup | 290 | 5 |
| Kraft Macaroni & Cheese Deluxe Dinner; as prep | ¾ cup | 260 | 20 |
| Kraft Spaghetti w/ Meat Sauce Dinner; as prep | 1 cup | 360 | 15 |
| Kraft Spiral Macaroni & Cheese Dinner; as prep | ¾ cup | 330 | 10 |
| Kraft Tangy Italian Style Spaghetti Dinner; as prep | 1 cup | 310 | 5 |
| Velveeta Shells and Cheese Dinner; as prep | ¾ cup | 260 | 25 |
| | | | |
| **FROZEN** | | | |
| Birds Eye Pasta Primavera Style International Recipe | ½ cup | 121 | 3 |

| FOOD | PORTION | CALORIES | CHOLESTEROL |
|---|---|---|---|
| Budget Gourmet Cheese Manicotti w/ Meat Sauce | 10 oz | 450 | 50 |
| Budget Gourmet Chicken w/ Fettucini | 10 oz | 400 | 100 |
| Budget Gourmet Italian Sausage Lasagne | 10 oz | 420 | 80 |
| Budget Gourmet Linguini w/ Shrimp | 10 oz | 330 | 75 |
| Budget Gourmet Pasta Alfredo w/ Broccoli | 5.5 oz | 200 | 25 |
| Budget Gourmet Pasta Shells & Beef | 10 oz | 340 | 35 |
| Budget Gourmet Slim Select Cheese Ravioli | 10 oz | 260 | 45 |
| Budget Gourmet Slim Select Fettucini w/ Meat Sauce | 10 oz | 290 | 25 |
| Budget Gourmet Slim Select Lasagne w/ Meat Sauce | 10 oz | 290 | 25 |
| Budget Gourmet Slim Select Linguini w/ Scallops & Clams | 9.5 oz | 280 | 60 |
| Budget Gourmet Three Cheese Lasagna | 10 oz | 400 | 65 |
| Lean Cuisine Linguini w/ Clam Sauce | 9⅝ oz | 260 | 30 |
| Lean Cuisine Tuna Lasagna w/ Spinach Noodles & Vegetables | 9¾ oz | 280 | 25 |
| Lean Cuisine Veal Lasagna | 10¼ oz | 280 | 75 |
| Lean Cuisine Veal Primavera | 9⅛ oz | 250 | 80 |
| Lean Cuisine Zucchini Lasagna | 11 oz | 260 | 20 |

| FOOD | PORTION | CALORIES | CHOLESTEROL |
|---|---|---|---|
| Macaroni & Cheese (Budget Gourmet) | 5.3 oz | 210 | 25 |
| OH Boy! Lasagna w/ Meat & Sauce | 6 oz | 230 | 35 |
| OH Boy! Spaghetti & Meatballs | 7 oz | 190 | 17 |
| Sensible Chef Fettucini Alfredo w/ Chicken Casserole | 9 oz | 410 | 56 |
| Sensible Chef Linguini w/ Shrimp & Clams Casserole | 9 oz | 190 | 46 |
| Tortellini, Cheese (Budget Gourmet) | 5.5 oz | 180 | 15 |
| HOME RECIPE lasagna | 1 piece 2½″ × 2½″ (8.8 oz) | 374 | 107 |
| macaroni & cheese | ¾ cup | 323 | 32 |
| manicotti | ¾ cup | 273 | 77 |
| noodle pudding | ½ cup | 132 | 27 |
| rigatoni w/ sausage sauce | ¾ cup | 260 | 59 |
| spaghetti w/ meatballs & cheese | 1 cup | 407 | 104 |
| spaghetti w/ meatballs & tomato sauce | 1 cup | 332 | 74 |

## PASTA SALAD

| FROZEN | | | |
|---|---|---|---|
| Italian Pasta Salad (Hanover) | ½ cup | 60 | 0 |
| Milano Pasta Salad (Hanover) | ½ cup | 60 | 0 |

| FOOD | PORTION | CALORIES | CHOLESTEROL |
|------|---------|----------|-------------|
| Oriental Pasta Salad (Hanover) | ½ cup | 80 | 0 |
| Primavera Pasta Salad (Hanover) | ½ cup | 50 | 0 |

## PÂTÉ

| | | | |
|------|---------|----------|-------------|
| CANNED | | | |
| goose liver, smoked | 1 oz | 131 | 43 |
| goose liver, smoked | 1 tbsp | 60 | 20 |

## PEACH

| | | | |
|------|---------|----------|-------------|
| CANNED | | | |
| Clingstone Halves (S&W) | ½ cup | 100 | 0 |
| Freestone Halves in Heavy Syrup (S&W) | ½ cup | 100 | 0 |
| Freestone Sliced in Heavy Syrup (S&W) | ½ cup | 100 | 0 |
| Yellow Cling Natural Lite (S&W) | ½ cup | 50 | 0 |
| Yellow Cling Natural Style (S&W) | ½ cup | 90 | 0 |
| Yellow Cling Sliced Premium in Heavy Syrup (S&W) | ½ cup | 100 | 0 |
| Yellow Cling Whole, Spiced, in Heavy Syrup (S&W) | ½ cup | 90 | 0 |
| halves in heavy syrup | 1 cup | 190 | 0 |
| halves in juice | 1 cup | 109 | 0 |

| FOOD | PORTION | CALORIES | CHOLESTEROL |
|------|---------|----------|-------------|
| halves in water pack | 1 cup | 58 | 0 |
| peaches, spiced, in heavy syrup | 1 cup | 180 | 0 |
| **DRIED**<br>Peaches<br>(Mariani) | ¼ cup | 140 | 0 |
| halves | 10 | 311 | 0 |
| **FRESH**<br>peach | 1 | 37 | 0 |
| **FROZEN**<br>peaches, sweetened, sliced | 1 cup | 235 | 0 |
| **JUICE**<br>Peach<br>(Smucker's) | 8 oz | 120 | 0 |
| Pure & Light<br>(Dole) | 6 oz | 102 | 0 |
| nectar | 1 cup | 134 | 0 |

## PEANUT BUTTER

| FOOD | PORTION | CALORIES | CHOLESTEROL |
|------|---------|----------|-------------|
| BAMA Creamy Peanut Butter | 2 Tbsp | 200 | 0 |
| BAMA Crunchy Peanut Butter | 2 Tbsp | 200 | 0 |
| BAMA Jelly & Peanut Butter | 2 Tbsp | 150 | 0 |
| Erewhon Chunky Salted | 2 Tbsp | 190 | 0 |
| Erewhon Chunky Unsalted | 2 Tbsp | 190 | 0 |
| Erewhon Creamy Salted | 2 Tbsp | 190 | 0 |
| Erewhon Creamy Unsalted | 2 Tbsp | 14 | 0 |
| Estee | 1 Tbsp | 100 | 0 |
| Health Valley Chunky | 1 Tbsp | 83 | 0 |

| FOOD | PORTION | CALORIES | CHOLESTEROL |
|---|---|---|---|
| Health Valley Chunky No Salt | 1 Tbsp | 83 | 0 |
| Health Valley Creamy | 1 Tbsp | 83 | 0 |
| Health Valley Creamy No Salt | 1 Tbsp | 83 | 0 |
| Home Brand Natural Lightly Salted | 2 Tbsp | 210 | 0 |
| Home Brand Natural Unsalted | 2 Tbsp | 210 | 0 |
| Home Brand No Sugar Added | 2 Tbsp | 180 | 0 |
| Home Brand Real Peanut Butter | 2 Tbsp | 210 | 0 |
| Jif Creamy | 2 Tbsp | 190 | 0 |
| Jif Crunchy | 2 Tbsp | 190 | 0 |
| Reese's Peanut Butter Flavored Chips (Hershey) | ¼ cup | 230 | 5 |
| Sexton Salt Free | 1 Tbsp | 98 | 0 |
| Skippy Creamy | 2 Tbsp | 190 | 0 |
| Skippy Creamy | 1 cup | 1540 | 0 |
| Skippy Creamy; w/ 2 slices white bread | 1 sandwich | 340 | 0 |
| Skippy Super Chunk | 2 Tbsp | 190 | 0 |
| Skippy Super Chunk | 1 cup | 1540 | 0 |
| Skippy Super Chunk; w/ 2 slices white bread | 1 sandwich | 340 | 0 |
| Smucker's Goober Grape | 2 Tbsp | 180 | 0 |
| Smucker's Goober Honey | 2 Tbsp | 180 | 0 |
| Smucker's Natural | 2 Tbsp | 200 | 0 |
| Smucker's Natural No Salt Added | 2 Tbsp | 200 | 0 |
| Teddie Natural Peanut Butter No Salt Added | 2 Tbsp | 200 | 0 |

| FOOD | PORTION | CALORIES | CHOLESTEROL |
|------|---------|----------|-------------|
| chunk style | 1 cup | 1520 | 0 |
| chunk style | 2 Tbsp | 188 | 0 |
| peanut butter | 1 Tbsp | 95 | 0 |
| peanut butter | 1 cup | 1526 | 0 |
| smooth style | 2 Tbsp | 188 | 0 |
| smooth style | 1 cup | 1517 | 0 |

## PEANUTS

| FOOD | PORTION | CALORIES | CHOLESTEROL |
|------|---------|----------|-------------|
| Cocktail, Oil Roasted (Planters) | 1 oz | 170 | 0 |
| Cocktail, Oil Roasted, Unsalted (Planters) | 1 oz | 170 | 0 |
| Dry Roasted (Guy's) | 1 oz | 170 | 0 |
| Dry Roasted (Lance) | 1⅛ oz | 190 | 0 |
| Dry Roasted (Planters) | 1 oz | 160 | 0 |
| Dry Roasted, Honey Roasted (Planters) | 1 oz | 160 | 0 |
| Dry Roasted, Unsalted (Planters) | 1 oz | 170 | 0 |
| Honey Roasted (Planters) | 1 oz | 170 | 0 |
| Honey Toasted P'nuts (Lance) | 1⅜ oz | 230 | 0 |
| Honey Toasted P'nuts (Lance) | 1¼ oz | 210 | 0 |
| Party Peanuts (Fisher) | 1 oz | 160 | 0 |

| FOOD | PORTION | CALORIES | CHOLESTEROL |
|---|---|---|---|
| Peanuts (Beer Nuts) | 1 oz | 180 | 0 |
| Redskin, Oil Roasted (Planters) | 1 oz | 170 | 0 |
| Redskin, Salted (Lance) | 1⅛ oz | 190 | 0 |
| Roasted w/ Shell (Lance) | 1¾ oz | 190 | 0 |
| Roasted-in-shell, Salted (Planters) | 1 oz | 160 | 0 |
| Roasted-in-shell, Unsalted (Planters) | 1 oz | 160 | 0 |
| Salted (Lance) | 1⅛ oz | 190 | 0 |
| Salted (Little Debbie) | 1 pkg (1.25 oz) | 230 | tr |
| Salted, Oil Roasted (Planters) | 1 oz | 170 | 0 |
| Spanish, Oil Roasted (Planters) | 1 oz | 170 | 0 |
| Spanish, Oil Roasted (Planters) | 1 cup | 851 | 0 |
| Spanish, Dry Roasted (Planters) | 1 oz | 160 | 0 |
| Spanish, Raw (Planters) | 1 oz | 150 | 0 |
| Spanish, Salted (Guy's) | 1 oz | 170 | 0 |
| Sweet 'N Crunchy (Planters) | 1 oz | 140 | 0 |

| FOOD | PORTION | CALORIES | CHOLESTEROL |
|---|---|---|---|
| boiled | ½ cup | 102 | 0 |
| dried | 1 oz | 161 | 0 |
| dry roasted | 1 cup | 855 | 0 |
| dry roasted | 1 oz | 164 | 0 |
| oil roasted | 1 oz | 165 | 0 |
| Valencia, oil roasted | 1 cup | 848 | 0 |
| Valencia, oil roasted | 1 oz | 165 | 0 |
| Virginia, oil roasted | 1 oz | 161 | 0 |
| Virginia, oil roasted | 1 cup | 826 | 0 |

## PEAR

| FOOD | PORTION | CALORIES | CHOLESTEROL |
|---|---|---|---|
| CANNED | | | |
| Bartlett Halves in Heavy Syrup (S&W) | ½ cup | 100 | 0 |
| Sliced Natural Style (S&W) | ½ cup | 80 | 0 |
| halves in light syrup | 1 cup | 144 | 0 |
| halves in water pack | 1 cup | 71 | 0 |
| pear halves in heavy syrup | 1 cup | 188 | 0 |
| pear halves in juice | 1 cup | 123 | 0 |
| DRIED | | | |
| Pears (Mariani) | ¼ cup | 150 | 0 |
| halves | 10 | 459 | 0 |
| FRESH | | | |
| pear | 1 | 98 | 0 |
| JUICE | | | |
| nectar | 1 cup | 149 | 0 |

| FOOD | PORTION | CALORIES | CHOLESTEROL |
|---|---|---|---|

## PEAS

**CANNED**

| FOOD | PORTION | CALORIES | CHOLESTEROL |
|---|---|---|---|
| Early June or Sweet (Owatonna) | ½ cup | 70 | 0 |
| Peas (Libby) | ½ cup | 60 | 0 |
| Peas (Seneca) | ½ cup | 60 | 0 |
| Peas Natural Pack (Libby) | ½ cup | 60 | 0 |
| Peas Natural Pack (Seneca) | ½ cup | 60 | 0 |
| Petit Pois (S&W) | ½ cup | 70 | 0 |
| Sweet Peas Perfection (S&W) | ½ cup | 70 | 0 |
| Sweet Peas Veri-Green (S&W) | ½ cup | 70 | 0 |
| peas, green | ½ cup | 61 | 0 |

**DRIED**

| FOOD | PORTION | CALORIES | CHOLESTEROL |
|---|---|---|---|
| Split Peas (Hurst Brand) | 1 cup | 277 | 0 |
| Whole Peas (Hurst Brand) | 1 cup | 272 | 0 |
| split, raw | 1 cup | 671 | 0 |
| split; cooked | 1 cup | 231 | 0 |

**FRESH**

| FOOD | PORTION | CALORIES | CHOLESTEROL |
|---|---|---|---|
| peas, edible-podded; cooked | ½ cup | 34 | 0 |
| peas, green, raw | ½ cup | 63 | 0 |
| peas, green; cooked | ½ cup | 67 | 0 |

| FOOD | PORTION | CALORIES | CHOLESTEROL |
|---|---|---|---|
| peas, raw | ½ cup | 30 | 0 |
| sprouts | ½ cup | 77 | 0 |
| FROZEN<br>Green<br>(Birds Eye) | ½ cup | 77 | 0 |
| Green; cooked<br>(Health Valley) | 5.6 oz | 126 | 0 |
| Peas w/ Cream Sauce<br>(Birds Eye) | ½ cup | 117 | tr |
| Petite Peas<br>(Hanover) | ½ cup | 70 | 0 |
| Snow Peas<br>(Hanover) | ½ cup | 35 | 0 |
| Sweet Peas<br>(Hanover) | ½ cup | 70 | 0 |
| Tiny Tender<br>(Birds Eye) | ½ cup | 62 | 0 |
| edible-podded; not prep | ½ cup | 30 | 0 |
| green; not prep | ½ cup | 55 | 0 |
| peas, edible-podded; cooked | ½ cup | 42 | 0 |
| peas, green; cooked | ½ cup | 63 | 0 |

## PECANS

| FOOD | PORTION | CALORIES | CHOLESTEROL |
|---|---|---|---|
| Chips, Halves or Pieces<br>(Planters) | 1 oz | 190 | 0 |
| dried | 1 oz | 190 | 0 |
| dry roasted | 1 oz | 187 | 0 |
| halves, dried | 1 cup | 721 | 0 |
| oil roasted | 1 oz | 195 | 0 |

| FOOD | PORTION | CALORIES | CHOLESTEROL |
|---|---|---|---|
| **PECTIN** | | | |
| Certo Fruit Pectin | 1 Tbsp | 2 | 0 |
| Sure-Jell Fruit Pectin | ¼ pkg | 38 | 0 |
| Sure-Jell Light Fruit Pectin | ¼ pkg | 33 | 0 |
| **PEPPER** | | | |
| CANNED | | | |
| chili, hot | 1 | 18 | 0 |
| green & red, sweet | ½ cup | 13 | 0 |
| jalapeno; chopped | ½ cup | 17 | 0 |
| DRIED | | | |
| green, freeze-dried | 1 Tbsp | 1 | 0 |
| red, freeze-dried | 1 Tbsp | 1 | 0 |
| FRESH | | | |
| green, raw | 1 | 18 | 0 |
| red, raw | 1 | 18 | 0 |
| red; chopped, cooked | ½ cup | 12 | 0 |
| FROZEN | | | |
| Green, Diced (Southland) | 2 oz | 10 | 0 |
| Sweet Red & Green, Cut (Southland) | 2 oz | 15 | 0 |
| green & red, sweet, chopped; not prep | 1 oz pkg | 6 | 0 |
| **PERCH** | | | |
| FRESH | | | |
| cooked | 1 fillet (1.6 oz) | 54 | 53 |

| FOOD | PORTION | CALORIES | CHOLESTEROL |
|---|---|---|---|
| cooked | 3 oz | 99 | 98 |
| ocean perch, Atlantic, raw | 3 oz | 80 | 36 |
| ocean perch, Atlantic, raw | 1 fillet (2.2 oz) | 60 | 27 |
| ocean perch, Atlantic; cooked | 1 fillet (1.8 oz) | 60 | 27 |
| ocean perch, Atlantic; cooked | 3 oz | 103 | 46 |
| raw | 3 oz | 77 | 76 |
| raw | 1 fillet (2.1 oz) | 55 | 54 |

## PERSIMMONS

| | | | |
|---|---|---|---|
| persimmons | 1 | 32 | 0 |

## PICKLE

| | | | |
|---|---|---|---|
| Bread 'N Butter Slices (Claussen) | 1 slice | 7 | 0 |
| Dill Spears (Claussen) | 1 spear | 4 | 0 |
| Kosher Halves (Claussen) | 1 half | 9 | 0 |
| Kosher Slices (Claussen) | 1 slice | 1 | 0 |
| Kosher Whole (Claussen) | 1 | 9 | 0 |
| No Garlic Dills (Claussen) | 1 | 17 | 0 |
| Relish (Claussen) | 1 Tbsp | 14 | 0 |

| FOOD | PORTION | CALORIES | CHOLESTEROL |
|---|---|---|---|
| **PIE** *(see also* PIE CRUST*)* | | | |
| CANNED FILLING | | | |
| pumpkin pie mix | 1 cup | 282 | 0 |
| FROZEN | | | |
| Apple (Mrs. Smith's) | 1/8 of 9⅝" pie | 390 | 10 |
| Apple Natural Juice (Mrs. Smith's) | 1/7 of 9" pie | 420 | 5 |
| Apple Streusel Natural Juice (Mrs. Smith's) | 1/7 of 9" pie | 420 | 5 |
| Blueberry (Mrs. Smith's) | 1/8 of 9⅝" pie | 380 | 10 |
| Cherry (Mrs. Smith's) | 1/8 of 9⅝" pie | 400 | 10 |
| Cherry Natural Juice (Mrs. Smith's) | 1/7 of 9" pie | 410 | 10 |
| Coconut Custard (Mrs. Smith's) | 1/8 of 9⅝" pie | 330 | 50 |
| Dutch Apple (Mrs. Smith's) | 1/8 of 9⅝" shell | 420 | 2 |
| Peach (Mrs. Smith's) | 1/8 of 9⅝" pie | 365 | 10 |
| Pecan Thaw 'N' Serve (Mrs. Smith's) | 1/8 of 9⅝" shell | 510 | 30 |
| Pumpkin Custard (Mrs. Smith's) | 1/8 of 9⅝" pie | 310 | 30 |
| HOME RECIPE | | | |
| apple | 1/7 of 9" pie | 402 | 7 |
| banana cream | 1/7 of 9" pie | 354 | 83 |

| FOOD | PORTION | CALORIES | CHOLESTEROL |
|------|---------|----------|-------------|
| blackberry | ⅓ of 9″ pie | 372 | 4 |
| blueberry | ⅓ of 9″ pie | 411 | 4 |
| butterscotch | ⅓ of 9″ pie | 417 | 108 |
| cherry | ⅓ of 9″ pie | 462 | 8 |
| chess | ⅓ of 9″ pie | 682 | 201 |
| chocolate chiffon | ⅓ of 9″ pie | 337 | 94 |
| chocolate meringue | ⅓ of 9″ pie | 371 | 83 |
| coconut custard | ⅓ of 9″ pie | 346 | 78 |
| custard | ⅓ of 9″ pie | 324 | 136 |
| grasshopper | ⅓ of 9″ pie | 396 | 179 |
| key lime | ⅓ of 9″ pie | 393 | 87 |
| lemon chiffon | ⅓ of 9″ pie | 381 | 145 |
| lemon meringue | ⅓ of 9″ pie | 399 | 91 |
| mince | ⅓ of 9″ pie | 441 | 6 |
| peach | ⅓ of 9″ pie | 409 | 8 |
| pecan | ⅓ of 9″ pie | 566 | 114 |

| FOOD | PORTION | CALORIES | CHOLESTEROL |
|---|---|---|---|
| pineapple chiffon | ⅟₇ of 9″ pie | 337 | 20 |
| pumpkin | ⅟₇ of 9″ pie | 287 | 84 |
| raisin | ⅟₇ of 9″ pie | 545 | 132 |
| rhubarb | ⅟₇ of 9″ pie | 414 | 7 |
| squash | ⅟₇ of 9″ pie | 311 | 87 |
| strawberry | ⅟₇ of 9″ pie | 282 | 0 |
| **MIX** | | | |
| Banana Cream No Bake Dessert; as prep (Jell-O) | ⅛ pie | 233 | 28 |
| Banana Cream; as prep w/ whole milk (Jell-O) | ⅙ of 8″ pie | 107 | 12 |
| Chocolate Mousse Pie No Bake Dessert; as prep (Jell-O) | ⅛ pie | 262 | 30 |
| Chocolate Cream Pie No Bake Dessert; as prep (Jell-O) | ⅛ pie | 260 | 29 |
| Coconut Cream; as prep w/ whole milk (Jell-O) | ⅙ of 8″ pie | 115 | 12 |
| Lemon; as prep (Jell-O) | ⅙ of 8″ pie | 180 | 94 |

| FOOD | PORTION | CALORIES | CHOLESTEROL |
|---|---|---|---|
| **SNACK** | | | |
| Apple (Hostess) | 1 | 403 | 19 |
| Berry (Hostess) | 1 | 391 | 19 |
| Blueberry (Hostess) | 1 | 378 | 19 |
| Cherry (Hostess) | 1 | 416 | 19 |
| Lemon (Hostess) | 1 | 416 | 32 |
| Marshmallow Pies, Banana (Little Debbie) | 1 pkg (1.4 oz) | 170 | tr |
| Marshmallow Pies, Banana (Little Debbie) | 1 pkg (3 oz) | 360 | tr |
| Marshmallow Pies, Chocolate (Little Debbie) | 1 pkg (1.38 oz) | 170 | tr |
| Marshmallow Pies, Chocolate (Little Debbie) | 1 pkg (3 oz) | 370 | tr |
| Oatmeal Creme Pies (Little Debbie) | 1 pkg (1.33 oz) | 160 | tr |
| Peach (Hostess) | 1 | 403 | 19 |
| Pecan Pie (Little Debbie) | 1 pkg (1.83 oz) | 170 | tr |
| Pecan Pie (Little Debbie) | 1 pkg (3 oz) | 280 | tr |
| Raisin Creme Pie (Little Debbie) | 1 pkg (1.17 oz) | 140 | tr |
| Raisin Creme Pie (Little Debbie) | 1 pkg (2.5 oz) | 290 | tr |

| FOOD | PORTION | CALORIES | CHOLESTEROL |
|------|---------|----------|-------------|

## PIE CRUST
(*see also* PIE)

| FOOD | PORTION | CALORIES | CHOLESTEROL |
|------|---------|----------|-------------|
| **FROZEN** | | | |
| Pie Shell (Mrs. Smith's) | ⅛ of 9⅝" shell | 130 | 5 |
| **HOME RECIPE** | | | |
| piecrust | 1 for 9" pie | 900 | 0 |

## PIEROGI

| FOOD | PORTION | CALORIES | CHOLESTEROL |
|------|---------|----------|-------------|
| **FROZEN** | | | |
| Potato Cheese (Mrs. T's) | 1 | 70 | 3 |
| Potato Onion (Mrs. T's) | 1 | 50 | 1 |
| Sauerkraut (Mrs. T's) | 1 | 60 | 2 |
| **HOME RECIPE** | | | |
| pierogi | ¾ cup | 307 | 49 |

## PIGEON PEAS

| FOOD | PORTION | CALORIES | CHOLESTEROL |
|------|---------|----------|-------------|
| **DRIED** | | | |
| cooked | ½ cup | 86 | 0 |
| cooked | 1 cup | 204 | 0 |
| raw | 1 cup | 704 | 0 |

## PIGNOLIA
(*see* PINE NUTS)

| FOOD | PORTION | CALORIES | CHOLESTEROL |
|------|---------|----------|-------------|
| **PIGS' EARS AND FEET** | | | |
| ears, frzn, raw | 1 ear (4 oz) | 263 | 93 |
| ears, frzn; simmered | 1 ear (3.7 oz) | 183 | 99 |
| feet, pickled | 1 oz | 58 | 26 |
| feet, pickled | 1 lb | 923 | 419 |
| feet, raw | 3.3 oz | 251 | 101 |
| feet; simmered | 2.5 oz | 138 | 71 |
| **PIKE** | | | |
| FRESH | | | |
| northern, raw | 3 oz | 75 | 33 |
| northern, raw | ½ fillet (6.9 oz) | 175 | 77 |
| northern; cooked | ½ fillet (5.4 oz) | 176 | 78 |
| northern; cooked | 3 oz | 96 | 43 |
| roe, raw | 3½ oz | 130 | 360 |
| walleye red, raw | 3 oz | 79 | 73 |
| walleye, raw | 1 fillet (5.6 oz) | 147 | 137 |
| **PINE NUTS** | | | |
| pignolia, dried | 1 oz | 146 | 0 |
| pignolia, dried | 1 Tbsp | 51 | 0 |
| pinyon, dried | 1 oz | 161 | 0 |
| **PINEAPPLE** | | | |
| CANDIED slices | 1 oz | 179 | 0 |

| FOOD | PORTION | CALORIES | CHOLESTEROL |
|---|---|---|---|
| **CANNED** | | | |
| All Cuts in Juice (Dole) | ½ cup | 70 | 0 |
| All Cuts in Syrup (Dole) | ½ cup | 95 | 0 |
| Hawaiian 100% Sliced (S&W) | 2 slices | 90 | 0 |
| Hawaiian 100% Sliced (S&W) | ½ cup | 70 | 0 |
| chunks in heavy syrup | 1 cup | 199 | 0 |
| chunks in juice | 1 cup | 150 | 0 |
| crushed | 1 cup | 199 | 0 |
| sliced in water pack | 1 slice | 19 | 0 |
| tidbits | 1 cup | 199 | 0 |
| tidbits in juice | 1 cup | 150 | 0 |
| tidbits in water pack | 1 cup | 79 | 0 |
| **FRESH** | | | |
| Chiquita | 1 cup | 90 | 0 |
| pineapple; diced | 1 cup | 77 | 0 |
| **FROZEN** | | | |
| chunks, sweetened | ½ cup | 104 | 0 |
| **JUICE** | | | |
| Pineapple (Dole) | 6 oz | 100 | 0 |
| Pineapple (Mott's) | 9.5 oz | 169 | 0 |
| Pineapple (Tree Top) | 6 oz | 100 | 0 |
| Unsweetened (S&W) | 6 oz | 100 | 0 |

| FOOD | PORTION | CALORIES | CHOLESTEROL |
|------|---------|----------|-------------|
| frzn; as prep | 1 cup | 129 | 0 |
| frzn; not prep | 6 oz container | 387 | 0 |
| pineapple juice | 1 cup | 139 | 0 |

## PINK BEANS

**DRIED**

| | | | |
|------|---------|----------|-------------|
| cooked | 1 cup | 252 | 0 |
| raw | 1 cup | 721 | 0 |

## PINTO BEANS

**CANNED**

| | | | |
|------|---------|----------|-------------|
| pinto | 1 cup | 186 | 0 |

**DRIED**

| | | | |
|------|---------|----------|-------------|
| Pinto (Hurst Brand) | 1 cup | 265 | 0 |
| cooked | 1 cup | 235 | 0 |
| raw | 1 cup | 656 | 0 |

**FROZEN**

| | | | |
|------|---------|----------|-------------|
| cooked | 3 oz | 152 | 0 |
| raw | 10 oz pkg | 484 | 0 |

**SPROUTS**

| | | | |
|------|---------|----------|-------------|
| cooked | 3½ oz | 22 | 0 |
| raw | 3½ oz | 62 | 0 |

## PINYON
(*see* PINE NUTS)

| FOOD | PORTION | CALORIES | CHOLESTEROL |
|---|---|---|---|
| **PISTACHIO** | | | |
| Dry Roasted (Planters) | 1 oz | 170 | 0 |
| Natural (Planters) | 1 oz | 170 | 0 |
| Pistachios (Lance) | 1⅛ oz | 180 | 0 |
| Red Pistachios (Planters) | 1 oz | 170 | 0 |
| Roasted Shelled Pistachios (Dole) | 1 oz | 163 | 0 |
| dried | 1 oz | 164 | 0 |
| dried | 1 cup | 739 | 0 |
| dry roasted | 1 oz | 172 | 0 |
| **PIZZA** | | | |
| (*see also* DOMINO'S PIZZA, SHAKEY'S) | | | |
| FROZEN Pizza Round (Lamb-Weston) | 4.8 oz | 370 | 10 |
| cheese | ½ of 10" pie | 140 | 23 |
| HOME RECIPE cheese & sausage | ⅛ of 14" pie | 266 | 35 |
| MIX Ragu Mix for Homemade Pizza Crust | ¼ crust | 170 | 0 |
| Ragu Mix for Homemade Pizza Crust; as prep pizza recipe | ¼ pizza | 300 | 25 |

| FOOD | PORTION | CALORIES | CHOLESTEROL |
|---|---|---|---|
| **SAUCE** | | | |
| Original Quick & Easy (Contadina) | ¼ cup | 30 | 0 |
| Pizza Sauce w/ Italian Cheese (Contadina) | ¼ cup | 30 | tr |
| Pizza Sauce w/ Pepperoni (Contadina) | ¼ cup | 40 | 2 |
| Ragu Pizza Quick Sauce Chunky Style | 3 Tbsp | 45 | 0 |
| Ragu Pizza Quick Sauce Chunky Style; as prep muffin recipe | 2 muffin halves | 220 | 15 |
| Ragu Pizza Quick Sauce Mushrooms | 3 Tbsp | 40 | 0 |
| Ragu Pizza Quick Sauce Mushrooms; as prep muffin recipe | 2 muffin halves | 220 | 15 |
| Ragu Pizza Quick Sauce Pepperoni | 3 Tbsp | 50 | 0 |
| Ragu Pizza Quick Sauce Pepperoni; as prep muffin recipe | 2 muffin halves | 230 | 15 |
| Ragu Pizza Quick Sauce Sausage | 3 Tbsp | 40 | 0 |
| Ragu Pizza Quick Sauce Sausage; as prep muffin recipe | 2 muffin halves | 220 | 15 |
| Ragu Pizza Quick Sauce Traditional | 3 Tbsp | 40 | 0 |
| Ragu Pizza Quick Sauce Traditional; as prep muffin recipe | 2 muffin halves | 220 | 15 |

| FOOD | PORTION | CALORIES | CHOLESTEROL |
|------|---------|----------|-------------|
| Ragu Pizza Sauce Extra Tomatoes | 3 Tbsp | 25 | 0 |
| Ragu Pizza Sauce Extra Tomatoes; as prep pizza recipe | ¼ pizza | 280 | 25 |

## PIZZA SAUCE
(*see* PIZZA, SAUCE; SPAGHETTI SAUCE; TOMATO)

## PLANTAINS

FRESH
| | | | |
|------|---------|----------|-------------|
| raw | 1 (6.3 oz) | 218 | 0 |
| sliced; cooked | ½ cup | 89 | 0 |

## PLUM

CANNED
| | | | |
|------|---------|----------|-------------|
| Purple Plums Halves Fancy Unpeeled in Extra Heavy Syrup (S&W) | ½ cup | 135 | 0 |
| Purple Plums Whole Fancy Unpeeled in Extra Heavy Syrup (S&W) | ½ cup | 135 | 0 |
| plums, purple in heavy syrup | 3 | 119 | 0 |
| plums, purple in juice | 3 | 55 | 0 |

FRESH
| | | | |
|------|---------|----------|-------------|
| plum | 1 | 36 | 0 |

| FOOD | PORTION | CALORIES | CHOLESTEROL |
|------|---------|----------|-------------|

# POI

FRESH
cooked | ½ cup | 134 | 0

# POKEBERRY SHOOTS

FRESH
cooked | ½ cup | 16 | 0
raw | ½ cup | 18 | 0

# POLLOCK

FRESH
Atlantic, raw | ½ fillet (6.8 oz) | 177 | 136
Atlantic, raw | 3 oz | 78 | 60
walleye, raw | 3 oz | 68 | 61
walleye, raw | 1 fillet (2.7 oz) | 62 | 55
walleye; cooked | 1 fillet (2.1 oz) | 68 | 58
walleye; cooked | 3 oz | 96 | 82

# POMEGRANATE

FRESH
pomegranates | 1 | 104 | 0

# POMPANO

FRESH
Florida, raw | 3 oz | 140 | 43

| FOOD | PORTION | CALORIES | CHOLESTEROL |
|------|---------|----------|-------------|
| Florida, raw | 1 fillet (3.9 oz) | 184 | 56 |
| Florida; cooked | 1 fillet (3.1 oz) | 185 | 56 |
| Florida; cooked | 3 oz | 179 | 54 |

## POPCORN
(*see also* CHIPS, PRETZELS, SNACKS)

| FOOD | PORTION | CALORIES | CHOLESTEROL |
|------|---------|----------|-------------|
| Bachman Popcorn | 1 oz | 160 | 0 |
| Jiffy Pop, Microwave Regular; as prep | 4 cups | 140 | 0 |
| Jiffy Pop, Microwave Butter Flavor; as prep | 4 cups | 140 | 0 |
| Jiffy Pop, Pan Butter Flavor; as prep | 4 cups | 130 | 0 |
| Jiffy Pop, Pan Regular; as prep | 4 cups | 130 | 0 |
| Lance Cheese Popcorn | 1 pkg (⅞ oz) | 130 | 5 |
| Lance Cheese Popcorn | 1 oz | 150 | 5 |
| Lance Plain | 1 pkg (1 oz) | 140 | 0 |
| air-popped | 1 cup | 30 | 0 |
| popped w/ vegetable oil | 1 cup | 55 | 0 |
| sugar syrup coated | 1 cup | 135 | 0 |

## POPOVER

| FOOD | PORTION | CALORIES | CHOLESTEROL |
|------|---------|----------|-------------|
| popover (home recipe) | 1 (1.4 oz) | 98 | 61 |

| FOOD | PORTION | CALORIES | CHOLESTEROL |
|------|---------|----------|-------------|

# PORK

(*see also* BACON, CANADIAN BACON, HAM, LUNCHEON MEATS/COLD CUTS, SAUSAGE)

The values for cooked pork may differ slightly from values for raw pork. When meat is cooked some moisture and fat is lost, changing the nutritive value slightly. As a rule of thumb, it can be assumed that a 4 oz raw portion will equal a 3 oz cooked portion of meat.

FRESH

| FOOD | PORTION | CALORIES | CHOLESTEROL |
|------|---------|----------|-------------|
| center loin chop, lean & fat, raw | 1 chop (4.4 oz) | 341 | 86 |
| center loin chop, lean & fat; braised | 1 chop (2.6 oz) | 266 | 81 |
| center loin chop, lean & fat; broiled | 1 chop (3.1 oz) | 275 | 84 |
| center loin chop, lean & fat; roasted | 1 chop (3.1 oz) | 268 | 80 |
| center loin chop, lean & fat; pan-fried | 1 chop (3.1 oz) | 333 | 92 |
| center loin chop, lean only, raw | 1 chop (3.4 oz) | 155 | 62 |
| center loin chop, lean only; braised | 1 chop (2.1 oz) | 166 | 68 |
| center loin chop, lean only; broiled | 1 chop (2.5 oz) | 166 | 71 |
| center loin chop, lean only; roasted | 1 chop (2.4 oz) | 180 | 68 |
| center loin chop, lean only; pan-fried | 1 chop (2.4 oz) | 178 | 71 |
| center loin, lean & fat; braised | 3 oz | 301 | 91 |
| center loin, lean & fat; broiled | 3 oz | 269 | 82 |

| FOOD | PORTION | CALORIES | CHOLESTEROL |
|---|---|---|---|
| center loin, lean & fat; roasted | 3 oz | 259 | 78 |
| center loin, lean & fat; pan-fried | 3 oz | 318 | 87 |
| center loin, lean only; broiled | 3 oz | 196 | 83 |
| center loin, lean only; roasted | 3 oz | 204 | 78 |
| center loin, lean only; pan-fried | 3 oz | 226 | 91 |
| ham, fresh, shank half, lean & fat; roasted | 3 oz | 258 | 78 |
| ham, fresh, shank half, lean only; roasted | 3 oz | 183 | 78 |
| ham, fresh, whole, lean & fat; roasted | 3 oz | 250 | 79 |
| ham, fresh, whole, lean only; roasted | 3 oz | 187 | 80 |
| ham, fresh, rump half, lean & fat; roasted | 3 oz | 233 | 81 |
| ham, fresh, rump half, lean only; roasted | 3 oz | 187 | 81 |
| leg, loin & shoulder, lean only; roasted | 3 oz | 198 | 79 |
| leg, rump half, lean & fat, raw | 3 oz | 198 | 57 |
| leg, rump half, lean only, raw | 3 oz | 87 | 51 |
| leg, shank half, lean & fat, raw | 3 oz | 240 | 57 |
| leg, shank half, lean only, raw | 3 oz | 117 | 51 |
| leg, whole, lean & fat, raw | 3 oz | 222 | 63 |
| leg, whole, lean only, raw | 3 oz | 117 | 57 |

| FOOD | PORTION | CALORIES | CHOLESTEROL |
|---|---|---|---|
| loin blade chop, lean & fat; braised | 1 chop (2.4 oz) | 275 | 72 |
| loin blade chop, lean & fat; braised | 1 chop (3.1 oz) | 321 | 79 |
| loin blade chop, lean & fat; pan-fried | 1 chop (3.1 oz) | 368 | 85 |
| loin blade chop, lean only: broiled | 1 chop (2.1 oz) | 177 | 59 |
| loin blade chop, lean only; braised | 1 chop (1.8 oz) | 156 | 57 |
| loin blade chop, lean only; roasted | 1 chop (2.5 oz) | 198 | 63 |
| loin blade chop, lean only; pan-fried | 1 chop (2.2 oz) | 175 | 60 |
| loin center rib chop, lean & fat, raw | 1 chop (3.9 oz) | 322 | 71 |
| loin center rib chop, lean only, raw | 1 chop (3 oz) | 138 | 47 |
| loin chop, lean & fat, raw | 1 chop (4 oz) | 345 | 81 |
| loin chop, lean & fat, raw | 1 chop (3.9 oz) | 356 | 79 |
| loin chop, lean & fat; braised | 1 chop (2.3 oz) | 267 | 67 |
| loin chop, lean & fat; braised | 1 chop (2.5 oz) | 261 | 73 |
| loin chop, lean & fat; pan-fried | 1 chop (2.9 oz) | 337 | 72 |
| loin chop, lean & fat; roasted | 1 chop (2.8 oz) | 274 | 68 |
| loin chop, lean & fat; roasted | 1 chop (2.9 oz) | 262 | 74 |

| FOOD | PORTION | CALORIES | CHOLESTEROL |
|------|---------|----------|-------------|
| loin chop, lean only, raw | 1 chop (3 oz) | 142 | 55 |
| loin chop, lean only; broiled | 1 chop (2.1 oz) | 165 | 60 |
| loin chop, lean only; pan-fried | 1 chop (2 oz) | 157 | 49 |
| loin chop, lean only; roasted | 1 chop (2.3 oz) | 167 | 54 |
| loin chop, lean & fat; broiled | 1 chop (2.7 oz) | 295 | 76 |
| loin chop, lean only; braised | 1 chop (1.8 oz) | 147 | 51 |
| loin, blade, lean & fat; braised | 3 oz | 348 | 92 |
| loin, blade, lean & fat; broiled | 3 oz | 334 | 83 |
| loin, blade, lean & fat; roasted | 3 oz | 310 | 76 |
| loin, blade, lean & fat; pan-fried | 3 oz | 352 | 81 |
| loin, blade, lean only; braised | 3 oz | 266 | 96 |
| loin, blade, lean only; broiled | 3 oz | 255 | 85 |
| loin, blade, lean only; roasted | 3 oz | 238 | 76 |
| loin, blade, lean only; pan-fried | 3 oz | 240 | 82 |
| loin, lean & fat; braised | 3 oz | 312 | 87 |
| loin, lean & fat; broiled | 3 oz | 294 | 80 |
| loin, lean & fat; roasted | 3 oz | 271 | 77 |
| loin, lean only; braised | 3 oz | 232 | 90 |
| loin, lean only; broiled | 3 oz | 218 | 81 |
| loin, lean only; roasted | 3 oz | 204 | 77 |

| FOOD | PORTION | CALORIES | CHOLESTEROL |
|---|---|---|---|
| lungs, raw | 3.5 oz | 83 | 314 |
| lungs; braised | 3 oz | 84 | 329 |
| pancreas, raw | 4 oz | 225 | 218 |
| pancreas; braised | 3 oz | 186 | 268 |
| rib chop, lean only; braised | 1 chop (1.8 oz) | 147 | 51 |
| rib chop, lean only; broiled | 1 chop (2.1 oz) | 162 | 69 |
| rib chop, lean only; pan-fried | 1 chop (2 oz) | 160 | 60 |
| rib chop, lean only; roasted | 1 chop (2.2 oz) | 162 | 52 |
| rib chop, lean & fat; braised | 1 chop (2.2 oz) | 246 | 64 |
| rib chop, lean & fat; broiled | 1 chop (2.6 oz) | 264 | 72 |
| rib chop, lean & fat; pan-fried | 1 chop (2.9 oz) | 343 | 74 |
| rib chop, lean & fat; roasted | 1 chop (2.6 oz) | 252 | 64 |
| salt pork | 1 oz | 212 | 25 |
| shoulder arm picnic, lean only, raw | 3 oz | 120 | 54 |
| shoulder arm picnic, lean & fat, raw | 3 oz | 231 | 60 |
| shoulder blade Boston steak, lean & fat; braised | 1 steak (5.6 oz) | 594 | 178 |
| shoulder blade Boston steak, lean & fat, raw | 1 steak (9.6 oz) | 737 | 193 |
| shoulder blade Boston steak, lean only, raw | steak (7.4 oz) | 346 | 142 |

| FOOD | PORTION | CALORIES | CHOLESTEROL |
|---|---|---|---|
| shoulder blade Boston steak, lean only; braised | 1 steak (4.6 oz) | 382 | 151 |
| shoulder blade Boston steak, lean only; broiled | 1 steak (5.3 oz) | 413 | 159 |
| shoulder blade Boston steak, lean only; roasted | 1 steak (5.5 oz) | 404 | 155 |
| shoulder blade Boston steak, lean & fat; broiled | 1 steak (6.5 oz) | 647 | 190 |
| shoulder blade Boston steak, lean & fat; roasted | 1 steak (6.5 oz) | 594 | 179 |
| shoulder whole, lean & fat, raw | 3 oz | 234 | 63 |
| shoulder whole, lean only, raw | 3 oz | 132 | 57 |
| shoulder, arm picnic, cured, lean & fat; roasted | 3 oz | 238 | 49 |
| shoulder, arm picnic, cured, lean only; roasted | 3 oz | 145 | 41 |
| shoulder, arm picnic, lean only; braised | 3 oz | 211 | 97 |
| shoulder, arm picnic, lean only; roasted | 3 oz | 194 | 81 |
| shoulder, arm picnic, lean & fat; braised | 3 oz | 293 | 93 |
| shoulder, arm picnic, lean & fat; roasted | 3 oz | 281 | 80 |
| shoulder, blade roll, cured, lean & fat; roasted | 3 oz | 244 | 57 |
| shoulder, Boston blade, lean only; braised | 3 oz | 250 | 99 |
| shoulder, Boston blade, lean only; broiled | 3 oz | 233 | 89 |

| FOOD | PORTION | CALORIES | CHOLESTEROL |
|---|---|---|---|
| shoulder, Boston blade, lean only; roasted | 3 oz | 218 | 83 |
| shoulder, Boston blade, lean & fat; braised | 3 oz | 316 | 95 |
| shoulder, Boston blade, lean & fat; broiled | 3 oz | 297 | 87 |
| shoulder, Boston blade, lean & fat; roasted | 3 oz | 273 | 82 |
| shoulder, whole, lean & fat; roasted | 3 oz | 277 | 81 |
| shoulder, whole, lean only; roated | 3 oz | 207 | 82 |
| sirloin chop, lean & fat, raw | 1 chop (4.2 oz) | 328 | 83 |
| sirloin chop, lean & fat; braised | 1 chop (2.4 oz) | 250 | 75 |
| sirloin chop, lean & fat; broiled | 1 chop (2.8 oz) | 278 | 81 |
| sirloin chop, lean & fat; roasted | 1 chop (2.8 oz) | 244 | 76 |
| sirloin chop, lean only, raw | 1 chop (3.2 oz) | 139 | 58 |
| sirloin chop, lean only; braised | 1 chop (1.9 oz) | 149 | 63 |
| sirloin chop, lean only; broiled | 1 chop (2.3 oz) | 165 | 67 |
| sirloin chop, lean only; roasted | 1 chop (2.5 oz) | 175 | 67 |
| spareribs, lean & fat, raw | 3 oz | 243 | 66 |
| spareribs, lean & fat; braised | 3 oz | 338 | 103 |

| FOOD | PORTION | CALORIES | CHOLESTEROL |
|---|---|---|---|
| spleen, raw | 4 oz | 113 | 410 |
| spleen; braised | 3 oz | 127 | 428 |
| tail, raw | 4 oz | 427 | 110 |
| tail; simmered | 3 oz | 336 | 110 |
| tenderloin, lean only, raw | 3 oz | 96 | 54 |
| tenderloin, lean only; roasted | 3 oz | 141 | 79 |
| top loin chop, lean & fat, raw | 1 chop (4 oz) | 360 | 77 |
| top loin chop, lean only, raw | 1 chop (3.1 oz) | 142 | 48 |

## POT PIE

| FOOD | PORTION | CALORIES | CHOLESTEROL |
|---|---|---|---|
| Beef (Banquet) | 7 oz | 500 | 25 |
| Beef (Morton) | 7 oz | 430 | 29 |
| Chicken (Banquet) | 7 oz | 540 | 35 |
| Chicken (Morton) | 7 oz | 415 | 35 |
| Tuna (Banquet) | 7 oz | 540 | 27 |
| Turkey (Banquet) | 7 oz | 500 | 37 |
| Turkey (Morton) | 7 oz | 420 | 38 |
| HOME RECIPE beef; baked | 4¼" diam | 558 | 48 |

| FOOD | PORTION | CALORIES | CHOLESTEROL |
|------|---------|----------|-------------|
| chicken | 1 (11 oz) | 706 | 118 |
| turkey | 1 (10.6 oz) | 710 | 122 |

## POTATO STARCH

| | | | |
|------|---------|----------|-------------|
| Potato Starch (Manischewitz) | 1 cup | 570 | 0 |

## POTATOES
(*see also* CHIPS)

| | | | |
|------|---------|----------|-------------|
| CANNED | | | |
| New Potatoes Extra Small (S&W) | ½ cup | 45 | 0 |
| Potatoes (Libby) | ½ cup | 45 | 0 |
| Potatoes (Seneca) | ½ cup | 45 | 0 |
| Scalloped Potatoes Flavored w/ Ham (Lunch Bucket) | 1 container (8.25 oz) | 250 | 35 |
| potatoes | ½ cup | 54 | 0 |
| FRESH | | | |
| Yukon Gold | 1 (5.3 oz) | 110 | 0 |
| baked, flesh only | 1 (5 oz) | 145 | 0 |
| baked, flesh & skin | 1 (6½ oz) | 220 | 0 |
| baked, skin only | skin from 1 potato | 115 | 0 |
| boiled | ½ cup | 68 | 0 |
| boiled | 1 (4.7 oz) | 119 | 0 |

| FOOD | PORTION | CALORIES | CHOLESTEROL |
|---|---|---|---|
| flesh & skin; microwaved | 1 (7 oz) | 212 | 0 |
| flesh only; microwaved | 1 (5.5 oz) | 156 | 0 |
| raw, flesh only | 1 (3.9 oz) | 88 | 0 |
| raw, skin only | 1 (1.3 oz) | 22 | 0 |
| FROZEN | | | |
| Bacon & Cheddar Baked Potato Entree (Idaho Original) | 11 oz | 982 | 21 |
| Cheddar Browns (Ore Ida) | 3 oz | 90 | 10 |
| Cheddared Potatoes (Budget Gourmet) | 5.5 oz | 230 | 35 |
| Cheddared Potatoes & Broccoli (Budget Gourmet) | 5 oz | 130 | 25 |
| Chicken & Almond Baked Potato Entree (Idaho Original) | 11 oz | 433 | 29 |
| Cottage Fries (Ore Ida) | 3 oz | 120 | 0 |
| Crinkle Cuts French Fries (Lamb-Weston) | 3 oz | 130 | 5 |
| Crinkle Cuts Lites (Ore Ida) | 3 oz | 90 | 0 |
| Crinkle Cuts Microwave (Ore Ida) | 3.5 oz | 180 | 0 |
| Crispers! (Ore Ida) | 3 oz | 230 | 0 |
| Crispy Crowns (Ore Ida) | 3 oz | 160 | 0 |
| Crispy Crowns w/ Onion (Ore Ida) | 3 oz | 170 | 0 |

| FOOD | PORTION | CALORIES | CHOLESTEROL |
|------|---------|----------|-------------|
| Deep Fries Crinkle Cuts (Heinz) | 3 oz | 150 | 0 |
| Deep Fries Shoestrings (Heinz) | 3 oz | 200 | 0 |
| French Fries (Heinz) | 3 oz | 160 | 0 |
| French Fries Golden Crinkles (Ore Ida) | 3 oz | 120 | 0 |
| French Fries Golden Fries (Ore Ida) | 3 oz | 120 | 0 |
| French Fries Lites (Ore Ida) | 3 oz | 90 | 0 |
| French Fries Pixie Crinkles (Ore Ida) | 3 oz | 140 | 0 |
| French Fries Shoestrings (Ore Ida) | 3 oz | 140 | 0 |
| Fries Country Style Dinner (Ore Ida) | 3 oz | 110 | 0 |
| Golden Patties (Ore Ida) | 2.5 oz | 140 | 0 |
| Hash Browns Microwave (Ore Ida) | 2 oz | 180 | 0 |
| Hash Browns Shredded (Ore Ida) | 3 oz | 70 | 0 |
| Hash Browns Southern Style w/ Butter & Onions (Heinz) | 3 oz | 110 | 5 |
| Hash Browns Southern Style (Ore Ida) | 3 oz | 70 | 0 |
| Home Browns Hash Browns (Lamb-Weston) | 1 piece (2.25 oz) | 150 | 10 |

| FOOD | PORTION | CALORIES | CHOLESTEROL |
|------|---------|----------|-------------|
| Italian Baked Potato Entree (Idaho Original) | 11 oz | 443 | 41 |
| MunchSkins (Lamb-Weston) | 3 oz | 120 | 5 |
| Nacho Potatoes (Budget Gourmet) | 5 oz | 180 | 30 |
| Natural Cuts Skin-On (Lamb-Weston) | 3 oz | 120 | 0 |
| Natural Slices Skin-On (Lamb-Weston) | 3 oz | 120 | 5 |
| Natural Trim Fries Skin-On (Lamb-Weston) | 3 oz | 140 | 5 |
| New Potatoes In Sour Cream Sauce (Budget Gourmet) | 5 oz | 120 | 20 |
| O'Brien Potatoes (Ore Ida) | 3 oz | 60 | 0 |
| Primavera Baked Potato Entree (Idaho Original) | 11 oz | 499 | 25 |
| Regular Cut French Fries (Lamb-Weston) | 3 oz | 130 | 5 |
| Shoestring French Fries (Lamb-Weston) | 3 oz | 140 | 5 |
| Shoestrings Lites (Ore Ida) | 3 oz | 90 | 0 |
| Steak House Fries (Lamb-Weston) | 3 oz | 120 | 5 |
| Stuffed Potatoes w/ Cheddar Cheese (OH Boy!) | 6 oz | 142 | 6 |

| FOOD | PORTION | CALORIES | CHOLESTEROL |
|---|---|---|---|
| Stuffed Potatoes w/ Real Bacon (OH Boy!) | 6 oz | 116 | 5 |
| Stuffed Potatoes w/ Sour Cream & Chives (OH Boy!) | 6 oz | 129 | 2 |
| Tater Puffs (Lamb-Weston) | 3 oz | 150 | 10 |
| Tater Tots (Ore Ida) | 3 oz | 140 | 0 |
| Tater Tots Microwave (Ore Ida) | 2 oz | 200 | 0 |
| Tater Tots w/ Bacon Flavored Vegetable Protein (Ore Ida) | 3 oz | 140 | 0 |
| Tater Tots w/ Onion (Ore Ida) | 3 oz | 140 | 0 |
| Tater Wedges (Lamb-Weston) | 2 pieces (4 oz) | 200 | 10 |
| Three Cheese Potatoes (Budget Gourmet) | 5.75 oz | 230 | 30 |
| Wedges Home Style (Ore Ida) | 3 oz | 100 | 0 |
| Western Style Baked Potato Entree (Idaho Original) | 11 oz | 567 | 33 |
| Whole Small (Ore Ida) | 3 oz | 70 | 0 |
| french fried; not prep | 10 strips | 107 | 0 |
| french-fried, cottage-cut; cooked | 10 strips | 109 | 0 |
| french-fried; cooked | 10 strips | 111 | 0 |
| potato puffs; as prep | ½ cup | 138 | 0 |

| FOOD | PORTION | CALORIES | CHOLESTEROL |
|---|---|---|---|
| whole; not prep | ½ cup | 71 | 0 |
| **HOME RECIPE** | | | |
| au gratin | ½ cup | 160 | 29 |
| au gratin w/ cheese | ½ cup | 178 | 18 |
| mashed | ½ cup | 111 | 2 |
| O'Brien | 1 cup | 157 | 7 |
| potato pancakes | 1 | 495 | 93 |
| scalloped | ½ cup | 105 | 14 |
| scalloped | ½ cup | 127 | 7 |
| **MIX** | | | |
| Mashed Idaho; as prep (French's) | ½ cup | 130 | 12 |
| Mashed Potato Buds; as prep (Betty Crocker) | ½ cup | 130 | 17 |
| Mashed; as prep (Hungry Jack) | ½ cup | 130 | 17 |
| Potato Pancakes; as prep (Frenchs) | 1 | 80 | 10 |
| mashed, dehydrated, flakes | ½ cup | 361 | 0 |
| mashed, dehydrated, flakes; as prep | ½ cup | 118 | 15 |
| mashed, granules; as prep w/ whole milk | ½ cup | 137 | 18 |
| mashed, granules not prep | ½ cup | 80 | 0 |
| **READY-TO-USE** | | | |
| salad | ½ cup | 179 | 86 |

## POUT

| | | | |
|---|---|---|---|
| **FRESH** | | | |
| ocean, raw | 3 oz | 67 | 44 |

| FOOD | PORTION | CALORIES | CHOLESTEROL |
|---|---|---|---|
| ocean, raw | ½ fillet (6.2 oz) | 140 | 92 |

## PRESERVE
(see JAM/JELLY/PRESERVE)

## PRETZELS
(see also CHIPS, POPCORN, SNACKS)

| FOOD | PORTION | CALORIES | CHOLESTEROL |
|---|---|---|---|
| Bachman Pretzel Rods | 1 rod (1 oz) | 110 | 0 |
| Estee Unsalted | 5 | 25 | 0 |
| J&J Soft Pretzels | 1 oz | 76 | 0 |
| Lance Pretzel Twist | 1½ oz | 150 | 0 |
| Lance Pretzels | 1 oz | 100 | 0 |
| Quinlan Artificial Butter Tiny Thins | 1 oz | 108 | 0 |
| Quinlan Beers | 1 oz | 110 | 0 |
| Quinlan Cheese Tiny Thins | 1 oz | 109 | 0 |
| Quinlan Logs | 1 oz | 103 | 0 |
| Quinlan Party Thins | 1 oz | 109 | 0 |
| Quinlan Philly Style | 1 oz | 107 | 0 |
| Quinlan Rods | 1 oz | 100 | 0 |
| Quinlan Sour Cheese Tiny Thins | 1 oz | 100 | 0 |
| Quinlan Sour Dough Thins Hard | 1 oz | 100 | 0 |
| Quinlan Sticks | 1 oz | 105 | 0 |
| Quinlan Thins | 1 oz | 104 | 0 |
| Quinlan Tiny Thins | 1 oz | 109 | 0 |
| Quinlan Tiny Thins No-Salt | 1 oz | 115 | 0 |

| FOOD | PORTION | CALORIES | CHOLESTEROL |
|---|---|---|---|
| Quinlan Ultra Thins | 1 oz | 106 | 0 |
| thin slim sticks | 47 pieces | 110 | 0 |
| twist, tiny | 14 pieces | 109 | 0 |

## PRUNE

CANNED
| | | | |
|---|---|---|---|
| prunes in heavy syrup | 5 | 90 | 0 |

DRIED
| | | | |
|---|---|---|---|
| Prunes, Pitted (Mariani) | ¼ cup | 140 | 0 |
| Prunes, Whole (Mariani) | ¼ cup | 140 | 0 |
| cooked w/o sugar | ½ cup | 113 | 0 |
| prunes | 10 | 201 | 0 |

JUICE
| | | | |
|---|---|---|---|
| Country Style (Mott's) | 6 oz | 130 | 0 |
| Prune (Mott's) | 6 oz | 130 | 0 |
| Unsweetened (S&W) | 6 oz | 120 | 0 |
| prune juice | 1 cup | 181 | 0 |

## PUDDING
(*see also* CUSTARD, PUDDING POPS)

HOME RECIPE
| | | | |
|---|---|---|---|
| bread w/ raisins | ½ cup | 180 | 77 |
| corn | ½ cup | 97 | 47 |
| corn | ⅔ cup | 181 | 230 |

| FOOD | PORTION | CALORIES | CHOLESTEROL |
|---|---|---|---|
| pumpkin | ½ cup | 170 | 105 |
| rice w/ raisins | ½ cup | 246 | 136 |
| tapioca | ½ cup | 169 | 111 |
| **MIX** | | | |
| Banana Creme Instant (Jell-O) | 1 pkg (3.5 oz) | 360 | tr |
| Butter Pecan Instant (Jell-O) | 1 pkg (3.5 oz) | 383 | tr |
| Butterscotch (Jell-O) | 1 pkg (3.6 oz) | 364 | 0 |
| Butterscotch Instant (Jell-O) | 1 pkg (3.5 oz) | 358 | tr |
| Butterscotch; as prep (Estee) | ½ cup | 70 | 2 |
| Chocolate (Jell-O) | 1 pkg (3.5 oz) | 346 | 0 |
| Chocolate Tapioca Americana (Jell-O) | 1 pkg (3.5 oz) | 378 | 0 |
| Chocolate Fudge (Jell-O) | 1 pkg (3.5 oz) | 345 | 0 |
| Chocolate; as prep (Estee) | ½ cup | 70 | 2 |
| Coconut Cream Instant (Jell-O) | 1 pkg (3.5 oz) | 416 | tr |
| French Vanilla (Jell-O) | 1 pkg (3.5 oz) | 365 | 0 |
| French Vanilla Instant (Jell-O) | 1 pkg (3.5 oz) | 360 | tr |
| Lemon Instant (Jell-O) | 1 pkg (3.5 oz) | 376 | tr |
| Lemon; as prep (Estee) | ½ cup | 70 | 2 |

| FOOD | PORTION | CALORIES | CHOLESTEROL |
|------|---------|----------|-------------|
| Milk Chocolate (Jell-O) | 1 pkg (3.5 oz) | 362 | 2 |
| Pineapple Cream Instant (Jell-O) | 1 pkg (3.5 oz) | 363 | tr |
| Pistachio Instant (Jell-O) | 1 pkg (3.5 oz) | 383 | tr |
| Vanilla Instant (Jell-O) | 1 pkg (3.5 oz) | 374 | tr |
| Vanilla; as prep (Estee) | ½ cup | 70 | 2 |
| **MIX WITH 2% MILK** | | | |
| Butterscotch Instant Sugar Free; as prep (Jell-O) | ½ cup | 88 | 9 |
| Chocolate Instant Sugar Free; as prep (Jell-O) | ½ cup | 96 | 9 |
| Chocolate Fudge Instant Sugar Free; as prep (Jell-O) | ½ cup | 100 | 9 |
| Chocolate Sugar Free; as prep (Jell-O) | ½ cup | 91 | 9 |
| Pistachio Instant Sugar Free; as prep (Jell-O) | ½ cup | 94 | 9 |
| Vanilla Instant Sugar Free; as prep (Jell-O) | ½ cup | 90 | 9 |
| Vanilla Sugar Free; as prep (Jell-O) | ½ cup | 82 | 9 |
| **MIX WITH SKIM MILK** | | | |
| Butterscotch (D-Zerta) | ½ cup | 69 | 2 |

| FOOD | PORTION | CALORIES | CHOLESTEROL |
|---|---|---|---|
| Butterscotch w/ NutraSweet; as prep (D-Zerta) | ½ cup | 69 | 2 |
| Chocolate w/ NutraSweet; as prep (D-Zerta) | ½ cup | 65 | 2 |
| Vanilla (D-Zerta) | ½ cup | 69 | 2 |
| Vanilla w/ NutraSweet; as prep (D-Zerta) | ½ cup | 69 | 2 |
| **MIX WITH WHOLE MILK** | | | |
| Banana Creme Instant; as prep (Jell-O) | ½ cup | 168 | 17 |
| Butter Pecan Instant; as prep (Jell-O) | ½ cup | 174 | 17 |
| Butterscotch Instant; as prep (Jell-O) | ½ cup | 168 | 17 |
| Butterscotch; as prep (Jell-O) | ½ cup | 171 | 17 |
| Chocolate Fudge Instant; as prep (Jell-O) | ½ cup | 174 | 17 |
| Chocolate Fudge; as prep (Jell-O) | ½ cup | 164 | 17 |
| Chocolate Instant; as prep (Jell-O) | ½ cup | 176 | 17 |
| Chocolate Tapioca Americana; as prep (Jell-O) | ½ cup | 173 | 17 |
| Chocolate; as prep (Jell-O) | ½ cup | 165 | 17 |

| FOOD | PORTION | CALORIES | CHOLESTEROL |
|---|---|---|---|
| Coconut Cream Instant; as prep (Jell-O) | ½ cup | 182 | 17 |
| French Vanilla Instant; as prep (Jell-O) | ½ cup | 168 | 17 |
| French Vanilla; as prep (Jell-O) | ½ cup | 171 | 17 |
| Golden Egg Custard Americana; as prep (Jell-O) | 1 pkg (3.5 oz) | 378 | 0 |
| Golden Egg Custard Americana; as prep (Jell-O) | ½ cup | 167 | 85 |
| Lemon Instant; as prep (Jell-O) | ½ cup | 172 | 17 |
| Milk Chocolate Instant; as prep (Jell-O) | ½ cup | 178 | 17 |
| Milk Chocolate; as prep (Jell-O) | ½ cup | 168 | 17 |
| Pineapple Cream Instant; as prep (Jell-O) | ½ cup | 168 | 17 |
| Pistachio Instant; as prep (Jell-O) | ½ cup | 172 | 17 |
| Rice Americana; as prep (Jell-O) | ½ cup | 177 | 17 |
| Vanilla Instant; as prep (Jell-O) | ½ cup | 171 | 17 |
| Vanilla Tapioca Americana; as prep (Jell-O) | ½ cup | 166 | 17 |

| FOOD | PORTION | CALORIES | CHOLESTEROL |
|---|---|---|---|
| Vanilla; as prep (Jell-O) | ½ cup | 162 | 17 |
| READY-TO-USE | | | |
| Banana Snack Pack (Hunt's) | 4.25 oz | 180 | 0 |
| Butterscotch Snack Pack (Hunt's) | 4.25 oz | 180 | 0 |
| Butterscotch Sugar Free (Diamond Crystal) | ½ cup | 80 | 3 |
| Chocolate Marshmallow Snack Pack (Hunt's) | 4.25 oz | 170 | 0 |
| Chocolate Snack Pack (Hunt's) | 4.25 oz | 180 | 0 |
| Chocolate Fudge Snack Pack (Hunt's) | 4.25 oz | 170 | 0 |
| Chocolate Sugar Free (Diamond Crystal) | ½ cup | 70 | 3 |
| German Chocolate Snack Pack (Hunt's) | 4.25 oz | 190 | 0 |
| Lemon Snack Pack (Hunt's) | 4.25 oz | 150 | 0 |
| Rice Snack Pack (Hunt's) | 4.25 oz | 190 | 0 |
| Tapicoa Snack Pack (Hunt's) | 4.25 oz | 120 | 0 |
| Vanilla Snack Pack (Hunt's) | 4.25 | 180 | 0 |
| Vanilla Sugar Free (Diamond Crystal) | ½ cup | 80 | 3 |

| FOOD | PORTION | CALORIES | CHOLESTEROL |
|------|---------|----------|-------------|

# PUDDING POPS
(*see also* ICE CREAM AND FROZEN DESSERTS, PUDDING)

| FOOD | PORTION | CALORIES | CHOLESTEROL |
|------|---------|----------|-------------|
| Chocolate Covered Chocolate Pudding Pops (Jell-O) | 1 pop | 130 | 2 |
| Chocolate Covered Vanilla Pudding Pops (Jell-O) | 1 pop | 130 | 2 |
| Chocolate Fudge Pudding Pops (Jell-O) | 1 pop | 73 | 1 |
| Chocolate Pudding Pops (Jell-O) | 1 pop | 80 | tr |
| Chocolate w/ Chocolate Chips Pudding Pops (Jell-O) | 1 pop | 82 | tr |
| Chocolate/Caramel Swirl Pudding Pops (Jell-O) | 1 pop | 78 | tr |
| Chocolate/Vanilla Swirl Pudding Pops (Jell-O) | 1 pop | 77 | tr |
| Double Chocolate Swirl Pudding Pops (Jell-O) | 1 pop | 74 | 1 |
| Milk Chocolate Pudding Pops (Jell-O) | 1 pop | 75 | 1 |
| Vanilla Pudding Pops (Jell-O) | 1 pop | 75 | tr |
| Vanilla w/ Chocolate Chips (Jell-O) | 1 pop | 82 | 1 |

| FOOD | PORTION | CALORIES | CHOLESTEROL |
|---|---|---|---|
| **PUMPKIN** | | | |
| CANNED | | | |
| Pumpkin (Owatonna) | ½ cup | 40 | 0 |
| Solid Pack (Libby's) | 1 cup | 80 | 0 |
| pumpkin | ½ cup | 41 | 0 |
| FRESH | | | |
| cooked; mashed | ½ cup | 24 | 0 |
| flowers, raw | 1 | 0 | 0 |
| flowers; cooked | ½ cup | 10 | 0 |
| raw; cubed | ½ cup | 15 | 0 |
| SEEDS | | | |
| seeds, dried | 1 oz | 154 | 0 |
| seeds, whole; roasted | 1 oz | 127 | 0 |
| **PURSLANE** | | | |
| FRESH | | | |
| cooked | ½ cup | 10 | 0 |
| raw | 1 cup | 7 | 0 |
| **QUAHOGS** (see CLAM) | | | |
| **QUICHE** | | | |
| lorraine (home recipe) | ⅙ of 9" pie | 379 | 159 |
| **RABBIT** | | | |
| stewed | 3.5 oz | 216 | 65 |

| FOOD | PORTION | CALORIES | CHOLESTEROL |
|------|---------|----------|-------------|

## RADISH

| | | | |
|------|---------|----------|-------------|
| DRIED | | | |
| oriental | ½ cup | 157 | 0 |
| seeds, sprouted, raw | ½ cup | 8 | 0 |
| FRESH | | | |
| Chinese; cooked | ½ cup | 13 | 0 |
| daikon; cooked | ½ cup | 13 | 0 |
| oriental, raw; sliced | ½ cup | 8 | 0 |
| raw | 10 | 7 | 0 |
| white icicle, raw; sliced | ½ cup | 7 | 0 |

## RAISINS

| | | | |
|------|---------|----------|-------------|
| California Seedless (Cinderella) | ½ cup | 250 | 0 |
| Golden Raisins (Dole) | ½ cup | 260 | 0 |
| Raisins (Dole) | ½ cup | 260 | 0 |
| raisins | 1 cup | 434 | 0 |
| raisins, golden | 1 cup | 437 | 0 |
| HOME RECIPE | | | |
| raisin sauce | 2 Tbsp | 51 | 0 |

## RASPBERRIES

| | | | |
|------|---------|----------|-------------|
| CANNED | | | |
| whole in heavy syrup | ½ cup | 117 | 0 |
| FRESH | | | |
| raspberries | 1 cup | 61 | 0 |

| FOOD | PORTION | CALORIES | CHOLESTEROL |
|---|---|---|---|
| FROZEN | | | |
| Red Raspberries Whole in Lite Syrup (Birds Eye) | ½ cup | 99 | 0 |
| raspberries, sweetened | 1 cup | 256 | 0 |
| JUICE | | | |
| Pure & Light (Dole) | 6 oz | 87 | 0 |
| Red Raspberry (Smucker's) | 8 oz | 120 | 0 |

## RELISH

| | | | |
|---|---|---|---|
| Sandwich Spred (Hellman's) | 1 Tbsp | 55 | 5 |
| chow chow (home recipe) | 1 Tbsp | 8 | 0 |
| chutney apple cranberry (home recipe) | 1 Tbsp | 16 | 0 |
| cranberry orange | ½ cup | 246 | 0 |

## RHUBARB

| | | | |
|---|---|---|---|
| FRESH | | | |
| rhubarb | 1 cup | 26 | 0 |

## RICE
(*see also* RICE CAKES)

| | | | |
|---|---|---|---|
| BROWN | | | |
| Pritikin Pilaf Brown Rice | ½ cup | 90 | 0 |
| Pritikin Spanish Brown Rice | ½ cup | 100 | 0 |
| S&W Quick Natural Long Grain; cooked | 2 oz | 63 | 0 |

| FOOD | PORTION | CALORIES | CHOLESTEROL |
|---|---|---|---|
| bran | 1 oz | 80 | 0 |
| **FROZEN** | | | |
| Birds Eye French Style International Rice | ½ cup | 106 | 0 |
| Birds Eye Italian Style International Rice | ½ cup | 119 | 0 |
| Birds Eye Rice & Peas w/ Mushrooms | ⅔ cup | 108 | 0 |
| Birds Eye Spanish Style International Rice | ½ cup | 111 | 0 |
| Budget Gourmet Oriental Rice & Vegetables | 5.75 oz | 210 | 20 |
| Budget Gourmet Rice Pilaf w/ Green Beans | 5.5 oz | 240 | 10 |
| **HOME RECIPE** | | | |
| pilaf | ½ cup | 84 | 22 |
| spanish | ¾ cup | 363 | 35 |
| **MIX, DRY** | | | |
| Chun King Stir-Fry Entree | .25 oz | 20 | 0 |
| Fried Rice Seasoning Mix (Kikkoman) | 1 oz pkg | 91 | tr |
| **WHITE** | | | |
| Minute Rice Drumstick; as prep (General Foods) | ½ cup | 143 | 10 |
| Minute Rice Fried; as prep (General Foods) | ½ cup | 164 | 0 |
| Minute Rice Long Grain & Wild; as prep (General Foods) | ½ cup | 149 | 10 |

| FOOD | PORTION | CALORIES | CHOLESTEROL |
|------|---------|----------|-------------|
| Minute Rice Rib Roast; as prep (General Foods) | ½ cup | 152 | 10 |
| Minute Rice; as prep (General Foods) | ⅔ cup | 142 | 5 |
| S&W Long Grain; cooked | 2 oz | 61 | 0 |

## RICE CAKES

| | | | |
|------|---------|----------|-------------|
| 7 Grain Rice Cakes (Pritikin Foods) | 1 | 35 | 0 |
| Crispy Rice Cakes Sodium Free (Chico-San) | 1 | 35 | 0 |
| Crispy Rice Cakes Very Low Sodium (Chico-San) | 1 | 35 | 0 |
| Plain Rice Cakes (Pritikin Foods) | 1 | 35 | 0 |
| Sesami Rice Cakes (Pritikin Foods) | 1 | 35 | 0 |

## ROCKFISH

FRESH
| Pacific, raw | 1 fillet (6.7 oz) | 180 | 66 |
|------|---------|----------|-------------|
| Pacific, raw | 3 oz | 80 | 29 |
| Pacific; cooked | 3 oz | 103 | 38 |
| Pacific; cooked | 1 fillet (5.2 oz) | 180 | 66 |

| FOOD | PORTION | CALORIES | CHOLESTEROL |
|------|---------|----------|-------------|

## ROE
(*see also individual fish names*)

FRESH
| | | | |
|------|---------|----------|-------------|
| raw | 1 oz | 39 | 105 |
| raw | 3 oz | 119 | 318 |

## ROLL
(*see also* BISCUIT, CROISSANT, ENGLISH MUFFIN, MUFFIN, POPOVER, SCONE)

| | | | |
|------|---------|----------|-------------|
| **HOME RECIPE** | | | |
| sweet roll | 1 (1.8 oz) | 143 | 18 |
| **READY-TO-EAT** | | | |
| Dark Bread (Hollywood) | 1 | 40 | 0 |
| Dinner (Roman Meal) | 1 | 45 | 0 |
| Hamburger Bun (Roman Meal) | 1 | 113 | 0 |
| Hamburger Bun (Shop 'n Save) | 1 | 120 | 0 |
| Hotdog Bun (Roman Meal) | 1 | 104 | 0 |
| Light Pan Dinner Rolls Special Formula (Hollywood) | 1 | 60 | 0 |
| Light Sliced Rolls Special Formula (Hollywood) | 1 | 80 | 0 |
| Potato Rolls (Martin's) | 1 | 130 | 0 |

| FOOD | PORTION | CALORIES | CHOLESTEROL |
|---|---|---|---|

## ROUGHY

| | | | |
|---|---|---|---|
| FRESH | | | |
| orange, raw | 3 oz | 107 | 17 |

## RUTABAGA

| | | | |
|---|---|---|---|
| FRESH | | | |
| cooked; mashed | ½ cup | 41 | 0 |
| raw; cubed | ½ cup | 25 | 0 |

## SABLEFISH

| | | | |
|---|---|---|---|
| FRESH | | | |
| raw | 3 oz | 166 | 42 |
| raw | ½ fillet (6.8 oz) | 377 | 95 |
| SMOKED | | | |
| sablefish | 1 oz | 72 | 18 |
| sablefish | 3 oz | 218 | 55 |

## SALAD
(see also PASTA SALAD)

| | | | |
|---|---|---|---|
| HOME RECIPE | | | |
| chef | 1½ cups | 386 | 244 |
| coleslaw | ½ cup | 59 | 0 |
| popeye | ½ cup | 204 | 75 |
| taco salad | 1 cup | 292 | 71 |
| tossed | 1 cup | 32 | 0 |
| waldorf | ½ cup | 79 | 8 |

| FOOD | PORTION | CALORIES | CHOLESTEROL |
|------|---------|----------|-------------|

## SALAD DRESSING

Salad dressings contain very small amounts of cholesterol in a one tablespoon portion. Some manufacturers' laboratory analysis information on cholesterol consider amounts less than 5 mg in a serving as either none or trace (tr). If you use portions larger than shown below, you may be getting a few milligrams of cholesterol.

| FOOD | PORTION | CALORIES | CHOLESTEROL |
|------|---------|----------|-------------|
| HOME RECIPE | | | |
| french | 2 Tbsp | 177 | 0 |
| vinegar & oil | 1 Tbsp | 72 | 0 |
| vinegar & oil | 2 Tbsp | 140 | 0 |
| MIXES | | | |
| Bleu Cheese & Herbs (Good Seasons) | 1 pkg | 4 | tr |
| Bleu Cheese & Herbs; as prep (Good Seasons) | 1 Tbsp | 72 | tr |
| Buttermilk Farm Style; as prep (Good Seasons) | 1 Tbsp | 58 | 5 |
| Cheese Garlic; as prep (Good Seasons) | 1 Tbsp | 72 | tr |
| Cheese Italian; as prep (Good Seasons) | 1 Tbsp | 72 | tr |
| Classic Herb; as prep (Good Seasons) | 1 Tbsp | 83 | 0 |
| Garlic & Herbs; as prep (Good Seasons) | 1 Tbsp | 84 | 0 |
| Italian Lite; as prep (Good Seasons) | 1 Tbsp | 27 | 0 |
| Italian Mild; as prep (Good Seasons) | 1 Tbsp | 73 | 0 |
| Italian No Oil; as prep (Good Seasons) | 1 Tbsp | 7 | 0 |

| FOOD | PORTION | CALORIES | CHOLESTEROL |
|---|---|---|---|
| Italian; as prep (Good Seasons) | 1 Tbsp | 71 | 0 |
| Lemon & Herbs; as prep (Good Seasons) | 1 Tbsp | 83 | 0 |
| Zesty Italian Lite; as prep (Good Seasons) | 1 Tbsp | 31 | 0 |
| Zesty Italian; as prep (Good Seasons) | 1 Tbsp | 71 | 0 |
| READY-TO-USE Bacon & Buttermilk (Kraft) | 1 Tbsp | 80 | 0 |
| Bacon & Tomato (Kraft) | 1 Tbsp | 70 | 0 |
| Blue Cheese (Diamond Crystal) | 1 Tbsp | 20 | 5 |
| Blue Cheese (Roka Brand) | 1 Tbsp | 60 | 10 |
| Blue Cheese Chunky (Kraft) | 1 Tbsp | 70 | 0 |
| Blue Cheese Lite (Wish-Bone) | 1 Tbsp | 38 | tr |
| Buttermilk Creamy (Kraft) | 1 Tbsp | 80 | 5 |
| Buttermilk & Chives Creamy (Kraft) | 1 Tbsp | 80 | 5 |
| Buttermilk Lite (Wish-Bone) | 1 Tbsp | 53 | 1 |
| Caesar Golden (Kraft) | 1 Tbsp | 70 | 0 |
| Ceasar (Wish-Bone) | 1 Tbsp | 78 | 1 |

| FOOD | PORTION | CALORIES | CHOLESTEROL |
|------|---------|----------|-------------|
| Coleslaw (Kraft) | 1 Tbsp | 70 | 10 |
| Creamy Italian (Pritikin Foods) | 1 Tbsp | 12 | 0 |
| Cucumber Creamy (Kraft) | 1 Tbsp | 70 | 0 |
| Dijon Classic Creamy (Wish-Bone) | 1 Tbsp | 62 | 4 |
| Dijon Classic Vinaigrette (Wish-Bone) | 1 Tbsp | 61 | tr |
| Famous Chef Style (Ott's) | 1 Tbsp | 40 | tr |
| French (Catalina) | 1 Tbsp | 70 | 0 |
| French (Kraft) | 1 Tbsp | 60 | 0 |
| French (Pritikin Foods) | 1 Tbsp | 10 | 0 |
| French Deluxe (Wish-Bone) | 1 Tbsp | 59 | 0 |
| French Lite (Wish-Bone) | 1 Tbsp | 31 | 0 |
| Garlic Creamy (Kraft) | 1 Tbsp | 50 | 10 |
| Garlic Creamy (Wish-Bone) | 1 Tbsp | 74 | 0 |
| Garlic French (Wish-Bone) | 1 Tbsp | 56 | 0 |
| Home Style (Diamond Crystal) | 1 Tbsp | 20 | 5 |
| Italian (Presto) | 1 Tbsp | 70 | 0 |

| FOOD | PORTION | CALORIES | CHOLESTEROL |
|---|---|---|---|
| Italian<br>(Pritikin Foods) | 1 Tbsp | 6 | 0 |
| Italian Chef Style<br>(Ott's) | 1 Tbsp | 80 | tr |
| Italian Creamy<br>(Wish-Bone) | 1 Tbsp | 56 | tr |
| Italian Creamy w/ Real Sour<br>Cream<br>(Kraft) | 1 Tbsp | 60 | 0 |
| Italian Herbal Classics<br>(Wish-Bone) | 1 Tbsp | 70 | 0 |
| Italian Oil-Free<br>(Kraft) | 1 Tbsp | 4 | 0 |
| Italian Robusto<br>(Wish-Bone) | 1 Tbsp | 70 | 0 |
| Oil & Vinegar<br>(Kraft) | 1 Tbsp | 70 | 0 |
| Onion & Chive<br>(Wish-Bone) | 1 Tbsp | 37 | 0 |
| Onion & Chives Creamy<br>(Kraft) | 1 Tbsp | 70 | 0 |
| Ranch<br>(Pritikin Foods) | 1 Tbsp | 18 | 0 |
| Ranch Lite<br>(Wish-Bone) | 1 Tbsp | 42 | 0 |
| Rancher's Choice Creamy<br>(Kraft) | 1 Tbsp | 80 | 5 |
| Red Wine Vinaigrette<br>(Wish-Bone) | 1 Tbsp. | 50 | 0 |
| Red Wine Vinegar & Oil<br>(Kraft) | 1 Tbsp | 50 | 0 |

| FOOD | PORTION | CALORIES | CHOLESTEROL |
|------|---------|----------|-------------|
| Romano & Parmesan Creamy (Wish-Bone) | 1 Tbsp | 89 | 6 |
| Russian (Kraft) | 1 Tbsp | 60 | 0 |
| Russian (Pritikin Foods) | 1 Tbsp | 12 | 0 |
| Russian (Wish-Bone) | 1 Tbsp | 47 | 0 |
| Russian Lite (Wish-Bone) | 1 Tbsp | 22 | 0 |
| Thousand Island & Bacon (Kraft) | 1 Tbsp | 60 | 0 |
| Thousand Island (Diamond Crystal) | 1 Tbsp | 20 | 5 |
| Thousand Island (Kraft) | 1 Tbsp | 60 | 5 |
| Thousand Island (Wish-Bone) | 1 Tbsp | 69 | 4 |
| Thousand Island Lite (Wish-Bone) | 1 Tbsp | 40 | 9 |
| Vinaigrette (Pritikin Foods) | 1 Tbsp | 10 | 0 |
| Zesty Italian (Kraft) | 1 Tbsp | 70 | 0 |
| Zesty Tomato (Pritikin Foods) | 1 Tbsp | 18 | 0 |

READY-TO-USE REDUCED CALORIE

| FOOD | PORTION | CALORIES | CHOLESTEROL |
|------|---------|----------|-------------|
| Bacon & Tomato Reduced Calorie (Kraft) | 1 Tbsp | 30 | 0 |

| FOOD | PORTION | CALORIES | CHOLESTEROL |
|---|---|---|---|
| Bacon Creamy Reduced Calorie (Kraft) | 1 Tbsp | 30 | 0 |
| Bacon & Tomato (Estee) | 1 Tbsp | 8 | 3 |
| Bleu Cheese (Walden Farms) | 1 Tbsp | 27 | 5 |
| Bleu Cheese Natural (Magic Mountain) | 1 Tbsp | 5 | tr |
| Blue Cheese (Estee) | 1 Tbsp | 8 | 10 |
| Blue Cheese Chunky Reduced Calorie (Kraft) | 1 Tbsp | 30 | 0 |
| Blue Cheese Reduced Calorie (Roka Brand) | 1 Tbsp | 14 | 5 |
| Buttermilk Creamy (Estee) | 1 Tbsp | 6 | 5 |
| Buttermilk Creamy Reduced Calorie (Kraft) | 1 Tbsp | 30 | 0 |
| Creamy Italian w/ Parmesan (Walden Farms) | 1 Tbsp | 35 | 4 |
| Cucumber Creamy Reduced Calorie (Kraft) | 1 Tbsp | 30 | 0 |
| Dijon Creamy (Estee) | 1 Tbsp | 8 | 30 |
| French (Walden Farms) | 1 Tbsp | 33 | 2 |
| French Reduced Calorie (Kraft) | 1 Tbsp | 25 | 0 |

| FOOD | PORTION | CALORIES | CHOLESTEROL |
|---|---|---|---|
| French Style Natural (Magic Mountain) | 1 Tbsp | 4 | 0 |
| Garlic Creamy w/ Red Wine Vinegar (Estee) | 1 Tbsp | 2 | 0 |
| Herb & Spice No Oil (Magic Mountain) | 1 Tbsp | 2 | 0 |
| Italian (Walden Farms) | 1 Tbsp | 9 | 0 |
| Italian Creamy (Estee) | 1 Tbsp | 4 | 5 |
| Italian Creamy Reduced Calorie (Kraft) | 1 Tbsp | 25 | 0 |
| Italian French (Estee) | 1 Tbsp | 4 | 5 |
| Italian No Sugar Added (Walden Farms) | 1 Tbsp | 6 | 0 |
| Italian Reduced Calorie (Kraft) | 1 Tbsp | 6 | 0 |
| Italian Sodium Free (Walden Farms) | 1 Tbsp | 9 | 0 |
| Northern Italian Natural (Magic Mountain) | 1 Tbsp | 2 | 0 |
| Ranch (Walden Farms) | 1 Tbsp | 35 | 8 |
| Rancher's Choice Creamy Reduced Calorie (Kraft) | 1 Tbsp | 30 | 5 |
| Reduced Calorie (Catalina) | 1 Tbsp | 16 | 0 |
| Russian Reduced Calorie (Kraft) | 1 Tbsp | 30 | 0 |

| FOOD | PORTION | CALORIES | CHOLESTEROL |
|---|---|---|---|
| Thousand Island (Estee) | 1 Tbsp | 6 | 5 |
| Thousand Island (Walden Farms) | 1 Tbsp | 24 | 8 |
| Thousand Island Reduced Calorie (Kraft) | 1 Tbsp | 30 | 5 |
| French | 1 Tbsp | 22 | 1 |
| Italian | 1 Tbsp | 16 | 1 |
| Russian | 1 Tbsp | 23 | 1 |
| Thousand Island | 1 Tbsp | 24 | 2 |

## SALMON

| FOOD | PORTION | CALORIES | CHOLESTEROL |
|---|---|---|---|
| CANNED | | | |
| Pink (Bumble Bee) | 3 oz | 137 | 45 |
| Pink Skinless (Bumble Bee) | 3.25 oz | 120 | 45 |
| Red (Bumble Bee) | 3 oz | 154 | 56 |
| chum w/ bone | 3 oz | 120 | 33 |
| chum w/ bone | 1 can (13.9 oz) | 521 | 144 |
| sockeye w/ bone | 3 oz | 130 | 37 |
| sockeye w/ bone | 1 can (12.9 oz) | 566 | 161 |
| FRESH | | | |
| Salmon Steak (Health Valley) | 3.5 oz | 220 | 0 |
| atlantic, raw | 3 oz | 121 | 47 |

| FOOD | PORTION | CALORIES | CHOLESTEROL |
|------|---------|----------|-------------|
| atlantic, raw | ½ fillet (6.9 oz) | 281 | 109 |
| chinook, raw | ½ fillet (6.9 oz) | 356 | 131 |
| chinook, raw | 3 oz | 153 | 56 |
| chum, raw | 3 oz | 102 | 63 |
| chum, raw | ½ fillet (6.9 oz) | 237 | 147 |
| coho, raw | ½ fillet (6.9 oz) | 289 | 77 |
| coho, raw | 3 oz | 124 | 33 |
| coho; cooked | 3 oz | 157 | 42 |
| coho; cooked | ½ fillet (5.4 oz) | 286 | 76 |
| pink, raw | ½ fillet (5.6 oz) | 185 | 83 |
| pink, raw | 3 oz | 99 | 44 |
| sockeye, raw | ½ fillet (6.9 oz) | 333 | 123 |
| sockeye, raw | 3 oz | 143 | 53 |
| sockeye; cooked | 3 oz | 183 | 74 |
| sockeye; cooked | ½ fillet (5.4 oz) | 334 | 135 |
| **HOME RECIPE** | | | |
| salmon cake | 3.4 oz | 241 | 104 |
| salmon casserole | ¾ cup | 416 | 91 |
| salmon rice loaf | 6.2 oz | 299 | 133 |
| **SMOKED** | | | |
| chinook | 1 oz | 33 | 7 |
| chinook | 3 oz | 99 | 20 |

| FOOD | PORTION | CALORIES | CHOLESTEROL |
|---|---|---|---|

## SALSIFY

| FRESH | | | |
|---|---|---|---|
| cooked; sliced | ½ cup | 46 | 0 |
| raw; sliced | ½ cup | 55 | 0 |

## SALT/SEASONED SALT
### (see also SALT SUBSTITUTE)

| Garlic Salt (Morton) | 1 tsp | 3 | 0 |
|---|---|---|---|
| Kosher Salt (Morton) | 1 tsp | 0 | 0 |
| Lite Salt Mixture (Morton) | 1 tsp | tr | 0 |
| Nature's Seasons Seasoning Blend (Morton) | 1 tsp | 3 | 0 |
| Salt Iodized (Morton) | 1 tsp | tr | 0 |
| Salt Non-Iodized (Morton) | 1 tsp | 0 | 0 |
| Seasoned Salt (Morton) | 1 tsp | 4 | 0 |

## SALT SUBSTITUTE

| Nu-Salt | 1 pkg (1 g) | 0 | 0 |
|---|---|---|---|
| Salt-It Salt Substitute (Estee) | ½ tsp | 0 | 0 |
| Salt Substitute (Morton) | 1 tsp | tr | 0 |
| Seasoned Salt Substitute (Morton) | 1 tsp | 2 | 0 |

| FOOD | PORTION | CALORIES | CHOLESTEROL |
|------|---------|----------|-------------|

# SAPODILLA

FRESH
| sapodilla | 1 | 140 | 0 |

# SARDINE

CANNED
| Atlantic in oil w/ bone | 1 can (3.2 oz) | 192 | 131 |
| Atlantic in oil w/ bone | 2 oz | 50 | 34 |
| Pacfic in brine & mustard | 1 large (.7 oz) | 39 | 24 |
| Pacific w/ tomato sauce w/ bone | 1 can (13 oz) | 658 | 225 |
| Pacific w/ tomato sauce w/ bone | 1 oz | 68 | 23 |

# SAUCE
(*see also* GRAVY, PIZZA, SPAGHETTI SAUCE, TOMATO)

DRY
| Bar-B-Q Sauce Mix (Diamond Crystal) | 2 oz | 35 | tr |
| Brown Sauce Mix (Diamond Crystal) | 2 oz | 15 | 2 |
| Cheese Sauce Mix (Diamond Crystal) | 2 oz | 50 | 2 |
| Cream Sauce Mix (Diamond Crystal) | 2 oz | 40 | 3 |
| Italian Sauce Mix (Diamond Crystal) | 3 oz | 50 | 0 |

| FOOD | PORTION | CALORIES | CHOLESTEROL |
|---|---|---|---|
| Marinade for Meat (Kikkoman) | 1 oz pkg | 64 | 0 |
| Sweet & Sour Sauce Mix (Kikkoman) | 2⅛ oz pkg | 228 | 0 |
| Sweet 'n Sour Entree Mix (Chun King) | 3.8 oz | 370 | 0 |
| Teriyaki Sauce Mix (Kikkoman) | 1½ oz pkg | 125 | 0 |
| bearnaise; as prep w/ milk & butter | 1 cup | 701 | 189 |
| bearnaise; not prep | 1 pkg (9 oz) | 90 | tr |
| cheese; as prep w/ milk | 1 cup | 307 | 53 |
| cheese; not prep | 1 pkg (1.2 oz) | 158 | 18 |
| curry; as prep w/ milk | 1 cup | 270 | 35 |
| curry; not prep | 1 pkg (1.2 oz) | 151 | tr |
| hollandaise w/ butterfat; as prep w/ water | 1 cup | 237 | 51 |
| hollandaise w/ butterfat; not prep | 1 pkg (1.2 oz) | 187 | 40 |
| hollandaise w/ oil; as prep w/ water | 1 cup | 703 | 189 |
| hollandaise w/ oil; not prep | 1 pkg (.9 oz) | 93 | tr |
| mushroom; as prep w/ milk | 1 cup | 228 | 34 |
| mushroom; not prep | 1 pkg (1 oz) | 99 | 0 |
| sour cream; as prep w/ milk | 1 cup | 509 | 91 |
| sour cream; not prep | 1 pkg (1.2 oz) | 180 | 28 |

| FOOD | PORTION | CALORIES | CHOLESTEROL |
|---|---|---|---|
| stroganoff; as prep w/ milk & water | 1 cup | 271 | 38 |
| stroganoff; not prep | 1 pkg (1.6 oz) | 161 | 12 |
| sweet & sour; as prep w/ water & vinegar | 1 cup | 294 | 0 |
| sweet & sour; not prep | 1 pkg (2 oz) | 220 | 0 |
| teriyaki; as prep w/ water | 1 cup | 131 | 0 |
| teriyaki; not prep | 1 pkg (1.6 oz) | 130 | 0 |
| white; as prep w/ milk | 1 cup | 241 | 34 |
| white; not prep | 1 pkg (1.7 oz) | 230 | tr |
| **HOME RECEIPE** hollandaise | 2 Tbsp | 130 | 16 |
| **JARRED** A-1 Steak Sauce (Heublein) | 1 Tbsp | 14 | 0 |
| Barbecue (Maull's) | 3.5 oz | 123 | 1 |
| Barbecue Beer Flavor, Non-Alcoholic (Maull's) | 3.5 oz | 128 | 1 |
| Barbecue Sauce (Estee) | 1 Tbsp | 18 | 0 |
| Barbecue Sauce (Kraft) | 2 Tbsp | 40 | 0 |
| Barbecue Sauce (Ott's) | 1 Tbsp | 14 | tr |

| FOOD | PORTION | CALORIES | CHOLESTEROL |
|---|---|---|---|
| Barbecue Sauce Garlic Flavored (Kraft) | 2 Tbsp | 40 | 0 |
| Barbecue Sauce Hickory Smoke (Open Pit) | 1 Tbsp | 25 | 0 |
| Barbecue Sauce Hickory Smoke Flavor (Kraft) | 2 Tbsp | 40 | 0 |
| Barbecue Sauce Hickory Smoke Flavored Onion Bits (Kraft) | 2 Tbsp | 50 | 0 |
| Barbecue Sauce Hot (Kraft) | 2 Tbsp | 40 | 0 |
| Barbecue Sauce Hot Hickory Smoke Flavored (Kraft) | 2 Tbsp | 40 | 0 |
| Barbecue Sauce Italian Seasoning (Kraft) | 2 Tbsp | 45 | 0 |
| Barbecue Sauce Kansas City Style (Kraft) | 2 Tbsp | 45 | 0 |
| Barbecue Sauce Mesquite Smoke (Kraft) | 2 Tbsp | 45 | 0 |
| Barbecue Sauce Onion Bits (Kraft) | 2 Tbsp | 50 | 0 |
| Barbecue Sauce Original (Bull's Eye) | 2 Tbsp | 50 | 0 |
| Barbecue Sauce Smoky (Ott's) | 1 Tbsp | 14 | tr |

| FOOD | PORTION | CALORIES | CHOLESTEROL |
|---|---|---|---|
| Barbecue Sauce Thick 'n Tangy Hickory (Open Pit) | 1 Tbsp | 25 | 0 |
| Barbecue Sauce Thick'n Spicy Chunky (Kraft) | 2 Tbsp | 50 | 0 |
| Barbecue Sauce Thick'n Spicy Hickory Smoked (Kraft) | 2 Tbsp | 50 | 0 |
| Barbecue Sauce Thick'n Spicy Kansas City Style (Kraft) | 2 Tbsp | 60 | 0 |
| Barbecue Sauce Thick'n Spicy Original (Kraft) | 2 Tbsp | 50 | 0 |
| Barbecue Sauce Thick'n Spicy w/ Honey (Kraft) | 2 Tbsp | 60 | 0 |
| Barbecue Smoky (Maull's) | 3.5 oz | 124 | 1 |
| Barbecue Sweet-N-Mild (Maull's) | 3.5 oz | 167 | 1 |
| Barbecue Sweet-N-Smoky (Maull's) | 3.5 oz | 160 | 1 |
| Barbecue w/ Onion Bits (Maull's) | 3.5 oz | 126 | 1 |
| Cocktail (Sauceworks) | 1 Tbsp | 12 | 0 |
| Cocktail Sauce (Estee) | 1 Tbsp | 10 | 0 |
| Rib Sauce (Gold's) | 1 oz | 60 | 0 |

| FOOD | PORTION | CALORIES | CHOLESTEROL |
|------|---------|----------|-------------|
| Steak Sauce (Estee) | ½ oz | 15 | 0 |
| Stir-Fry Sauce (Kikkoman) | 1 tsp | 6 | 0 |
| Sweet & Sour Sauce (Kikkoman) | 1 Tbsp | 18 | 0 |
| Sweet 'N Sour (Sauceworks) | 1 Tbsp | 20 | 0 |
| Sweet 'n Sour (Contadina) | ½ cup | 150 | 0 |
| Tartar Sauce (Best Foods) | 1 Tbsp | 70 | 5 |
| Tartar Sauce (Bright Day) | 1 Tbsp | 50 | 0 |
| Tartar Sauce (Hellman's) | 1 Tbsp | 70 | 5 |
| Tartar Sauce (Kraft) | 1 Tbsp | 70 | 5 |
| Tartar Sauce (Sauceworks) | 1 Tbsp | 70 | 5 |
| Tartar Sauce Natural Lemon & Herb Flavor (Sauceworks) | 1 Tbsp | 70 | 5 |
| Teriyaki Sauce (Kikkoman) | 1 Tbsp | 15 | tr |
| Tobasco (McIlhenny) | ¼ tsp | tr | 0 |
| Worchestershire (Lea & Perrins) | 1 Tbsp | 59 | 0 |
| barbecue | 1 cup | 188 | 0 |
| teriyaki | 1 Tbsp | 15 | 0 |
| teriyaki | 1 oz | 30 | 0 |

| FOOD | PORTION | CALORIES | CHOLESTEROL |
|------|---------|----------|-------------|

## SAUERKRAUT

| FOOD | PORTION | CALORIES | CHOLESTEROL |
|------|---------|----------|-------------|
| **CANNED** | | | |
| Sauerkraut (Claussen) | ½ cup | 17 | 0 |
| Sauerkraut (Libby) | ½ cup | 20 | 0 |
| Sauerkraut (Seneca) | ½ cup | 20 | 0 |
| canned | ½ cup | 22 | 0 |
| **JUICE** | | | |
| Sauerkraut Juice (S&W) | 5 oz | 14 | 0 |

## SAUSAGE
(*see also* HOT DOG, SAUSAGE SUBSTITUTE)

| FOOD | PORTION | CALORIES | CHOLESTEROL |
|------|---------|----------|-------------|
| Breakfast Sausage, Turkey (Bil Mar Foods) | 1 oz | 58 | 16 |
| Knockwurst (Health Valley) | 3.5 oz | 280 | 56 |
| Knockwurst (Hebrew National) | 1 (3 oz) | 260 | 26 |
| Oscar Mayer Bratwurst Smoked | 1 (2.7 oz) | 237 | 40 |
| Oscar Mayer Italian Smoked Cooked Cured | 1 (2.6 oz) | 264 | 39 |
| Oscar Mayer Kielbasa | 1 oz | 83 | 14 |
| Oscar Mayer Little Friers Pork; cooked | 1 (.7 oz) | 82 | 17 |
| Oscar Mayer Polish | 1 (2.7 oz) | 229 | 31 |
| Oscar Mayer Smoked | 1 oz | 83 | 15 |

| FOOD | PORTION | CALORIES | CHOLESTEROL |
|---|---|---|---|
| Oscar Mayer Smokies, Beef | 1 (1.5 oz) | 123 | 27 |
| Oscar Mayer Smokies, Cheese | 1 (1.5 oz) | 127 | 29 |
| Oscar Mayer Smokies Links | 1 (1.5 oz) | 124 | 28 |
| Oscar Mayer Smokies, Little | 1 (.3 oz) | 28 | 6 |
| Polish Kielbasa (Mr. Turkey) | 3 oz | 177 | 44 |
| Pork Breakfast Patties (Jones) | 1 (2 oz) | 136 | 42 |
| Pork Brown & Serve Links (Jones) | 1 (.8 oz) | 55 | 17 |
| Pork Brown & Serve Patties (Jones) | 1 (2 oz) | 136 | 42 |
| Pork, Light Breakfast Links (Jones) | 1 (.8 oz) | 55 | 17 |
| Pork, Light Breakfast Links (Jones) | 1 (2 oz) | 136 | 42 |
| Smoked Sausage (Bil Mar Foods) | 3 oz | 142 | 57 |
| bratwurst, pork; cooked | 1 link (85 g) | 256 | 51 |
| bratwurst, pork; cooked | 1 oz | 85 | 17 |
| bratwurst, pork & beef | 1 link (70 g) | 226 | 44 |
| bratwurst, pork & beef | 1 oz | 92 | 18 |
| country-style, pork; cooked | 1 patty (1 oz) | 100 | 22 |
| country-style, pork; cooked | 1 link (½ oz) | 48 | 11 |
| Italian, pork, raw | 1 link (2.3 oz) | 315 | 69 |

| FOOD | PORTION | CALORIES | CHOLESTEROL |
|---|---|---|---|
| Italian, pork, raw | 1 link (4 oz) | 391 | 86 |
| Italian, pork; cooked | 1 link (67 g) | 216 | 52 |
| Italian, pork; cooked | 1 link (83 g) | 268 | 65 |
| kielbasa | 1 oz | 88 | 19 |
| kielbasa, pork | 1 slice (26 g) | 81 | 17 |
| knockwurst, pork & beef | 1 link (68 g) | 209 | 39 |
| knockwurst, pork & beef | 1 oz | 87 | 16 |
| Polish, pork | 1 link (8 oz) | 739 | 158 |
| Polish, pork | 1 oz | 92 | 20 |
| pork, country-style, raw | 1 patty (2 oz) | 238 | 39 |
| pork, country-style, raw | 1 link (1 oz) | 118 | 19 |
| pork, raw | 1 patty (2 oz) | 238 | 39 |
| pork, raw | 1 link (1 oz) | 118 | 19 |
| pork; cooked | 1 patty (1 oz) | 100 | 22 |
| pork; cooked | 1 link (½ oz) | 48 | 11 |
| smoked, beef; cooked | 1 sausage (1.4 oz) | 134 | 29 |
| smoked, pork | 1 link (2⅓ oz) | 256 | 46 |

| FOOD | PORTION | CALORIES | CHOLESTEROL |
|------|---------|----------|-------------|
| smoked, pork | 1 sm link (½ oz) | 62 | 11 |
| smoked, pork & beef | 1 link (2⅓ oz) | 229 | 48 |
| smoked, pork & beef | 1 sm link (½ oz) | 54 | 11 |
| Vienna, canned, beef & pork | 1 sausage (½ oz) | 45 | 8 |

## SAUSAGE SUBSTITUTE

| FOOD | PORTION | CALORIES | CHOLESTEROL |
|------|---------|----------|-------------|
| Grillers, frzn (Morningstar Farms) | 3.5 oz | 290 | 2 |
| Linketts (Loma Linda) | 2 (2.6 oz) | 150 | 0 |
| Links, frzn (Morningstar Farms) | 3.5 oz | 237 | 1 |
| Little Links (Loma Linda) | 2 (1.6 oz) | 80 | 0 |

## SCALLOP

| FOOD | PORTION | CALORIES | CHOLESTEROL |
|------|---------|----------|-------------|
| **FRESH** | | | |
| raw | 3 oz | 75 | 28 |
| raw | 2 lg | 26 | 10 |
| raw | 5 sm | 26 | 10 |
| **FROZEN** | | | |
| Lightly Breaded Scallops (King & Prince) | 3.5 oz | 120 | 14 |
| **HOME RECIPE** | | | |
| breaded & fried | 2 lg | 67 | 19 |

| FOOD | PORTION | CALORIES | CHOLESTEROL |
|------|---------|----------|-------------|

## SCONE

HOME RECIPE

| apricot scone | 1 | 232 | 34 |
|------|---------|----------|-------------|
| scone | 1 (1.4 oz) | 130 | 56 |

## SCROD

FROZEN

| Ready-to-Bake Scrod (King & Prince) | 5 oz | 252 | 32 |
|------|---------|----------|-------------|
| Ready-to-Bake Scrod (King & Prince) | 8 oz | 403 | 52 |

## SEA BASS
(*see* BASS)

## SEATROUT
(*see* TROUT)

## SEASONING

| Herb Seasoning (American Heart Association) | ¼ tsp | tr | 0 |
|------|---------|----------|-------------|
| Instead of Salt All Purpose (Health Valley) | ¾ tsp | 11 | 0 |
| Instead of Salt Chicken (Health Valley) | ¾ tsp | 8 | 0 |
| Instead of Salt Fish (Health Valley) | ¾ tsp | 11 | 0 |
| Instead of Salt Steak & Hamburger (Health Valley) | ½ tsp | 6 | 0 |

| FOOD | PORTION | CALORIES | CHOLESTEROL |
|------|---------|----------|-------------|
| Instead of Salt Vegetable (Health Valley) | 1 tsp | 13 | 0 |
| Lemon Herb Seasoning (American Heart Association) | ¼ tsp | tr | 0 |
| Original Herb Seasoning (American Heart Association) | ¼ tsp | tr | 0 |
| Savorex (Loma Linda) | 1 tsp | 16 | 0 |

## SEEDS
(*see individual names*)

## SESAME

| | | | |
|------|---------|----------|-------------|
| Sesame Nut Mix Oil Roasted (Planters) | 1 oz | 160 | 0 |
| Sesame Nut Mix Dry Roasted (Planters) | 1 oz | 160 | 0 |
| seeds | 1 tsp | 16 | 0 |
| seeds, dried | 1 Tbsp | 52 | 0 |
| seeds, dried | 1 cup | 825 | 0 |
| seeds, roasted & toasted | 1 oz | 161 | 0 |
| sesame butter | 1 Tbsp | 95 | 0 |
| tahini, from roasted & toasted kernels | 1 Tbsp | 89 | 0 |
| tahini, from unroasted kernels | 1 Tbsp | 85 | 0 |

## SHAD

FRESH
| | | | |
|------|---------|----------|-------------|
| roe, raw | 3½ oz | 130 | 360 |

| FOOD | PORTION | CALORIES | CHOLESTEROL |
|---|---|---|---|
| **SHALLOT** | | | |
| DRIED | | | |
| freeze-dried | 1 Tbsp | 3 | 0 |
| FRESH | | | |
| chopped | 1 Tbsp | 7 | 0 |
| **SHARK** | | | |
| FRESH | | | |
| raw | 3 oz | 111 | 43 |
| HOME RECIPE | | | |
| batter-dipped & fried | 3 oz | 194 | 50 |

## SHELLFISH
(*see individual names*, SHELLFISH SUBSTITUTE)

## SHELLFISH SUBSTITUTE

| FOOD | PORTION | CALORIES | CHOLESTEROL |
|---|---|---|---|
| Crab Delights (Louis Kemp) | 2 oz | 60 | 10 |
| Kibun Sea Pasta w/ Shrimp w/ dressing | ½ pkg | 210 | 30 |
| Kibun Sea Pasta w/ Shrimp w/o dressing | ½ pkg | 140 | 30 |
| Kibun Sea Pasta w/ dressing | ½ pkg | 220 | 10 |
| Kibun Sea Pasta w/o dressing | ½ pkg | 110 | 10 |
| Kibun Sea Stix Salad Style | 4 oz | 110 | 20 |
| Kibun Sea Stix Whole Leg | 4 oz | 110 | 20 |
| Kibun Sea Tails | 4 oz | 110 | 15 |
| SeaLegs Imitation Lobster Meat | 3 oz | 80 | 10 |

| FOOD | PORTION | CALORIES | CHOLESTEROL |
|---|---|---|---|
| crab, imitation | 3 oz | 87 | 17 |
| scallop, imitation | 3 oz | 84 | 18 |
| shrimp, imitation | 3 oz | 86 | 31 |
| surimi | 1 oz | 28 | 8 |
| surimi | 3 oz | 84 | 25 |

## SHELLIE BEANS

| | | | |
|---|---|---|---|
| CANNED<br>shellie beans | ½ cup | 37 | 0 |

## SHRIMP

| | | | |
|---|---|---|---|
| CANNED | | | |
| canned | 1 cup | 154 | 222 |
| canned | 3 oz | 102 | 147 |
| FRESH | | | |
| cooked | 4 lg | 22 | 43 |
| cooked | 3 oz | 84 | 166 |
| raw | 3 oz | 90 | 130 |
| raw | 4 lg | 30 | 43 |
| FROZEN | | | |
| Cooked in the Shell<br>(King & Prince) | 4 oz | 70 | 91 |
| Cooked in the Shell<br>(King & Prince) | 3.5 oz | 65 | 77 |
| Gourmet Hand Breaded<br>Shrimp Butterfly<br>(King & Prince) | 3.5 oz | 150 | 56 |
| Gourmet Hand Breaded<br>Shrimp Round<br>(King & Prince) | 3.5 oz | 150 | 56 |

| FOOD | PORTION | CALORIES | CHOLESTEROL |
|------|---------|----------|-------------|
| Shrimp Del Ray (King & Prince) | 3 oz | 85 | 38 |
| Shrimp Del Ray (King & Prince) | 1.5 oz | 43 | 19 |
| Shrimp a la Monterey (King & Prince) | 3.5 oz | 190 | 65 |
| Shrimp a la Monterey (King & Prince) | 2 oz | 107 | 37 |
| Supreme Hand Breaded Shrimp Butterfly (King & Prince) | 3.5 oz | 130 | 55 |
| Supreme Hand Breaded Shrimp Round (King & Prince) | 3.5 oz | 140 | 65 |
| Western Style Breaded Shrimp (King & Prince) | 3.5 oz | 115 | 70 |
| HOME RECIPE | | | |
| jambalaya | ¾ cup | 188 | 50 |
| shrimp; breaded & fried | 3 oz | 206 | 150 |
| shrimp; breaded & fried | 4 lg | 73 | 53 |
| stew | 1 cup | 207 | 79 |
| READY-TO-USE | | | |
| Fried Shrimp (American Original Foods) | 4 oz | 253 | 27 |

## SMELT

| FOOD | PORTION | CALORIES | CHOLESTEROL |
|------|---------|----------|-------------|
| FRESH | | | |
| rainbow, raw | 3 oz | 83 | 60 |
| rainbow; cooked | 3 oz | 106 | 76 |

| FOOD | PORTION | CALORIES | CHOLESTEROL |
|---|---|---|---|

## SNACKS
(*see also* CHIPS; FRUIT SNACKS; NUTS, MIXED; POPCORN; PRETZELS)

| FOOD | PORTION | CALORIES | CHOLESTEROL |
|---|---|---|---|
| Cheddar Lites (Health Valley) | .2 oz | 40 | tr |
| Cheddar Lites w/ Green Onion (Health Valley) | .2 oz | 40 | 0 |
| Cheese Balls (Lance) | 1 pkg (1⅛ oz) | 190 | 5 |
| Cheese Balls (Lance) | 1 oz | 160 | 5 |
| Cheetos Crunchy Cheese Flavored | 1 oz | 160 | tr |
| Cheetos Puffed Balls Cheese Flavored | 1 oz | 160 | tr |
| Cheetos Puffs Cheese Flavored | 1 oz | 160 | tr |
| Cornnuts, Barbecue | 1 oz | 110 | 0 |
| Cornnuts, Nacho Cheese | 1 oz | 110 | 0 |
| Cornnuts, Original | 1 oz | 120 | 0 |
| Cornnuts, Unsalted | 1 oz | 120 | 0 |
| Crunchy Cheese Twists (Lance) | 1 pkg (1½ oz) | 230 | 0 |
| Crunchy Cheese Twists (Lance) | 1 oz | 150 | tr |
| Funyuns (Frito-Lay) | 1 oz | 140 | 0 |
| Gold-N-Chee (Lance) | 1⅜ oz | 180 | 5 |
| Gold-N-Chee (Lance) | 1 oz | 130 | 0 |
| Munchos | 1 oz | 150 | 0 |

| FOOD | PORTION | CALORIES | CHOLESTEROL |
|------|---------|----------|-------------|
| Pork Skins (Lance) | ½ oz | 80 | 20 |
| Pork Skins Regular (Lance) | ½ oz | 80 | 20 |
| Tostada Nacho (Lance) | 1 oz | 140 | tr |
| Tostada Regular (Lance) | 1 oz | 150 | 0 |
| Wheat Snax (Estee) | 1 oz | 110 | 0 |

## SNAIL
(see WHELK)

## SNAP BEANS

| | | | |
|------|---------|----------|-------------|
| CANNED | | | |
| seasoned | ½ cup | 18 | 0 |
| snap beans | ½ cup | 18 | 0 |
| FRESH | | | |
| cooked | ½ cup | 22 | 0 |
| raw | ½ cup | 17 | 0 |
| FROZEN | | | |
| snap beans | ½ cup | 18 | 0 |

## SNAPPER

| | | | |
|------|---------|----------|-------------|
| FRESH | | | |
| cooked | 1 fillet (6 oz) | 217 | 80 |
| cooked | 3 oz | 109 | 40 |

| FOOD | PORTION | CALORIES | CHOLESTEROL |
|---|---|---|---|
| raw | 3 oz | 85 | 31 |
| raw | 1 fillet (7.6 oz) | 217 | 81 |

## SODA
(*see also* DRINK MIXER)

| FOOD | PORTION | CALORIES | CHOLESTEROL |
|---|---|---|---|
| 7-Up | 1 oz | 12 | 0 |
| 7-Up Cherry | 1 oz | 13 | 0 |
| 7-Up Cherry Diet | 1 oz | tr | 0 |
| 7-Up Diet | 1 oz | tr | 0 |
| 7-Up Gold | 1 oz | 13 | 0 |
| 7-Up Gold Diet | 1 oz | tr | 0 |
| Apple Sparkling (Welch's) | 12 oz | 180 | 0 |
| Birch Beer Diet (Shasta) | 12 oz | 4 | 0 |
| Black Cherry (Shasta) | 12 oz | 162 | 0 |
| Cherry Cola (Shasta) | 12 oz | 140 | 0 |
| Citrus Mist (Shasta) | 12 oz | 170 | 0 |
| Club (Schweppes) | 6 oz | 0 | 0 |
| Club Soda (Shasta) | 12 oz | 0 | 0 |
| Coca-Cola | 6 oz | 77 | 0 |
| Coca-Cola Caffeine-Free | 6 oz | 77 | 0 |
| Coca-Cola Cherry | 6 oz | 76 | 0 |
| Coca-Cola Classic | 6 oz | 72 | 0 |

| FOOD | PORTION | CALORIES | CHOLESTEROL |
|---|---|---|---|
| Cola (Shasta) | 8 oz | 98 | 0 |
| Cola (Shasta) | 12 oz | 147 | 0 |
| Cola Diet (Shasta) | 8 oz | 0 | 0 |
| Collins (Shasta) | 12 oz | 118 | 0 |
| Creme (Shasta) | 12 oz | 154 | 0 |
| Diet Cherry Coca-Cola | 6 oz | tr | 0 |
| Diet Coke | 6 oz | tr | 0 |
| Diet Coke Caffeine-Free | 6 oz | tr | 0 |
| Diet Minute Maid Lemon-Lime | 6 oz | 10 | 0 |
| Diet Minute Maid Orange | 6 oz | 4 | 0 |
| Diet Sprite | 6 oz | 2 | 0 |
| Dr Pepper | 1 oz | 13 | 0 |
| Dr Pepper Diet | 1 oz | tr | 0 |
| Dr. Diablo (Shasta) | 12 oz | 140 | 0 |
| Fanta Ginger Ale | 6 oz | 63 | 0 |
| Fanta Grape | 6 oz | 86 | 0 |
| Fanta Orange | 6 oz | 88 | 0 |
| Fanta Root Beer | 6 oz | 78 | 0 |
| Fresca | 6 oz | 2 | 0 |
| Fruit Punch (Shasta) | 12 oz | 173 | 0 |
| Ginger Ale (Health Valley) | 13 oz | 153 | 0 |

| FOOD | PORTION | CALORIES | CHOLESTEROL |
| --- | --- | --- | --- |
| Ginger Ale (Schweppes) | 6 oz | 63 | 0 |
| Ginger Ale (Shasta) | 8 oz | 80 | 0 |
| Ginger Ale (Shasta) | 12 oz | 120 | 0 |
| Ginger Ale Diet (Schweppes) | 6 oz | tr | 0 |
| Ginger Ale Diet (Shasta) | 8 oz | 0 | 0 |
| Ginger Beer (Schweppes) | 6 oz | 68 | 0 |
| Grape (Schweppes) | 6 oz | 92 | 0 |
| Grape (Shasta) | 12 oz | 177 | 0 |
| Grape Sparkling (Welch's) | 12 oz | 180 | 0 |
| Grapefruit (Schweppes) | 6 oz | 77 | 0 |
| Lemon-Lime (Schweppes) | 6 oz | 71 | 0 |
| Lemon-Lime (Shasta) | 8 oz | 97 | 0 |
| Lemon-Lime (Shasta) | 12 oz | 146 | 0 |
| Lemon-Lime Diet (Shasta) | 8 oz | 0 | 0 |
| Like Cola | 1 oz | 13 | 0 |
| Like Cola Sugar Free | 1 oz | tr | 0 |
| Mello Yellow | 6 oz | 87 | 0 |

| FOOD | PORTION | CALORIES | CHOLESTEROL |
|------|---------|----------|-------------|
| Minute Maid Lemon-Lime | 6 oz | 71 | 0 |
| Minute Maid Orange | 6 oz | 87 | 0 |
| Mr. PIBB | 6 oz | 71 | 0 |
| Orange (Shasta) | 12 oz | 177 | 0 |
| Orange Sparkling (Welch's) | 12 oz | 180 | 0 |
| Orange Sparkling (Schweppes) | 6 oz | 86 | 0 |
| Pepper Free | 1 oz | 12 | 0 |
| Pepper Free Diet | 1 oz | tr | 0 |
| Ramblin' Root Beer | 6 oz | 88 | 0 |
| Red Berry (Shasta) | 12 oz | 158 | 0 |
| Red Pop (Shasta) | 12 oz | 158 | 0 |
| Root Beer (Health Valley) | 13 oz | 120 | 0 |
| Root Beer (Schweppes) | 6 oz | 75 | 0 |
| Root Beer (Shasta) | 12 oz | 154 | 0 |
| Sarsaparilla (Health Valley) | 13 oz | 153 | 0 |
| Seltzer (Schweppes) | 6 oz | 0 | 0 |
| Seltzer Flavored (Schweppes) | 6 oz | 0 | 0 |
| Seltzer Light Black Cherry Cider (Crystal Geyser) | 6 oz | 60 | 0 |

| FOOD | PORTION | CALORIES | CHOLESTEROL |
|---|---|---|---|
| Seltzer Light Cranberry-Raspberry (Crystal Geyser) | 6 oz | 60 | 0 |
| Seltzer Light Kiwi Lemonade (Crystal Geyser) | 6 oz | 60 | 0 |
| Seltzer Light Natural Peach (Crystal Geyser) | 6 oz | 60 | 0 |
| Seltzer Light Vanilla Creme (Crystal Geyser) | 6 oz | 60 | 0 |
| Seltzer No Salt Added No Calories (Manischewitz) | 8 oz | 0 | 0 |
| Shasta Free Cola | 12 oz | 151 | 0 |
| Sprite | 6 oz | 71 | 0 |
| Strawberry (Shasta) | 12 oz | 147 | 0 |
| Strawberry, Sparkling (Welch's) | 12 oz | 180 | 0 |
| TAB | 6 oz | tr | 0 |
| TAB Caffeine-Free | 6 oz | tr | 0 |
| Tonic Water (Shasta) | 12 oz | 0 | 0 |
| Wild Berry (Health Valley) | 13 oz | 142 | 0 |
| club | 12 oz | 0 | 0 |
| cola | 12 oz | 151 | 0 |
| cream | 12 oz | 191 | 0 |
| ginger ale | 12 oz can | 124 | 0 |
| grape | 12 oz | 161 | 0 |
| lemon-lime | 12 oz | 149 | 0 |

| FOOD | PORTION | CALORIES | CHOLESTEROL |
|---|---|---|---|
| orange | 12 oz | 177 | 0 |
| root beer | 12 oz | 152 | 0 |
| tonic water | 12 | 125 | 0 |

## SOLE

FROZEN
| | | | |
|---|---|---|---|
| Sole a la Monterey (King & Prince) | 6 oz | 221 | 11 |
| Sole a la Monterey (King & Prince) | 8 oz | 295 | 15 |

## SOUFFLE

HOME RECIPE
| | | | |
|---|---|---|---|
| cheese | 1 cup | 308 | 196 |
| grand marnier | 1 cup | 109 | 139 |
| lemon, chilled | 1 cup | 176 | 2 |
| raspberry, chilled | 1 cup | 173 | 3 |
| spinach souffle | 1 cup | 218 | 184 |

## SOUP

CANNED
| | | | |
|---|---|---|---|
| 5 Bean Chunky (Health Valley) | 7.5 oz | 80 | 0 |
| Barley w/ Beef; as prep w/ water (Campbell) | 1 cup | 86 | tr |
| Bean (Health Valley) | 4 oz | 115 | 0 |
| Bean w/ Bacon, Special Request (Campbell's) | 8 oz | 120 | 5 |

| FOOD | PORTION | CALORIES | CHOLESTEROL |
|---|---|---|---|
| Bean w/ Bacon, Special Request (Campbell's) | 8 oz | 120 | 5 |
| Beef Broth (Pritikin Foods) | 6⅞ oz | 20 | <5 |
| Borscht (Gold's) | 8 oz | 100 | 0 |
| Borscht Low Calorie (Manischewitz) | 8 oz | 20 | 0 |
| Borscht w/ Beets (Manischewitz) | 8 oz | 80 | 0 |
| Borscht, Lo-Cal (Gold's) | 8 oz | 20 | 0 |
| Chicken Vegetable Soup (Pritikin Foods) | 7¼ oz | 70 | 0 |
| Chicken Broth (Health Valley) | 4 oz | 15 | 4 |
| Chicken Broth (Pritikin Foods) | 6⅞ oz | 14 | 0 |
| Chicken Gumbo (Pritikin Foods) | 7⅜ oz | 60 | 5 |
| Chicken Soup w/ Ribbon Pasta (Pritikin Foods) | 7¼ oz | 60 | 0 |
| Chicken w/ Rice, Special Request (Campbell's) | 8 oz | 60 | 10 |
| Clam Chowder (Health Valley) | 4 oz | 80 | 7 |
| Country Vegetable (Lunch Bucket) | 1 container (8.25 oz) | 90 | 0 |
| Lentil (Health Valley) | 4 oz | 90 | 0 |

| FOOD | PORTION | CALORIES | CHOLESTEROL |
|------|---------|----------|-------------|
| Lentil Soup (Pritikin Foods) | 7⅜ oz | 100 | 0 |
| Manhattan Clam Chowder (Pritikin Foods) | 7⅜ oz | 70 | 2 |
| Minestrone (Health Valley) | 7.5 oz | 90 | 0 |
| Minestrone Chunky (Health Valley) | 4 oz | 70 | 0 |
| Minestrone Soup (Pritikin Foods) | 7⅜ oz | 110 | 0 |
| Mushroom (Health Valley) | 4 oz | 70 | 0 |
| Mushroom (Pritikin Foods) | 7⅜ oz | 60 | 2 |
| Navy Bean (Pritikin Foods) | 7⅜ oz | 130 | 2 |
| New England Chowder (American Original Foods) | 4 oz | 64 | 5 |
| New England Clam Chowder (Pritikin Foods) | 7⅜ oz | 118 | 2 |
| Potato (Health Valley) | 4 oz | 70 | 0 |
| Schav (Gold's) | 8 oz | 25 | 15 |
| Split Pea Soup (Pritikin Foods) | 7½ oz | 130 | 5 |
| Split Pea Green (Health Valley) | 4 oz | 70 | 0 |
| Tomato (Health Valley) | 4 oz | 60 | 0 |
| Tomato Soup w/ Tomato Pieces (Pritikin Foods) | 7¼ oz | 70 | 0 |

| FOOD | PORTION | CALORIES | CHOLESTEROL |
|------|---------|----------|-------------|
| Turkey Vegetable Soup w/ Ribbon Pasta (Pritikin Foods) | 7⅜ oz | 50 | 5 |
| Vegetable (Health Valley) | 7.5 oz | 80 | 0 |
| Vegetable Beef (Lunch Bucket) | 1 container (8.25 oz) | 140 | 15 |
| Vegetable Chicken Chunky (Health Valley) | 4 oz | 120 | 12 |
| Vegetable Soup (Pritikin Foods) | 7⅜ oz | 70 | 0 |
| asparagus, cream of; as prep w/ milk | 1 cup | 161 | 22 |
| asparagus, cream of; as prep w/ water | 1 cup | 87 | 5 |
| bean w/ frankfurters; as prep w/ water | 1 cup | 187 | 12 |
| bean w/ frankfurters; not prep | 1 can (11¼ oz) | 454 | 29 |
| bean black; as prep w/ water | 1 cup | 116 | 0 |
| bean black; not prep | 1 can (11 oz) | 285 | 0 |
| bean w/ bacon; not prep | 1 can (11½ oz) | 420 | 6 |
| bean w/ bacon; as prep w/ water | 1 cup | 173 | 3 |
| bean w/ ham, chunky, ready-to-serve | 1 can (19¼ oz) | 519 | 49 |
| bean w/ ham, chunky, ready-to-serve | 1 cup | 231 | 22 |
| beef broth, ready-to-serve | 1 can (14 oz) | 27 | 1 |

| FOOD | PORTION | CALORIES | CHOLESTEROL |
|---|---|---|---|
| beef broth, ready-to-serve | 1 cup | 16 | tr |
| beef, chunky, ready-to-serve | 1 cup | 171 | 14 |
| beef, chunky, ready-to-serve | 1 can (19 oz) | 383 | 32 |
| beef noodle; as prep w/ water | 1 cup | 84 | 5 |
| beef noodle; not prep | 1 can (10¾ oz) | 204 | 12 |
| black bean turtle soup | 1 cup | 218 | 0 |
| celery, cream of; as prep w/ milk | 1 can (10¾ oz) | 400 | 78 |
| celery, cream of; as prep w/ milk | 1 cup | 165 | 32 |
| celery, cream of; as prep w/ water | 1 cup | 90 | 15 |
| celery, cream of; not prep | 1 can (10¾ oz) | 219 | 34 |
| cheese; as prep w/ milk | 1 cup | 230 | 48 |
| cheese; as prep w/ milk | 1 can (11 oz) | 558 | 116 |
| cheese; as prep w/ water | 1 can (11 oz) | 377 | 72 |
| cheese; as prep w/ water | 1 cup | 155 | 30 |
| cheese; not prep | 1 can (11 oz) | 377 | 72 |
| chicken vegetable, chunky, ready-to-serve | 1 can (19 oz) | 374 | 38 |
| chicken vegetable, chunky, ready-to-serve | 1 cup | 167 | 17 |
| chicken vegetable; as prep w/ water | 1 cup | 74 | 10 |

| FOOD | PORTION | CALORIES | CHOLESTEROL |
|------|---------|----------|-------------|
| chicken vegetable; not prep | 1 can (10½ oz) | 181 | 21 |
| chicken & dumplings; as prep w/ water | 1 cup | 406 | 34 |
| chicken & dumplings; not prep | 1 can (10½ oz) | 236 | 80 |
| chicken broth; as prep w/ water | 1 can (10¾ oz) | 95 | 2 |
| chicken broth; as prep w/ water | 1 cup | 39 | 1 |
| chicken broth; not prep | 1 can (10¾ oz) | 94 | 3 |
| chicken, chunky, ready-to-serve | 1 cup | 178 | 30 |
| chicken, chunky, ready-to-serve | 1 can (10¾ oz) | 216 | 37 |
| chicken, cream of; as prep w/ milk | 1 cup | 191 | 27 |
| chicken, cream of; as prep w/ water | 1 can (10¾ oz) | 464 | 66 |
| chicken, cream of; as prep w/ water | 1 cup | 116 | 10 |
| chicken, cream of; not prep | 1 can (10¾ oz) | 283 | 24 |
| chicken gumbo; as prep w/ water | 1 cup | 56 | 5 |
| chicken gumbo; not prep | 1 can (10¾ oz) | 137 | 9 |
| chicken noodle w/ meatballs, ready-to-serve | 1 cup | 99 | 10 |
| chicken noodle w/ meatballs, ready-to-serve | 1 can (20 oz) | 227 | 23 |

| FOOD | PORTION | CALORIES | CHOLESTEROL |
|---|---|---|---|
| chicken noodle; as prep w/ water | 1 cup | 75 | 7 |
| chicken noodle; not prep | 1 can (10½ oz) | 182 | 15 |
| chicken rice, chunky, ready-to-serve | 1 can (19 oz) | 286 | 27 |
| chicken rice, chunky, ready-to-serve | 1 cup | 127 | 12 |
| chicken rice; as prep w/ water | 1 cup | 251 | 7 |
| chicken rice; not prep | 1 can (10½ oz) | 146 | 15 |
| chicken rice; not prep | 1 can (10½ oz) | 146 | 15 |
| chili beef; as prep w/ water | 1 cup | 169 | 12 |
| chili beef; not prep | 1 can (11¼ oz) | 411 | 32 |
| clam chowder, Manhattan, chunky, ready-to-serve | 1 cup | 133 | 14 |
| clam chowder, Manhattan, chunky, ready-to-serve | 1 can (19 oz) | 299 | 32 |
| clam chowder, Manhattan; as prep w/ water | 1 cup | 78 | 2 |
| clam chowder, Manhattan; not prep | 1 can (10¾ oz) | 187 | 6 |
| clam chowder, New England; as prep w/ milk | 1 cup | 163 | 22 |
| clam chowder, New England; as prep w/ water | 1 cup | 95 | 5 |
| clam chowder, New England; not prep | 1 can (10¾ oz) | 214 | 12 |
| consomme w/ gelatin; as prep w/ water | 1 cup | 29 | 0 |

| FOOD | PORTION | CALORIES | CHOLESTEROL |
|---|---|---|---|
| consomme w/ gelatin; not prep | 1 can (10½ oz) | 71 | 0 |
| crab, ready-to-serve | 1 cup | 76 | 10 |
| crab, ready-to-serve | 1 can (13 oz) | 114 | 10 |
| escarole, ready-to-serve | 1 can (19½ oz) | 61 | 6 |
| escarole, ready-to-serve | 1 cup | 27 | 2 |
| gazpacho, ready-to-serve | 1 cup | 57 | 0 |
| gazpacho, ready-to-serve | 1 can (13 oz) | 87 | 0 |
| lentil w/ ham, ready-to-serve | 1 can (20 oz) | 320 | 17 |
| lentil w/ ham, ready-to-serve | 1 cup | 140 | 7 |
| minestrone, chunky, ready-to-serve | 1 cup | 127 | 5 |
| minestrone, chunky, ready-to-serve | 1 can (19 oz) | 285 | 11 |
| minestrone; as prep w/ water | 1 cup | 83 | 2 |
| minestrone; not prep | 1 can (10½ oz) | 202 | 3 |
| mushroom w/ beef stock; as prep w/ water | 1 can (10¾ oz) | 208 | 18 |
| mushroom w/ beef stock; as prep w/ water | 1 cup | 85 | 7 |
| mushroom w/ beef stock; not prep | 1 can (10¾ oz) | 208 | 18 |
| mushroom, cream of; as prep w/ milk | 1 can (10¾ oz) | 494 | 48 |
| mushroom, cream of; as prep w/ milk | 1 cup | 203 | 20 |

| FOOD | PORTION | CALORIES | CHOLESTEROL |
|------|---------|----------|-------------|
| mushroom, cream of; as prep w/ water | 1 cup | 129 | 2 |
| mushroom, cream of; not prep | 1 can (10¾ oz) | 313 | 3 |
| onion; as prep w/ water | 1 cup | 57 | 0 |
| onion; not prep | 1 can (10½ oz) | 138 | 0 |
| oyster stew; as prep w/ milk | 1 cup | 134 | 32 |
| oyster stew; as prep w/ milk | 1 can (10½ oz) | 325 | 77 |
| oyster stew; as prep w/ water | 1 cup | 59 | 14 |
| oyster stew; not prep | 1 can (10½ oz) | 144 | 33 |
| pea, green; as prep w/ milk | 1 can (11¼ oz) | 579 | 43 |
| pea, green; as prep w/ milk | 1 cup | 239 | 18 |
| pea, green; as prep w/ water | 1 cup | 164 | 0 |
| pea, green; not prep | 1 can (11¼ oz) | 398 | 0 |
| pepperpot; as prep w/ water | 1 cup | 103 | 10 |
| pepperpot; not prep | 1 can (10½ oz) | 251 | 24 |
| potato, cream of; as prep w/ milk | 1 can (10¾ oz) | 360 | 54 |
| potato, cream of; as prep w/ milk | 1 cup | 148 | 22 |
| potato, cream of; as prep w/ water | 1 cup | 73 | 5 |
| potato, cream of; not prep | 1 can (10¾ oz) | 178 | 15 |

| FOOD | PORTION | CALORIES | CHOLESTEROL |
|---|---|---|---|
| scotch broth; not prep | 1 can (10½ oz) | 195 | 12 |
| scotch broth; as prep w/ water | 1 cup | 80 | 5 |
| shrimp, cream of; as prep w/ milk | 1 can (10¾ oz) | 400 | 84 |
| shrimp, cream of; as prep w/ milk | 1 cup | 165 | 35 |
| shrimp, cream of; as prep w/ water | 1 cup | 90 | 17 |
| shrimp, cream of; not prep | 1 can (10¾ oz) | 219 | 40 |
| split pea w/ ham, chunky, ready-to-serve | 1 cup | 184 | 7 |
| split pea w/ ham, chunky, ready-to-serve | 1 can (19 oz) | 413 | 16 |
| split pea w/ ham; as prep w/ water | 1 cup | 189 | 8 |
| split pea w/ ham; not prep | 1 can (11½ oz) | 459 | 20 |
| stockpot; as prep w/ water | 1 cup | 100 | 5 |
| stockpot; not prep | 1 can (11 oz) | 242 | 9 |
| tomato beef w/ noodle; as prep w/ water | 1 cup | 140 | 5 |
| tomato beef w/ noodle; not prep | 1 can (10¾ oz) | 341 | 9 |
| tomato bisque; as prep w/ milk | 1 can (11 oz) | 481 | 53 |
| tomato bisque; as prep w/ milk | 1 cup | 198 | 22 |

| FOOD | PORTION | CALORIES | CHOLESTEROL |
|---|---|---|---|
| tomato bisque; as prep w/ water | 1 cup | 123 | 4 |
| tomato bisque; not prep | 1 can (11 oz) | 300 | 11 |
| tomato rice; as prep w/ water | 1 cup | 120 | 2 |
| tomato rice; not prep | 1 can (11 oz) | 291 | 3 |
| tomato; as prep w/ milk | 1 can (10¾ oz) | 389 | 42 |
| tomato; as prep w/ milk | 1 cup | 160 | 17 |
| tomato; as prep w/ water | 1 cup | 86 | 0 |
| tomato; not prep | 1 can (10¾ oz) | 208 | 0 |
| turkey, chunky, ready-to-serve | 1 can (18¾ oz) | 306 | 21 |
| turkey, chunky, ready-to-serve | 1 cup | 136 | 9 |
| turkey noodle; as prep w/ water | 1 cup | 69 | 5 |
| turkey noodle; not prep | 1 can (10¾ oz) | 168 | 12 |
| turkey vegetable; as prep w/ water | 1 cup | 74 | 2 |
| turkey vegetable; not prep | 1 can (10½ oz) | 179 | 3 |
| vegetable, chunky, ready-to-serve | 1 cup | 122 | 0 |
| vegetable, chunky, ready-to-serve | 1 can (19 oz) | 274 | 0 |
| vegetable w/ beef broth; as prep w/ water | 1 cup | 81 | 2 |

| FOOD | PORTION | CALORIES | CHOLESTEROL |
|---|---|---|---|
| vegetable w/ beef broth; not prep | 1 can (10½ oz) | 197 | 6 |
| vegetable w/ beef; as prep w/ water | 1 cup | 79 | 5 |
| vegetable w/ beef; not prep | 1 can (10¾ oz) | 192 | 12 |
| vegetarian vegetable; as prep w/ water | 1 cup | 72 | 0 |
| vegetarian vegetable; not prep | 1 can (10½ oz) | 176 | 0 |
| vichyssoise | 1 cup | 148 | 22 |
| vichyssoise | 1 can (10¾ oz) | 360 | 54 |
| **DRY** | | | |
| Beef Flavor Noodle; as prep w/ water (Cup-a-Soup) | 6 oz | 10 | 0 |
| Beef Noodle; as prep (Estee) | 6 oz | 20 | 1 |
| Beef; as prep (Diamond Crystal) | 6 oz | 30 | tr |
| Beefy Tomato; as prep w/ water (Cup-a-Soup Trim) | 6 oz | 10 | 0 |
| Chicken Vegetable; as prep w/ water (Cup-a-Soup) | 8 oz | 40 | 5 |
| Chicken Flavor; as prep w/ water (Cup-a-Soup) | 6 oz | 25 | 5 |
| Chicken Flavored; as prep w/ water (Lots-a-Noodles) | 7 oz | 120 | 30 |

| FOOD | PORTION | CALORIES | CHOLESTEROL |
|------|---------|----------|-------------|
| Chicken Noodle Instant; as prep (Estee) | 6 oz | 25 | 4 |
| Chicken Noodle; as prep w/ water (Cup-a-Soup) | 6 oz | 90 | 15 |
| Chicken w/ Rice; as prep w/ water (Cup-a-Soup) | 6 oz | 45 | 5 |
| Chicken; as prep w/ water (Cup-a-Soup Trim) | 6 oz | 10 | 0 |
| Chicken; as prep (Diamond Crystal) | 6 oz | 30 | 2 |
| Cream of Mushroom; as prep w/ water (Cup-a-Soup) | 6 oz | 80 | 0 |
| Cream of Chicken; as prep w/ water (Cup-a-Soup) | 6 oz | 80 | 0 |
| Cream of Chicken; as prep w/ water (Lots-a-Noodles) | 7 oz | 150 | 35 |
| Cream; as prep (Diamond Crystal) | 6 oz | 90 | 5 |
| French Onion; as prep w/ water (Cup-a-Soup Trim) | 6 oz | 10 | 0 |
| Green Pea; as prep w/ water (Cup-a-Soup) | 6 oz | 120 | 0 |
| Herb Chicken; as prep w/ water (Cup-a-Soup Trim) | 6 oz | 10 | 0 |
| Minestrone Soup Mix; as prep (Manischewitz) | 6 oz | 50 | 0 |

| FOOD | PORTION | CALORIES | CHOLESTEROL |
|---|---|---|---|
| Mushroom Instant; as prep (Estee) | 6 oz | 40 | 1 |
| Onion Instant; as prep (Estee) | 6 oz | 25 | 1 |
| Onion; as prep w/ water (Cup-a-Soup) | 6 oz | 30 | 0 |
| Split Pea Soup Mix; as prep (Manischewitz) | 6 oz | 45 | 0 |
| Tomato Instant; as prep (Estee) | 6 oz | 40 | 0 |
| Tomato; as prep w/ water (Cup-a-Soup) | 6 oz | 80 | 0 |
| Tomato; as prep (Diamond Crystal) | 6 oz | 70 | 3 |
| asparagus, cream of; as prep w/ water | 1 cup | 59 | tr |
| asparagus, cream of; not prep | 1 pkg (2.2 oz) | 234 | 1 |
| bean w/ bacon; as prep w/ water | 1 cup | 105 | 3 |
| bean w/ bacon; not prep | 1 pkg (1 oz) | 105 | 3 |
| beef broth cube; as prep w/ water | 1 cup | 8 | tr |
| beef broth; as prep w/ water | 1 cup | 19 | 1 |
| beef broth; as prep w/ water | 1 cube | 6 | tr |
| beef broth; not prep | 1 pkg (.2 oz) | 14 | 1 |
| beef noodle; as prep w/ water | 6 oz | 30 | 1 |
| beef noodle; as prep w/ water | 1 cup | 41 | 2 |

| FOOD | PORTION | CALORIES | CHOLESTEROL |
|---|---|---|---|
| beef noodle; not prep | 1 pkg (.3 oz) | 30 | 1 |
| cauliflower; as prep w/ water | 1 cup | 68 | tr |
| cauliflower; not prep | 1 pkg (.7 oz) | 68 | tr |
| celery, cream of; as prep w/ water | 1 cup | 63 | 1 |
| celery, cream of; not prep | 1 pkg (.6 oz) | 62 | 1 |
| chicken vegetable; as prep w/ water | 1 cup | 49 | 3 |
| chicken vegetable; not prep | 1 pkg (.4 oz) | 37 | 2 |
| chicken broth cube; as prep w/ water | 1 cup | 13 | 1 |
| chicken broth cube; not prep | 1 cube | 9 | 1 |
| chicken broth; as prep w/ water | 1 cup | 21 | 1 |
| chicken broth; not prep | 1 pkg (.2 oz) | 16 | 1 |
| chicken, cream of; as prep w/ water | 1 cup | 107 | 3 |
| chicken, cream of; not prep | 1 pkg (.6 oz) | 80 | 2 |
| chicken noodle; as prep w/ water | 1 cup | 53 | 3 |
| chicken noodle; not prep | 1 pkg (2.6 oz) | 257 | 10 |
| chicken rice; as prep w/ water | 1 cup | 60 | 3 |
| chicken rice; not prep | 1 pkg (.6 oz) | 60 | 3 |

| FOOD | PORTION | CALORIES | CHOLESTEROL |
|---|---|---|---|
| clam chowder, Manhattan; not prep | 1 pkg (.7 oz) | 65 | 0 |
| clam chowder, New England; not prep | 1 pkg (.8 oz) | 95 | 1 |
| consomme, w/ gelatin; as prep w/ water | 1 cup | 17 | 0 |
| consomme, w/ gelatin; not prep | 1 pkg (2 oz) | 77 | 0 |
| leek; as prep w/ water | 1 cup | 71 | 3 |
| leek; not prep | 1 pkg (2.7 oz) | 294 | 9 |
| minestrone; as prep w/ water | 1 cup | 79 | 3 |
| minestrone; not prep | 1 pkg (2.7 oz) | 279 | 6 |
| mushroom, instant; not prep | 1 pkg (.6 oz) | 74 | 0 |
| mushroom; as prep w/ water | 1 cup | 96 | 1 |
| mushroom; not prep | 1 pkg (2.6 oz) | 328 | 2 |
| onion, French; not prep | 1 pkg (1.4 oz) | 115 | 2 |
| onion; as prep w/ water | 1 cup | 28 | 0 |
| onion; not prep | 1 pkg (1.4 oz) | 115 | 2 |
| oxtail; as prep w/ water | 1 cup | 71 | 3 |
| oxtail; not prep | 1 pkg (2.6 oz) | 280 | 11 |
| pea, green; as prep w/ water | 1 cup | 133 | 3 |
| pea, green; not prep | 1 pkg (4 oz) | 402 | 1 |

| FOOD | PORTION | CALORIES | CHOLESTEROL |
|---|---|---|---|
| pea, split; as prep w/ water | 1 cup | 133 | 3 |
| pea, split; not prep | 1 pkg (4 oz) | 402 | 1 |
| tomato vegetable; as prep w/ water | 1 cup | 55 | tr |
| tomato vegetable; not prep | 1 pkg (1.4 oz) | 125 | 1 |
| tomato; as prep w/ water | 1 cup | 102 | 1 |
| tomato; not prep | 1 pkg (.7 oz) | 77 | 1 |
| vegetable, beef; as prep w/ water | 1 cup | 53 | 1 |
| vegetable, beef; not prep | 1 pkg (2.6 oz) | 256 | 6 |
| vegetable, cream of; as prep w/ water | 1 cup | 105 | 0 |
| vegetable, cream of; not prep | 1 pkg (.62 oz) | 79 | 0 |
| HOME RECIPE | | | |
| black bean turtle soup | 1 cup | 241 | 0 |
| corn & cheese chowder | ¾ cup | 215 | 66 |
| corn chowder | 1 cup | 233 | 75 |
| gazpacho | 1 cup | 46 | 0 |
| greek | ¾ cup | 63 | 83 |
| hot & sour | 1 cup | 74 | 70 |
| lentil | 1 cup | 175 | 0 |
| mock turtle | 1 cup | 256 | 164 |
| potato | 1 cup | 201 | 37 |

| FOOD | PORTION | CALORIES | CHOLESTEROL |
|------|---------|----------|-------------|
| seafood chowder | 1 cup | 170 | 68 |
| vegetable | 1 cup | 70 | 0 |
| vegetable beef | 1 cup | 320 | 54 |
| wonton | 1 cup | 205 | 89 |

# SOUR CREAM
(*see also* SOUR CREAM SUBSTITUTE)

| | | | |
|------|---------|----------|-------------|
| **LOWFAT** | | | |
| Lean Cream (Land O'Lakes) | 1 Tbsp | 20 | 4 |
| Lean Cream w/ Chives (Land O'Lakes) | 1 Tbsp | 20 | 4 |
| Lite Delite (Friendship) | 2 Tbsp | 35 | 8 |
| **REGULAR** | | | |
| Friendship | 2 Tbsp | 55 | 42 |
| Sour Cream (Land O'Lakes) | 1 Tbsp | 32 | 7 |
| Sour Cream (Land O'Lakes) | 1 Tbsp | 25 | 5 |
| half & half | 1 Tbsp | 20 | 6 |
| sour cream | 1 Tbsp | 26 | 5 |
| sour cream | 1 cup | 493 | 102 |

# SOUR CREAM SUBSTITUTE

| | | | |
|------|---------|----------|-------------|
| Formagg Sour Sour Cream Style | 1 oz | 40 | 0 |

| FOOD | PORTION | CALORIES | CHOLESTEROL |
|---|---|---|---|
| imitation, non-dairy | 1 oz | 59 | 0 |
| imitation, non-dairy | 1 cup | 479 | 0 |
| sour cream, non-butterfat | 1 Tbsp | 21 | 1 |
| sour cream, non-butterfat | 1 cup | 417 | 13 |

## SOY
(*see also* ICE CREAM, NON-DAIRY; TEXTURED VEGETABLE PROTEIN; TOFU)

| FOOD | PORTION | CALORIES | CHOLESTEROL |
|---|---|---|---|
| Soo Moo Soybean Milk (Health Valley) | 8.5 oz | 120 | 0 |
| Soy Sauce (Kikkoman) | 1 Tbsp | 10 | tr |
| Soy Sauce Lite (Kikkoman) | 1 Tbsp | 11 | tr |
| Soy Sauce Mix (Diamond Crystal) | 1 tsp | 5 | 0 |
| lecithin | 1 Tbsp | 120 | 0 |
| milk | 1 cup | 79 | 0 |
| soy sauce | 1 Tbsp | 7 | 0 |
| soy sauce, shoyu | 1 Tbsp | 9 | 0 |
| soy sauce, tamari | 1 Tbsp | 11 | 0 |
| soybean sprouts | ½ cup | 45 | 0 |
| soybean, roasted & toasted | 1 oz | 129 | 0 |
| soybeans, roasted | ½ cup | 405 | 0 |
| soybeans, dry-roasted | ½ cup | 387 | 0 |
| soybeans, raw | 1 cup | 774 | 0 |
| soybeans; cooked | 1 cup | 298 | 0 |

| FOOD | PORTION | CALORIES | CHOLESTEROL |
|------|---------|----------|-------------|

# SPAGHETTI
(*see* PASTA, SPAGHETTI SAUCE)

# SPAGHETTI SAUCE
(*see also* PIZZA, TOMATO)

JARRED

| FOOD | PORTION | CALORIES | CHOLESTEROL |
|------|---------|----------|-------------|
| Estee Spaghetti Sauce | 4 oz | 70 | 0 |
| Pritikin Foods Spaghetti Sauce | 4 oz | 60 | 0 |
| Pritikin Foods Spaghetti Sauce w/ Mushrooms | 4 oz | 60 | 0 |
| Ragu Chunky Gardenstyle Extra Tomatoes, Garlic & Onions | 4 oz | 80 | 0 |
| Ragu Chunky Gardenstyle Extra Tomatoes, Garlic & Onions w/ pasta | 4 oz + 5 oz pasta | 290 | 0 |
| Ragu Chunky Gardenstyle Green Peppers & Mushrooms | 4 oz | 80 | 0 |
| Ragu Chunky Gardenstyle Green Peppers & Mushrooms w/ pasta | 4 oz + 5 oz pasta | 290 | 0 |
| Ragu Chunky Gardenstyle Italian Garden Combination | 4 oz | 80 | 0 |
| Ragu Chunky Gardenstyle Italian Garden Combination w/ pasta | 4 oz + 5 oz pasta | 290 | 0 |
| Ragu Chunky Gardenstyle Mushrooms & Onions | 4 oz | 80 | 0 |
| Ragu Chunky Gardenstyle Mushrooms & Onions w/ pasta | 4 oz + 5 oz pasta | 290 | 0 |

| FOOD | PORTION | CALORIES | CHOLESTEROL |
|------|---------|----------|-------------|
| Ragu Chunky Gardenstyle Sweet Green & Red Peppers | 4 oz | 80 | 0 |
| Ragu Chunky Gardenstyle Sweet Green & Red Peppers w/ pasta | 4 oz + 5 oz pasta | 290 | 0 |
| Ragu Extra Thick & Zesty Flavored w/ Meat | 4 oz | 100 | 2 |
| Ragu Extra Thick & Zesty Flavored w/ Meat w/ pasta | 4 oz + 5 oz pasta | 310 | 2 |
| Ragu Extra Thick & Zesty Plain | 4 oz | 100 | 0 |
| Ragu Extra Thick & Zesty Plain w/ pasta | 4 oz + 5 oz pasta | 310 | 0 |
| Ragu Extra Thick & Zesty w/ Mushrooms | 4 oz | 110 | 0 |
| Ragu Extra Thick & Zesty w/ Mushrooms w/ pasta | 4 oz + 5 oz pasta | 320 | 0 |
| Ragu Homestyle Flavored w/ Meat | 4 oz | 70 | 2 |
| Ragu Homestyle Flavored w/ Meat w/ pasta | 4 oz + 5 oz pasta | 280 | 2 |
| Ragu Homestyle Plain | 4 oz | 70 | 0 |
| Ragu Homestyle Plain w/ pasta | 4 oz + 5 oz pasta | 280 | 0 |
| Ragu Homestyle w/ Mushrooms | 4 oz | 70 | 0 |
| Ragu Homestyle w/ Mushrooms w/ pasta | 4 oz + 5 oz pasta | 280 | 0 |
| Ragu Old World Style Flavored w/ Meat | 4 oz | 80 | 2 |
| Ragu Old World Style Flavored w/ Meat w/ pasta | 4 oz + 5 oz pasta | 290 | 2 |

| FOOD | PORTION | CALORIES | CHOLESTEROL |
|------|---------|----------|-------------|
| Ragu Old World Style Marinara Sauce | 4 oz | 90 | 0 |
| Ragu Old World Style Marinara Sauce w/ pasta | 4 oz + 5 oz pasta | 300 | 0 |
| Ragu Old World Style Plain | 4 oz | 80 | 0 |
| Ragu Old World Style Plain w/ pasta | 4 oz + 5 oz pasta | 290 | 0 |
| Ragu Old World Style w/ Extra Cheese | 4 oz | 80 | 1 |
| Ragu Old World Style w/ Extra Cheese w/ pasta | 4 oz + 5 oz pasta | 290 | 1 |
| Ragu Old World Style w/ Extra Garlic | 4 oz | 80 | 0 |
| Ragu Old World Style w/ Extra Garlic w/ pasta | 4 oz + 5 oz pasta | 290 | 0 |
| Ragu Old World Style w/ Mushrooms | 4 oz | 80 | 0 |
| Ragu Old World Style w/ Mushrooms w/ pasta | 4 oz + 5 oz pasta | 290 | 0 |
| Ragu Thick & Hearty Flavored w/ Leaner Ground Beef | 4 oz | 120 | 2 |
| Ragu Thick & Hearty Flavored w/ Leaner Ground Beef w/ pasta | 4 oz + 5 oz pasta | 330 | 2 |
| Ragu Thick & Hearty Marinara | 4 oz | 110 | 0 |
| Ragu Thick & Hearty Marinara w/ pasta | 4 oz + 5 oz pasta | 320 | 0 |
| Ragu Thick & Hearty Plain | 4 oz | 110 | 0 |
| Ragu Thick & Hearty Plain w/ pasta | 4 oz + 5 oz pasta | 320 | 0 |

| FOOD | PORTION | CALORIES | CHOLESTEROL |
|------|---------|----------|-------------|
| Ragu Thick & Hearty w/ Mushrooms | 4 oz | 110 | 0 |
| Ragu Thick & Hearty w/ Mushrooms w/ pasta | 4 oz + 5 oz pasta | 320 | 0 |
| marinara sauce | 1 cup | 171 | 0 |
| spaghetti sauce | 15½ oz jar | 479 | 0 |
| **MIX** | | | |
| spaghetti sauce; not prep | 1 pkg 1.5 oz | 118 | 0 |
| w/mushrooms; not prep | 1 pkg 1.4 oz | 118 | 11 |

# SPICES
(*see* HERBS/SPICES)

# SPINACH

| FOOD | PORTION | CALORIES | CHOLESTEROL |
|------|---------|----------|-------------|
| **CANNED** | | | |
| Northwest Premium (S&W) | ½ cup | 25 | 0 |
| Spinach (Libby) | ½ cup | 25 | 0 |
| Spinach (Seneca) | ½ cup | 25 | 0 |
| spinach | ½ cup | 25 | 0 |
| **FRESH** | | | |
| cooked | ½ cup | 21 | 0 |
| raw; chopped | ½ cup | 6 | 0 |

| FOOD | PORTION | CALORIES | CHOLESTEROL |
|---|---|---|---|
| **FROZEN** | | | |
| Chopped (Birds Eye) | ⅓ cup | 22 | 0 |
| Chopped; cooked (Health Valley) | 7.2 oz | 57 | 0 |
| Creamed (Birds Eye) | ⅓ cup | 59 | tr |
| Leaf (Birds Eye) | ⅓ cup | 22 | 0 |
| Leaf; cooked (Health Valley) | 6.7 oz | 53 | 0 |
| Spinach Au Gratin (Budget Gourmet) | 6 oz | 120 | 40 |
| frzn; cooked | ½ cup | 27 | 0 |
| frzn; not prep | 10 oz pkg | 68 | 0 |

## SPORTS DRINKS

| | | | |
|---|---|---|---|
| thirst quencher | 1 cup | 60 | 0 |

## SQUAB

| | | | |
|---|---|---|---|
| **FRESH** | | | |
| breast, raw | 3.5 oz | 135 | 91 |

## SQUASH
(*see also* ZUCCHINI)

| | | | |
|---|---|---|---|
| **CANNED** | | | |
| crookneck; sliced | ½ cup | 14 | 0 |
| **FRESH** | | | |
| acorn; cooked, mashed | ½ cup | 41 | 0 |

| FOOD | PORTION | CALORIES | CHOLESTEROL |
|---|---|---|---|
| acorn; cubed, baked | ½ cup | 57 | 0 |
| butternut; baked | ½ cup | 41 | 0 |
| crookneck, iced; cooked | ½ cup | 18 | 0 |
| hubbard; baked | ½ cup | 51 | 0 |
| hubbard; cooked, mashed | ½ cup | 35 | 0 |
| scallop; cooked | ½ cup | 14 | 0 |
| spaghetti; cooked | ½ cup | 23 | 0 |
| summer, all varieties, raw; sliced | ½ cup | 13 | 0 |
| summer; sliced, cooked | ½ cup | 18 | 0 |
| winter, all varieties, raw; cubed | ½ cup | 21 | 0 |
| winter; cubed, cooked | ½ cup | 39 | 0 |
| FROZEN Butternut (Southland) | 4 oz | 45 | 0 |
| Winter Cooked (Birds Eye) | ⅓ cup | 45 | 0 |
| butternut; cooked, mashed | ½ cup | 47 | 0 |
| crookneck; sliced, cooked | ½ cup | 24 | 0 |
| SEEDS seeds, dried | 1 oz | 154 | 0 |
| seeds, whole, roasted | 1 oz | 127 | 0 |

# SQUID

| FRESH fried | 3 oz | 149 | 221 |
| raw | 3 oz | 78 | 198 |

| FOOD | PORTION | CALORIES | CHOLESTEROL |
|------|---------|----------|-------------|

# STRAWBERRY

**FRESH**

| | | | |
|------|---------|----------|-------------|
| strawberries | 1 cup | 45 | 0 |

**FROZEN**

| | | | |
|------|---------|----------|-------------|
| Strawberries Halved Quick Thaw (Birds Eye) | ½ cup | 119 | 0 |
| Strawberries Halved in Lite Syrup (Birds Eye) | ½ cup | 87 | 0 |
| Strawberries Whole in Lite Syrup (Birds Eye) | ½ cup | 81 | 0 |
| strawberries, sweetened | 1 cup | 200 | 0 |
| strawberries, unsweetened | 1 cup | 52 | 0 |

**JUICE**

| | | | |
|------|---------|----------|-------------|
| Strawberry (Smucker's) | 8 oz | 130 | 0 |

# STUFFING/DRESSING

| | | | |
|------|---------|----------|-------------|
| Beef (Stove Top) | ½ cup | 165 | 19 |
| Chicken (Stove Top) | ½ cup | 181 | 22 |
| Chicken Flexible Serve (Stove Top) | ½ cup | 180 | 17 |
| Chicken w/ Rice (Stove Top) | ½ cup | 184 | 22 |
| Cornbread (Stove Top) | ½ cup | 163 | 19 |

| FOOD | PORTION | CALORIES | CHOLESTEROL |
|------|---------|----------|-------------|
| Cornbread Flexible Serve (Stove Top) | ½ cup | 180 | 17 |
| Herb Homestyle Flexible Serve (Stove Top) | ½ cup | 180 | 17 |
| Long Grain & Wild Rice (Stove Top) | ½ cup | 184 | 22 |
| Pork (Stove Top) | ½ cup | 179 | 21 |
| San Francisco Style Americana (Stove Top) | ½ cup | 162 | 19 |
| Savory Herbs (Stove Top) | ½ cup | 180 | 22 |
| Select Chicken Florentine (Stove Top) | ½ cup | 203 | 31 |
| Select Garden Herb (Stove Top) | ½ cup | 219 | 34 |
| Select Vegetable & Almond (Stove Top) | ½ cup | 227 | 34 |
| Select Wild Rice & Mushroom (Stove Top) | ½ cup | 172 | 21 |
| Turkey (Stove Top) | ½ cup | 179 | 21 |
| **HOME RECIPE** | | | |
| bread; as prep w/ water & fat | ½ cup | 251 | tr |
| bread; as prep w/ water, egg & fat | ½ cup | 107 | 75 |
| sausage | ½ cup | 292 | 12 |

| FOOD | PORTION | CALORIES | CHOLESTEROL |
|------|---------|----------|-------------|

## SUCKER

**FRESH**

| | | | |
|------|---------|----------|-------------|
| white, raw | 3 oz | 79 | 35 |
| white, raw | 1 fillet (5.6 oz) | 147 | 66 |

## SUGAR
(*see also* FRUCTOSE, SUGAR SUBSTITUTE, SYRUP)

| | | | |
|------|---------|----------|-------------|
| brown | 1 cup | 836 | 0 |
| cube | 1 cube | 27 | 0 |
| powdered | 1 cup | 493 | 0 |
| white | 1 cup | 770 | 0 |

## SUGAR SUBSTITUTE
(*see also* FRUCTOSE)

| | | | |
|------|---------|----------|-------------|
| Adolph's | 1 tsp | 0 | 0 |
| Diamond | 1 tsp | tr | 0 |
| Spoon for Spoon | 1 tsp | 2 | 0 |
| Sucaryl | 1 tsp | 0 | 0 |
| Sugar Twin | 1 tsp | tr | 0 |
| Sweet'n Low Brown Sugar Substitute | 1/10 tsp | 2 | 0 |
| Sweet'n Low Granulated | 1 pkg (1 g) | 4 | 0 |
| Sweet'n Low Liquid | 10 drops | 0 | 0 |
| Sweet'n Low | 1 tsp | 12 | 0 |
| Sweet'n It (Estee) | 6 drops | 0 | 0 |

| FOOD | PORTION | CALORIES | CHOLESTEROL |
|---|---|---|---|

## SUNDAE TOPPINGS
(*see* ICE CREAM TOPPINGS)

## SUNFISH

FRESH
pumpkinseed, raw | 3 oz | 76 | 57

## SUNFLOWER SEEDS

| Sunflower (Planters) | 1 oz | 160 | 0 |
| Sunflower Nuts, Oil Roasted (Planters) | 1 oz | 170 | 0 |
| Sunflower Nuts, Dry Roasted (Planters) | 1 oz | 160 | 0 |
| Sunflower Nuts, Dry Roasted, Unsalted (Planters) | 1 oz | 170 | 0 |
| dried | 1 oz | 162 | 0 |
| dry roasted | 1 oz | 165 | 0 |
| oil roasted | 1 oz | 175 | 0 |
| sunflower butter | 1 Tbsp | 93 | 0 |
| toasted | 1 oz | 176 | 0 |

## SWEET POTATO
(*see also* YAM)

| CANNED Surf (American Original Foods) | 4 oz | 100 | 20 |
| Surf (American Original Foods) | 4 oz | 90 | 40 |
| in syrup pack | ½ cup | 106 | 0 |

| FOOD | PORTION | CALORIES | CHOLESTEROL |
|------|---------|----------|-------------|
| mashed | ½ cup | 233 | 0 |
| pieces | 1 cup | 183 | 0 |
| FRESH | | | |
| baked in skin | 1 (3½ oz) | 118 | 0 |
| mashed | ½ cup | 172 | 0 |
| raw | 1 (4.6 oz) | 136 | 0 |
| FROZEN | | | |
| frzn; baked | ½ cup | 88 | 0 |

## SWISS CHARD

| | | | |
|------|---------|----------|-------------|
| FRESH | | | |
| cooked | ½ cup | 18 | 0 |
| raw; chopped | ½ cup | 3 | 0 |

## SWORDFISH

| | | | |
|------|---------|----------|-------------|
| FRESH | | | |
| cooked | 1 piece (3.7 oz) | 164 | 53 |
| cooked | 3 oz | 132 | 43 |
| raw | 3 oz | 103 | 33 |
| raw | 1 piece (4.8 oz) | 164 | 54 |

## SYRUP
(*see also* ICE CREAM TOPPINGS, PANCAKE/WAFFLE SYRUP)

| | | | |
|------|---------|----------|-------------|
| All Flavors Fruit Syrup (Smucker's) | 2 Tbsp | 100 | 0 |
| Blueberry (Estee) | 1 Tbsp | 4 | 0 |

| FOOD | PORTION | CALORIES | CHOLESTEROL |
|------|---------|----------|-------------|
| Corn Syrup Light (Karo) | 1 Tbsp | 60 | 0 |
| Corn Syrup Light (Karo) | 1 cup | 960 | 0 |
| Corn Syrup Dark (Karo) | 1 Tbsp | 60 | 0 |
| Corn Syrup Dark (Karo) | 1 cup | 975 | 0 |
| Fruit Flavored, All Varieties (Smucker's) | 1 Tbsp | 50 | 0 |
| Maple Rich (Home Brands) | 1 oz | 110 | 0 |

## TAHINI
(*see* SESAME)

## TAMARIND

FRESH
| tamarind | 1 | 5 | 0 |

## TANGERINE

FRESH
| tangerine | 1 | 37 | 0 |

JUICE
| Mandarin Tangerine (Dole) | 6 oz | 97 | 0 |
| frzn, sweetened; as prep | 1 cup | 110 | 0 |
| frzn; not prep | 6 oz can | 344 | 0 |
| sweetened | 1 cup | 125 | 0 |

| FOOD | PORTION | CALORIES | CHOLESTEROL |
|------|---------|----------|-------------|

## TAPIOCA

| Minute Tapioca (General Foods) | 1 Tbsp | 35 | 0 |

## TEA/HERBAL TEA

HERBAL

| Almond Orange (Bigelow) | 5 oz | tr | 0 |
| Almond Sunset (Celestial Seasonings) | 1 cup | 3 | 0 |
| Apple Orchard (Bigelow) | 1 cup | 5 | 0 |
| Apple Spice (Bigelow) | 5 oz | tr | 0 |
| Chamomile (Bigelow) | 5 oz | tr | 0 |
| Chamomile (Celestial Seasonings) | 1 cup | 2 | 0 |
| Chamomile Mint (Bigelow) | 5 oz | tr | 0 |
| Cinnamon Apple Spice (Celestial Seasonings) | 1 cup | 3 | 0 |
| Cinnamon Orange (Bigelow) | 5 oz | tr | 0 |
| Cinnamon Rose (Celestial Seasonings) | 1 cup | 2 | 0 |
| Country Peach Spice (Celestial Seasonings) | 1 cup | 3 | 0 |
| Cranberry Cove (Celestial Seasonings) | 1 cup | 3 | 0 |
| Early Riser (Bigelow) | 1 cup | 3 | 0 |

| FOOD | PORTION | CALORIES | CHOLESTEROL |
|------|---------|----------|-------------|
| Emperor's Choice (Celestial Seasonings) | 1 cup | 4 | 0 |
| Feeling Free (Bigelow) | 1 cup | 1 | 0 |
| Fruit & Almond (Bigelow) | 1 cup | 1 | 0 |
| Ginseng Plus (Celestial Seasonings) | 1 cup | 3 | 0 |
| Grandma's Tummy Mints (Celestial Seasonings) | 1 cup | 2 | 0 |
| Hibiscus & Rose Hips (Bigelow) | 5 oz | 1 | 0 |
| I Love Lemon (Bigelow) | 1 cup | 1 | 0 |
| Lemon & C (Bigelow) | 5 oz | tr | 0 |
| Lemon Mist (Celestial Seasonings) | 1 cup | 2 | 0 |
| Lemon Zinger (Celestial Seasonings) | 1 cup | 4 | 0 |
| Looking Good (Bigelow) | 1 cup | 1 | 0 |
| Mandarin Orange Spice (Celestial Seasonings) | 1 cup | 5 | 0 |
| Mellow Mint (Celestial Seasonings) | 1 cup | 2 | 0 |
| Mint Blend (Bigelow) | 5 oz | tr | 0 |
| Mint Magic (Celestial Seasonings) | 1 cup | 1 | 0 |
| Mint Medley (Bigelow) | 1 cup | 1 | 0 |

| FOOD | PORTION | CALORIES | CHOLESTEROL |
|---|---|---|---|
| Mo's 24 (Celestial Seasonings) | 1 cup | 2 | 0 |
| Nice Over Ice (Bigelow) | 1 cup | 1 | 0 |
| Orange & C (Bigelow) | 5 oz | tr | 0 |
| Orange & Spice (Bigelow) | 1 cup | 1 | 0 |
| Orange Zinger (Celestial Seasonings) | 1 cup | 5 | 0 |
| Peppermint (Bigelow) | 5 oz | tr | 0 |
| Peppermint (Celestial Seasonings) | 1 cup | 2 | 0 |
| Raspberry Patch (Celestial Seasonings) | 1 cup | 4 | 0 |
| Red Zinger (Celestial Seasonings) | 1 cup | 4 | 0 |
| Roastaroma (Celestial Seasonings) | 1 cup | 11 | 0 |
| Roasted Grain & Carob (Bigelow) | 5 oz | 3 | 0 |
| Sleepytime (Celestial Seasonings) | 1 cup | 5 | 0 |
| Spearmint (Bigelow) | 5 oz | tr | 0 |
| Spearmint (Celestial Seasonings) | 1 cup | 5 | 0 |
| Strawberry Fields (Celestial Seasonings) | 1 cup | 4 | 0 |
| Sunburst C (Celestial Seasonings) | 1 cup | 3 | 0 |

| FOOD | PORTION | CALORIES | CHOLESTEROL |
|------|---------|----------|-------------|
| Sweet Dreams (Bigelow) | 1 cup | 1 | 0 |
| Take-A-Break (Bigelow) | 1 cup | 3 | 0 |
| Wild Forest Blueberry (Celestial Seasonings) | 1 cup | 2 | 0 |
| **REGULAR** Amaretto Nights (Celestial Seasonings) | 1 cup | 3 | 0 |
| Apple Spice and Tea (Celestial Seasonings) | 1 cup | tr | 0 |
| Bavarian Chocolate Orange (Celestial Seasonings) | 1 cup | 7 | 0 |
| Caffeine-Free (Celestial Seasonings) | 1 cup | 4 | 0 |
| Chinese Fortune (Bigelow) | 1 cup | 1 | 0 |
| Cinnamon Stick (Bigelow) | 1 cup | 1 | 0 |
| Cinnamon Vienna (Celestial Seasonings) | 1 cup | 2 | 0 |
| Classic English Breakfast (Celestial Seasonings) | 1 cup | 3 | 0 |
| Constant Comment (Bigelow) | 1 cup | 1 | 0 |
| Darjeeling Gardens (Celestial Seasonings) | 1 cup | 3 | 0 |
| Darjeeling Blend (Bigelow) | 1 cup | 1 | 0 |
| Earl Grey (Bigelow) | 1 cup | 1 | 0 |

| FOOD | PORTION | CALORIES | CHOLESTEROL |
|------|---------|----------|-------------|
| English Teatime (Bigelow) | 1 cup | 1 | 0 |
| Extraordinary Earl Grey (Celestial Seasonings) | 1 cup | 3 | 0 |
| Fruit Tea Fruit Cooler; as prep (Lipton) | 8 oz | 87 | 0 |
| Iced Berry Tea; as prep (Crystal Light) | 8 oz | 3 | 0 |
| Iced Tea (SIPPS) | 8.45 oz | 100 | 0 |
| Iced Tea (Shasta) | 12 oz | 124 | 0 |
| Irish Cream Mist (Celestial Seasonings) | 1 cup | 3 | 0 |
| Lemon Lift (Bigelow) | 1 cup | 1 | 0 |
| Lemons and Tea (Celestial Seasonings) | 1 cup | tr | 0 |
| Morning Thunder (Celestial Seasonings) | 1 cup | 3 | 0 |
| Orange Pekoe (Bigelow) | 1 cup | 1 | 0 |
| Orange Spice and Tea (Celestial Seasonings) | 1 cup | tr | 0 |
| Peppermint Stick (Bigelow) | 1 cup | 1 | 0 |
| Plantation Mint (Bigelow) | 1 cup | 1 | 0 |
| Raspberries and Tea (Celestial Seasonings) | 1 cup | 2 | 0 |
| Raspberry Royale (Bigelow) | 1 cup | 1 | 0 |

| FOOD | PORTION | CALORIES | CHOLESTEROL |
|---|---|---|---|
| Swiss Mint (Celestial Seasonings) | 1 cup | tr | 0 |
| instant, sugar sweetened, lemon flavor powder; as prep w/ water | 9 oz | 87 | 0 |
| instant, unsweetened powder; as prep w/ water | 8 oz | 2 | 0 |
| instant, unsweetened, lemon flavor powder; as prep w/ water | 8 oz | 4 | 0 |
| tea | 6 oz | 2 | 0 |

## TEMPEH

| | | | |
|---|---|---|---|
| tempeh | ½ cup | 165 | 0 |

## TEXTURED VEGETABLE PROTEIN
(see also MEAT SUBSTITUTE, SOY)

| | | | |
|---|---|---|---|
| simulated meat products | 1 oz | 88 | 0 |

## TOFU
(see also ICE CREAM, NON-DAIRY)

| | | | |
|---|---|---|---|
| fried | 1 piece (½ oz) | 35 | 0 |
| fuyu, salted & fermented | 1 block (⅓ oz) | 13 | 0 |
| koyadofu, dried, frozen | 1 piece (½ oz) | 82 | 0 |
| raw, firm | ¼ block (3 oz) | 118 | 0 |
| raw, regular | ¼ block (4 oz) | 88 | 0 |

| FOOD | PORTION | CALORIES | CHOLESTEROL |
|------|---------|----------|-------------|

# TOFUTTI
(see ICE CREAM, NON-DAIRY)

# TOMATO
(see also PIZZA, SPAGHETTI SAUCE)

| FOOD | PORTION | CALORIES | CHOLESTEROL |
|------|---------|----------|-------------|
| CANNED | | | |
| Aspic Supreme (S&W) | ½ cup | 60 | 0 |
| California Sliced (Contadina) | ½ cup | 40 | 0 |
| Crushed Tomatoes in Tomato Puree (Contadina) | ½ cup | 30 | 0 |
| Diced Tomatoes in Rich Puree (S&W) | ½ cup | 35 | 0 |
| Italian Paste (Contadina) | 2 oz | 65 | tr |
| Italian Stewed (S&W) | ½ cup | 35 | 0 |
| Italian Style (Contadina) | ½ cup | 25 | 0 |
| Italian Style Stewed (Cantadina) | ½ cup | 35 | 0 |
| Italian Style w/ Basil (S&W) | ½ cup | 25 | 0 |
| Kosher Tomatoes (Claussen) | 1 | 9 | 0 |
| Paste (Contadina) | 2 oz | 50 | 0 |
| Paste (S&W) | 6 oz | 150 | 0 |

| FOOD | PORTION | CALORIES | CHOLESTEROL |
|------|---------|----------|-------------|
| Peeled Ready Cut (S&W) | ½ cup | 25 | 0 |
| Puree (Contadina) | ½ cup | 40 | 0 |
| Puree (S&W) | ½ cup | 60 | 0 |
| Sauce (S&W) | ½ cup | 40 | 0 |
| Sauce, Thick & Zesty (Contadina) | ½ cup | 40 | 0 |
| Stewed (Contadina) | ½ cup | 35 | 0 |
| Stewed Tomatoes (S&W) | ½ cup | 35 | 0 |
| Stewed Tomatoes 50% Salt Reduced (S&W) | ½ cup | 35 | 0 |
| Tomato Sauce (Health Valley) | 4 oz | 30 | 0 |
| Tomato Sauce No Salt Added (Health Valley) | 4 oz | 30 | 0 |
| Whole Peeled (Contadina) | ½ cup | 25 | 0 |
| Whole Peeled (S&W) | ½ cup | 25 | 0 |
| red, whole | 1 cup | 47 | 0 |
| sauce, spanish style | ½ cup | 40 | 0 |
| stewed | 1 cup | 68 | 0 |
| tomato paste | ½ cup | 110 | 0 |
| tomato puree | 1 cup | 102 | 0 |

| FOOD | PORTION | CALORIES | CHOLESTEROL |
|---|---|---|---|
| tomato sauce | 1 cup | 74 | 0 |
| tomato sauce w/ mushrooms | 1 cup | 85 | 0 |
| tomato sauce w/ onion | ½ cup | 50 | 0 |
| tomato sauce w/ tomato tidbits | ½ cup | 39 | 0 |
| wedges in tomato juice | 1 cup | 67 | 0 |
| FRESH green | 1 | 30 | 0 |
| red | 1 | 24 | 0 |
| scalloped | ½ cup | 88 | 8 |
| stewed | 1 cup | 59 | 0 |
| JUICE California (S&W) | 5½ oz | 35 | 0 |
| tomato juice | 6 fl oz | 32 | 0 |

## TONGUE

| | | | |
|---|---|---|---|
| beef, raw | 4 oz | 252 | 98 |
| beef; simmered | 3 oz | 241 | 91 |
| pork, raw | 4 oz | 254 | 114 |
| pork; braised | 3 oz | 230 | 124 |

## TOPPINGS
(*see* ICE CREAM TOPPINGS)

## TORTILLA CHIPS
(*see* CHIPS)

| FOOD | PORTION | CALORIES | CHOLESTEROL |
|---|---|---|---|
| **TROUT** | | | |
| **FRESH** | | | |
| rainbow, raw | 3 oz | 100 | 48 |
| rainbow, raw | 1 fillet (2.8 oz) | 93 | 45 |
| rainbow; cooked | 1 fillet (2.1 oz) | 94 | 45 |
| rainbow; cooked | 3 oz | 129 | 62 |
| seatrout, raw | 1 fillet (8.4 oz) | 248 | 198 |
| seatrout, raw | 3 oz | 88 | 71 |
| **TUNA** | | | |
| (*see also* TUNA DISHES) | | | |
| **CANNED** | | | |
| Chunk Light in Oil (Bumble Bee) | 3 oz | 200 | 30 |
| Chunk Light in Water (Bumble Bee) | 3 oz | 90 | 30 |
| Chunk White in Oil (Bumble Bee) | 3 oz | 200 | 30 |
| Chunk White in Water (Bumble Bee) | 3 oz | 90 | 30 |
| Solid White in Oil (Bumble Bee) | 3 oz | 190 | 30 |
| Solid White in Water (Bumble Bee) | 3 oz | 90 | 30 |
| Tuna (Health Valley) | 6.5 oz | 180 | 30 |
| Tuna Diet No Salt (Health Valley) | 6.5 oz | 200 | 30 |

| FOOD | PORTION | CALORIES | CHOLESTEROL |
|---|---|---|---|
| Tuna Salad (The Spreadables) | ¼ can | 90 | 13 |
| light in oil | 3 oz | 169 | 15 |
| light in oil | 1 can (6 oz) | 399 | 30 |
| white in oil | 3 oz | 158 | 26 |
| white in oil | 1 can (6.2 oz) | 331 | 55 |
| white in water | 1 can (6 oz) | 234 | 72 |
| white in water | 3 oz | 116 | 35 |
| FRESH bluefin, raw | 3 oz | 122 | 32 |
| bluefin; cooked | 3 oz | 157 | 42 |
| skipjack, raw | 3 oz | 88 | 40 |
| skipjack, raw | ½ fillet (6.9 oz) | 204 | 93 |
| yellowfin, raw | 3 oz | 92 | 38 |
| READY-TO-USE Salad (Wampler Longacre) | 1 oz | 61 | 7 |
| tuna salad | 3 oz | 159 | 11 |
| tuna salad | 1 cup | 383 | 27 |

# TUNA DISHES

| | | | |
|---|---|---|---|
| Tuna Sandwich (Micrwave Chefwich) | 1 (5 oz) | 380 | 28 |
| HOME RECIPE pattie | 1 (3 oz) | 228 | 69 |

| FOOD | PORTION | CALORIES | CHOLESTEROL |
|------|---------|----------|-------------|
| stuffed green pepper | 1 (9.9 oz) | 261 | 59 |
| tuna casserole | ¾ cup | 299 | 56 |

# TURKEY
(*see also* DINNER, HOT DOG, TURKEY DISHES, TURKEY SUBSTITUTE)

| FOOD | PORTION | CALORIES | CHOLESTEROL |
|------|---------|----------|-------------|
| CANNED | | | |
| Turkey Salad (The Spreadables) | ¼ can | 100 | 20 |
| FRESH | | | |
| Breast (Land O'Lakes) | 3 oz | 100 | 50 |
| Breast Boneless Roast, Fresh Young; cooked (Perdue) | 3 oz | 162 | 63 |
| Breast, Fresh Young, meat only; cooked | 3 oz | 162 | 63 |
| Breast Half, Fresh Young, meat only; cooked (Perdue) | 3 oz | 162 | 63 |
| Breast Hen w/ Wing; cooked (Louis Rich) | 1 oz | 53 | 16 |
| Breast Hen w/o Back; cooked (Louis Rich) | 1 oz | 47 | 17 |
| Breast Hen w/o Wing; cooked (Louis Rich) | 1 oz | 53 | 11 |
| Breast Roast; cooked (Louis Rich) | 1 oz | 41 | 18 |
| Breast Slices; cooked (Louis Rich) | 1 oz | 44 | 13 |
| Breast Steak Fresh Young; cooked (Perdue) | 3 oz | 115 | 71 |

| FOOD | PORTION | CALORIES | CHOLESTEROL |
|---|---|---|---|
| Breast Steaks; cooked (Louis Rich) | 1 oz | 40 | 19 |
| Breast Tender-loins, Fresh Young; cooked (Perdue) | 3 oz | 115 | 71 |
| Breast Tender-loins; cooked (Louis Rich) | 1 oz | 41 | 11 |
| Breast; cooked (Louis Rich) | 1 oz | 50 | 12 |
| Drumsticks, Fresh Young, meat only; cooked (Perdue) | 3 oz | 173 | 73 |
| Drumsticks; cooked (Louis Rich) | 1 oz | 55 | 33 |
| Ground Lean 90% Fat Free; cooked (Louis Rich) | 3.5 oz | 183 | 85 |
| Ground Lean 90% Fat Free; cooked (Louis Rich) | 1 oz | 51 | 24 |
| Ground Turkey (Bil Mar Foods) | 3 oz | 163 | 60 |
| Ground; cooked (Louis Rich) | 1 oz | 61 | 24 |
| Ground; cooked (Louis Rich) | 3.5 oz | 217 | 87 |
| Thighs Boneless, Fresh Young; cooked (Perdue) | 3 oz | 153 | 70 |
| Thighs, Fresh Young, meat only; cooked (Perdue) | 3 oz | 211 | 73 |
| Thighs; cooked (Louis Rich) | 1 oz | 65 | 28 |

| FOOD | PORTION | CALORIES | CHOLESTEROL |
|---|---|---|---|
| Whole, Fresh Young, meat only; cooked (Perdue) | 3 oz | 178 | 70 |
| Whole; cooked (Louis Rich) | 3.5 oz | 200 | 18 |
| Whole; cooked (Louis Rich) | 1 oz | 56 | 18 |
| Wing Drumettes; cooked (Louis Rich) | 1 oz | 52 | 20 |
| Wings, Fresh Young, meat only; cooked (Perdue) | 3 oz | 196 | 69 |
| Wings Drummettes, Fresh Young, meat only; cooked (Perdue) | 3 oz | 196 | 69 |
| Wing Portions, Fresh Young, meat only; cooked (Perdue) | 3 oz | 196 | 69 |
| Wings; cooked (Louis Rich) | 1 oz | 54 | 26 |
| Young Whole (Land O'Lakes) | 3 oz | 130 | 65 |
| Young, Whole, Butter Basted (Land O'Lakes) | 3 oz | 140 | 85 |
| Young, Whole, Self-Basting (Land O'Lakes) | 3 oz | 120 | 77 |
| back, meat & skin, raw | ½ back (1.1 lbs) | 940 | 416 |
| back, meat & skin, raw | 1.6 oz | 81 | 36 |
| back, meat & skin; roasted | ½ back (13.3 oz) | 903 | 358 |
| breast, meat & skin, raw | ½ breast (3.9 lbs) | 2700 | 1195 |

| FOOD | PORTION | CALORIES | CHOLESTEROL |
|---|---|---|---|
| breast, meat & skin, raw | 5.4 oz | 234 | 103 |
| breast, meat & skin; roasted | 4 oz | 217 | 87 |
| breast, meat & skin; roasted | ½ breast (2.9 lbs) | 2510 | 1002 |
| dark meat w/ skin, raw | 5.3 oz | 232 | 117 |
| dark meat w/ skin, raw | ½ turkey (3.9 lbs) | 2681 | 1355 |
| dark meat w/ skin; roasted | ½ turkey (2.6 lbs) | 2553 | 1081 |
| dark meat w/ skin; roasted | 3.6 oz | 222 | 94 |
| dark meat w/o skin, raw | 4.7 oz | 163 | 99 |
| dark meat w/o skin, raw | ½ turkey (3.4 lbs) | 1879 | 1142 |
| dark meat w/o skin; roasted | 1 cup | 260 | 123 |
| dark meat w/o skin; roasted | 3.2 oz | 167 | 79 |
| flesh & skin, raw | ½ turkey (8.5 lbs) | 6013 | 2796 |
| flesh & skin, raw | 11.9 oz | 522 | 243 |
| flesh & skin; roasted | ½ turkey (6 lbs) | 5545 | 2265 |
| flesh & skin; roasted | 8.4 oz | 482 | 197 |
| flesh, raw | ½ turkey (7.2 lbs) | 3867 | 2240 |
| flesh, raw | 10 oz | 335 | 194 |
| flesh; roasted | 7.2 oz | 345 | 159 |
| flesh; roasted | 1 cup | 235 | 108 |
| leg, meat & skin, raw | 2.7 lbs | 1736 | 939 |
| leg, meat & skin, raw | 3.8 oz | 150 | 81 |
| leg, meat & skin; roasted | 2.5 oz | 144 | 63 |

| FOOD | PORTION | CALORIES | CHOLESTEROL |
|---|---|---|---|
| leg, meat & skin; roasted | 1.8 lbs | 1660 | 727 |
| light meat w/ skin, raw | 6.5 oz | 288 | 125 |
| light meat w/ skin, raw | ½ turkey (4.7 lbs) | 3331 | 1439 |
| light meat w/ skin; roasted | ½ turkey (3.4 lbs) | 2992 | 1182 |
| light meat w/ skin; roasted | 4.8 oz | 260 | 103 |
| light meat w/o skin, raw | 5.4 oz | 176 | 95 |
| light meat w/o skin, raw | ½ turkey (3.9 lbs) | 2023 | 1097 |
| light meat w/o skin; roasted | 1 cup | 2153 | 97 |
| light meat w/o skin; roasted | 4.1 oz | 180 | 81 |
| neck, meat, raw | 1 neck (6.3 oz) | 243 | 142 |
| neck, meat; simmered | 1 neck (5.3 oz) | 274 | 186 |
| skin, raw | ½ turkey (1.3 lbs) | 2180 | 564 |
| skin, raw | 1.8 oz | 188 | 49 |
| skin; roasted | ½ turkey (13.1 oz) | 1578 | 436 |
| skin; roasted | 1 oz | 135 | 37 |
| whole, flesh, skin, giblets & neck, raw | 18.4 lbs | 12799 | 6826 |
| whole, flesh, skin, giblets & neck; roasted | 13.1 lbs | 11873 | 5745 |
| whole, flesh, skin, giblets & neck; roasted | 10 oz | 514 | 249 |
| wing, meat & skin, raw | 1 oz | 57 | 22 |

| FOOD | PORTION | CALORIES | CHOLESTEROL |
|---|---|---|---|
| wing, meat & skin, raw | 12.2 oz | 656 | 250 |
| wing, meat & skin; roasted | 8.3 oz | 524 | 192 |
| roast, boneless, seasoned, light & dark meat, raw | 10 oz | 340 | |
| **FROZEN PREPARED** | | | |
| Kibun Turkey Pasta Salad w/ dressing | ½ pkg | 250 | 15 |
| Kibun Turkey Pasta Salad w/o dressing | ½ pkg | 140 | 10 |
| **READY-TO-USE** | | | |
| Baked Ham (Wampler Longacre) | 1 oz | 38 | 22 |
| Baked Ham w/ 12% water (Wampler Longacre) | 1 oz | 33 | 19 |
| Baked Ham w/ 20% water (Wampler Longacre) | 1 oz | 39 | 16 |
| Bologna (Louis Rich) | 1 slice (28 g) | 59 | 20 |
| Bologna (Wampler Longacre) | 1 oz | 56 | 22 |
| Bologna Mild (Louis Rich) | 1 slice (28 g) | 61 | 13 |
| Bologna Red Rind (Mr. Turkey) | 1 oz | 63 | 20 |
| Bologna Sliced (Wampler Longacre) | 1 oz | 57 | 21 |
| Breast Barbecued (Louis Rich) | 1 oz | 36 | 11 |
| Breast & White Turkey Deli Chef (Wampler Longacre) | 1 oz | 35 | 12 |

| FOOD | PORTION | CALORIES | CHOLESTEROL |
|------|---------|----------|-------------|
| Breast & White Turkey No Skin Covering (Wampler Longacre) | 1 oz | 39 | 11 |
| Breast BBQ Quarter (Mr. Turkey) | 1 oz | 34 | 11 |
| Breast Fillets w/ Cheese (Land O'Lakes) | 5 oz | 300 | 35 |
| Breast Gourmet (Wampler Longacre) | 1 oz | 31 | 10 |
| Breast Gourmet Browned & Roasted (Wampler Longacre) | 1 oz | 35 | 16 |
| Breast Gourmet Browned & Glazed (Wampler Longacre) | 1 oz | 28 | 11 |
| Breast Gourmet Skinless (Wampler Longacre) | 1 oz | 28 | 10 |
| Breast Hickory Smoked (Louis Rich) | 1 oz | 31 | 12 |
| Breast Honey Roasted (Louis Rich) | 1 slice (28 g) | 29 | 11 |
| Breast Mini Gourmet (Wampler Longacre) | 1 oz | 35 | 15 |
| Breast Oven Roasted (Louis Rich) | 1 slice (28 g) | 31 | 11 |
| Breast Oven Roasted (Louis Rich) | 1 oz | 30 | 11 |
| Breast Oven Roasted Oven Lite (Wampler Longacre) | 1 oz | 35 | 14 |
| Breast Oven Roasted Quarter (Mr. Turkey) | 1 oz | 34 | 12 |

| FOOD | PORTION | CALORIES | CHOLESTEROL |
|---|---|---|---|
| Breast Premium (Wampler Longacre) | 1 oz | 29 | 11 |
| Breast Premium Browned & Glazed (Wampler Longacre) | 1 oz | 29 | 11 |
| Breast Premium Skinless (Wampler Longacre) | 1 oz | 26 | 8 |
| Breast Premium Skinless Browned & Roasted (Wampler Longacre) | 1 oz | 26 | 8 |
| Breast Roll Sliced (Wampler Longacre) | 1 oz | 37 | 10 |
| Breast Salt Watchers (Wampler Longacre) | 1 oz | 35 | 19 |
| Breast Skinless Gourmet High Yield (Wampler Longacre) | 1 oz | 28 | 10 |
| Breast Smoked (Bil Mar Foods) | 1 oz | 31 | 10 |
| Breast Smoked Chunk (Louis Rich) | 1 oz | 34 | 11 |
| Breast Smoked Gourmet (Wampler Longacre) | 1 oz | 37 | 15 |
| Breast Smoked Lean-Lite (Wampler Longacre) | 1 oz | 38 | 16 |
| Breast Smoked Mini Gourmet (Wampler Longacre) | 1 oz | 37 | 15 |
| Breast Smoked Quarter (Mr. Turkey) | 1 oz | 35 | 10 |
| Breast Smoked Sliced (Louis Rich) | 1 slice (21 g) | 21 | 7 |
| Breast Smoked Sliced (Wampler Longacre) | 1 oz | 27 | 9 |

| FOOD | PORTION | CALORIES | CHOLESTEROL |
|---|---|---|---|
| Breasts, Bronze Label (Land O'Lakes) | 3 oz | 100 | 50 |
| Breasts, Gold Label, Browned (Land O'Lakes) | 3 oz | 120 | 55 |
| Breasts, Gold Label, Skin On (Land O'Lakes) | 3 oz | 120 | 55 |
| Breasts, Gold Label, Skinless (Land O'Lakes) | 3 oz. | 90 | 50 |
| Breasts, Silver Label (Land O'Lakes) | 3 oz | 100 | 50 |
| Cheese Patties (Bil Mar Foods) | 3 oz | 213 | 37 |
| Chunk Ham w/ 12% water (Wampler Longacre) | 1 oz | 36 | 20 |
| Chunk Ham w/ 20% water (Wampler Longacre) | 1 oz | 39 | 16 |
| Chunk Pastrami (Wampler Longacre) | 1 oz | 35 | 24 |
| Cotto Salami (Louis Rich) | 1 slice (28 g) | 52 | 22 |
| Cotto Salami (Mr. Turkey) | 1 oz | 45 | 16 |
| Dark Smoked Cured (Wampler Longacre) | 1 oz | 45 | 21 |
| Diced Combination Roll (Wampler Longacre) | 1 oz | 43 | 14 |
| Diced Ham w/ 20% water (Wampler Longacre) | 1 oz | 39 | 16 |
| Diced White Roll (Wampler Longacre) | 1 oz | 43 | 12 |
| Diced, White/Dark Mixed (Land O'Lakes) | 3 oz | 120 | 35 |

| FOOD | PORTION | CALORIES | CHOLESTEROL |
|------|---------|----------|-------------|
| Ham (Land O'Lakes) | 3 oz | 100 | 55 |
| Ham Chopped (Louis Rich) | 1 slice (28 g) | 42 | 17 |
| Ham Cured Thigh Meat (Louis Rich) | 1 slice (28 g) | 34 | 19 |
| Ham Cured Thigh Meat Square (Louis Rich) | 1 slice (21 g) | 24 | 12 |
| Ham Cured Thigh Meat Water Added (Louis Rich) | 1 slice (28 g) | 34 | 18 |
| Ham Honey Cured (Louis Rich) | 1 slice (21 g) | 25 | 15 |
| Ham Lean-Lite (Wampler Longacre) | 1 oz | 36 | 6 |
| Ham Sliced (Wampler Longacre) | 1 oz | 37 | 17 |
| Ham Smoked Breakfast (Mr. Turkey) | 1 oz | 33 | 16 |
| Ham Smoked Buffet Style (Bil Mar Foods) | 1 oz | 32 | 17 |
| Luncheon Loaf (Louis Rich) | 1 slice (28 g) | 43 | 14 |
| Luncheon Loaf Square Spiced (Bil Mar Foods) | 1 slice (1 oz) | 51 | 11 |
| Nuggets (Mr. Turkey) | 1 nugget | 33 | 6 |
| Nuggets White Breaded Fully Cooked (Wampler Longacre) | 1 oz | 87 | 13 |

| FOOD | PORTION | CALORIES | CHOLESTEROL |
|---|---|---|---|
| Oscar Mayer Breast Oven Roasted | 1 slice (21 g) | 22 | 9 |
| Oscar Mayer Breast Smoked | 1 slice (21 g) | 20 | 9 |
| Pastrami (Bil Mar Foods) | 1 slice (1 oz) | 28 | 17 |
| Pastrami (Louis Rich) | 1 slice (28 g) | 33 | 14 |
| Pastrami (Wampler Longacre) | 1 oz | 35 | 24 |
| Pastrami Sliced (Wampler Longacre) | 1 oz | 34 | 20 |
| Pastrami Square (Louis Rich) | 1 slice (23 g) | 23 | 13 |
| Patties (Land O'Lakes) | 2¼ oz | 170 | 30 |
| Patties (Mr. Turkey) | 3 oz | 195 | 36 |
| Roast White w/ Gravy (Land O'Lakes) | 3 oz | 110 | 20 |
| Roast White/Dark w/ Gravy (Land O'Lakes) | 3 oz | 120 | 20 |
| Roasted Thighs (Wampler Longacre) | 1 oz | 38 | 18 |
| Roll Breast & White Turkey (Deli Chef) | 1 oz | 39 | 10 |
| Roll Combination Turkey (Wampler Longacre) | 1 oz | 43 | 14 |
| Roll White Turkey (Wampler Longacre) | 1 oz | 43 | 12 |

| FOOD | PORTION | CALORIES | CHOLESTEROL |
|---|---|---|---|
| Roll, Blue Label, Mixed (Land O'Lakes) | 3 oz | 120 | 50 |
| Roll, Blue Label, White (Land O'Lakes) | 3 oz | 110 | 50 |
| Roll, Red Label, Mixed (Land O'Lakes) | 3 oz | 110 | 50 |
| Roll, Red Label, White (Land O'Lakes) | 3 oz | 110 | 50 |
| Salad (Wampler Longacre) | 1 oz | 71 | 15 |
| Salami (Louis Rich) | 1 slice (28 g) | 52 | 20 |
| Salami (Wampler Longacre) | 1 oz | 45 | 21 |
| Salami Sliced (Wampler Longacre) | 1 oz | 46 | 25 |
| Smoked (Louis Rich) | 1 slice (28 g) | 33 | 12 |
| Sticks (Mr. Turkey) | 1 stick | 65 | 12 |
| Summer Sausage (Louis Rich) | 1 slice (28 g) | 52 | 22 |
| Turkey (Carl Buddig) | 1 oz | 50 | 6 |
| Turkey Bologna (Mr. Turkey) | 1 oz | 63 | 20 |
| Turkey Breakfast Sausage; cooked (Louis Rich) | 1 (1 oz) | 59 | 22 |
| Turkey Breast (Bil Mar Foods) | 1 slice (1 oz) | 31 | 10 |

| FOOD | PORTION | CALORIES | CHOLESTEROL |
|---|---|---|---|
| Turkey Breast Smoked Sliced (Bil Mar Foods) | 1 oz | 31 | 10 |
| Turkey Ham (Carl Buddig) | 1 oz | 40 | 19 |
| Turkey Ham Smoked (Bil Mar Foods) | 1 oz | 32 | 18 |
| Turkey Ham Square Chopped (Bil Mar Foods) | 1 slice (1 oz) | 37 | 17 |
| Turkey Ham w/ 20% Water (Wampler Longacre) | 1 oz | 39 | 16 |
| Turkey Salami (Carl Buddig) | 1 oz | 40 | 19 |
| Turkey Smoked Sausage w/ Cheese; cooked (Louis Rich) | 1 (1 oz) | 58 | 19 |
| Turkey Smoked Sausage; cooked (Louis Rich) | 1 (1 oz) | 55 | 19 |
| Turkey Sticks (Land O'Lakes) | 2 (1 oz each) | 150 | 25 |
| White Meat, Diced (Mr. Turkey) | 2 oz | 84 | 32 |
| Whole Smoked (Wampler Longacre) | 1 oz | 40 | 16 |
| bologna, turkey | 1 slice (28 g) | 57 | 28 |
| breast | 1 slice (21 g) | 23 | 9 |
| breast | 1 oz | 47 | 17 |

| FOOD | PORTION | CALORIES | CHOLESTEROL |
|------|---------|----------|-------------|
| poultry salad sandwich spread | 1 Tbsp | 109 | 4 |
| poultry salad sandwich spread | 1 oz | 238 | 9 |
| prebasted breast, meat & skin; roasted | 3.8 lbs | 2175 | 718 |
| prebasted breast, meat & skin; roasted | ½ breast (1.9 lbs) | 1087 | 359 |
| prebasted thigh, meat & skin; roasted | 11 oz | 494 | 194 |
| prebasted thigh, meat & skin; roasted | 2 thighs (1.4 lbs) | 990 | 389 |
| roll, light & dark meat | 1 slice (28 g) | 42 | 16 |
| roll, light meat | 1 slice (28 g) | 42 | 12 |
| salami, cooked | 1 pkg (8 oz) | 446 | 186 |
| salami, cooked | 1 slice (28 g) | 56 | 23 |
| turkey loaf, breast meat | 2 slices (1.5 oz) | 47 | 17 |
| turkey loaf, breast meat | 1 pkg (6 oz) | 187 | 69 |

# TURKEY DISHES

(*see also* DINNER, TURKEY SUBSTITUTE)

**HOME RECIPE**

| | | | |
|------|------|------|------|
| stew | ¾ cup | 336 | 138 |

| FOOD | PORTION | CALORIES | CHOLESTEROL |
|------|---------|----------|-------------|
| turkey loaf | 1 slice (4.7 oz) | 263 | 138 |

## TURKEY SUBSTITUTE

| | | | |
|------|---------|----------|-------------|
| Meatless Turkey (Loma Linda) | 2 slices (2 oz) | 95 | 0 |
| Smoked Turkey, frzn (Worthington) | 3.5 oz | 239 | 2 |

## TURNIP

| | | | |
|------|---------|----------|-------------|
| CANNED | | | |
| greens | ½ cup | 17 | 0 |
| FRESH | | | |
| greens, raw; chopped | ½ cup | 7 | 0 |
| greens; chopped, cooked | ½ cup | 15 | 0 |
| raw; cubed | ½ cup | 18 | 0 |
| FROZEN | | | |
| frzn; not prep | 10 oz pkg | 44 | 0 |
| greens & turnips; not prep | 10 oz pkg | 59 | 0 |
| greens; cooked | ½ cup | 24 | 0 |
| greens; not prep | 10 oz pkg | 62 | 0 |

## VANILLA EXTRACT

| | | | |
|------|---------|----------|-------------|
| Pure Vanilla Extract (Virginia Dare) | 1 tsp | 10 | 0 |

| FOOD | PORTION | CALORIES | CHOLESTEROL |
|---|---|---|---|

# VEAL
(*see also* BEEF, VEAL DISHES)

FRESH

| FOOD | PORTION | CALORIES | CHOLESTEROL |
|---|---|---|---|
| cutlet, w/ bone, lean & fat; cooked | 3 oz | 184 | 86 |
| loin chop, w/ bone, lean & fat; cooked | 1 sm (2.9 oz) | 190 | 82 |
| loin chop, w/ bone, lean & fat; cooked | 1 med (3.9 oz) | 257 | 111 |
| loin chop, w/ bone, lean only; cooked | 1 sm (2.4 oz) | 143 | 68 |
| loin chop, w/ bone, lean only; cooked | 1 med (3.3 oz) | 194 | 93 |
| loin roast, w/ bone, lean & fat; roasted | 3 oz | 199 | 86 |
| loin roast, w/ bone, lean only; roasted | 3 oz | 130 | 84 |
| rib chop, w/bone, lean & fat; cooked | 1 med (3.5 oz) | 269 | 99 |
| round, lean & fat; chopped, cooked | ½ cup | 151 | 71 |
| round, lean & fat; ground, cooked | ½ cup | 119 | 56 |
| round, patty; cooked | 3 oz | 184 | 86 |
| shoulder arm roast, w/o bone, lean & fat; braised | 3 oz | 200 | 86 |
| shoulder arm roast, w/o bone, lean only; braised | 3 oz | 170 | 84 |
| shoulder arm steak, w/ bone, lean only; cooked | 3.5 oz | 196 | 97 |

| FOOD | PORTION | CALORIES | CHOLESTEROL |
|---|---|---|---|

## VEAL DISHES

HOME RECIPE
| parmigiana | 4.2 oz | 279 | 136 |
| veal loaf | 1 slice (4.7 oz) | 270 | 135 |

## VEGETABLES, MIXED
(*see also individual vegetables*)

| | | | |
|---|---|---|---|
| CANNED | | | |
| Beets Pickled w/ Onions (Libby) | ½ cup | 80 | 0 |
| Beets Pickled w/ Onions (Seneca) | ½ cup | 80 | 0 |
| Garden Salad Marinated (S&W) | ½ cup | 60 | 0 |
| Green Beans & Wax Beans (S&W) | ½ cup | 20 | 0 |
| Mixed Vegetables (Hanover) | ½ cup | 110 | 0 |
| Mixed Vegetables (Libby) | ½ cup | 40 | 0 |
| Mixed Vegetables (Seneca) | ½ cup | 40 | 0 |
| Mixed Vegetables Old Fashioned Harvest Time (S&W) | ½ cup | 35 | 0 |
| Okra Creole Gumbo (Trappey's) | ½ cup | 25 | 0 |
| Okra Cut & Tomatoes (Trappey's) | ½ cup | 25 | 0 |

| FOOD | PORTION | CALORIES | CHOLESTEROL |
|------|---------|----------|-------------|
| Okra Cut, Tomatoes & Corn (Trappey's) | ½ cup | 25 | 0 |
| Peas & Carrots (Libby) | ½ cup | 50 | 0 |
| Peas & Carrots (Seneca) | ½ cup | 50 | 0 |
| Succotash (Libby) | ½ cup | 80 | 0 |
| Succotash (Seneca) | ½ cup | 80 | 0 |
| Succotash Country Style (S&W) | ½ cup | 80 | 0 |
| Sweet Peas & Diced Carrots (S&W) | ½ cup | 50 | 0 |
| Sweet Peas w/ Tiny Pearl Onions (S&W) | ½ cup | 60 | 0 |
| Vegetable Salad (Hanover) | ½ cup | 90 | 0 |
| corn w/ red & green peppers | ½ cup | 86 | 0 |
| mixed vegetables | ½ cup | 44 | 0 |
| peas and carrots | ½ cup | 48 | 0 |
| peas and onions | ½ cup | 30 | 0 |
| succotash | ½ cup | 102 | 0 |
| FROZEN Broccoli Cut & Cauliflower Cut (Hanover) | ½ cup | 20 | 0 |
| Broccoli, Carrots & Pasta Twists in Lightly Seasoned Sauce (Birds Eye) | ⅔ cup | 87 | 0 |

| FOOD | PORTION | CALORIES | CHOLESTEROL |
|---|---|---|---|
| Broccoli, Cauliflower & Carrots Farm Fresh Mixtures (Birds Eye) | ¾ cup | 33 | 0 |
| Broccoli, Cauliflower w/ Creamy Italian Cheese Sauce (Birds Eye) | ½ cup | 89 | 14 |
| Broccoli, Cauliflower, Carrots w/ Cheese Sauce (Birds Eye) | ½ cup | 99 | 4 |
| Broccoli, Baby Carrots & Water Chestnuts Farm Fresh Mixtures (Birds Eye) | ¾ cup | 45 | 0 |
| Broccoli, Corn & Red Peppers Farm Fresh Mixtures (Birds Eye) | ⅔ cup | 60 | tr |
| Brussels Sprouts, Cauliflower & Carrots Farm Fresh Mixtures (Birds Eye) | ¾ cup | 40 | 0 |
| Caribbean Blend (Hanover) | ½ cup | 20 | 0 |
| Carrots, Baby Whole Sweet Peas & Onions Deluxe Vegetable (Birds Eye) | ½ cup | 48 | 0 |
| Cauliflower, Baby Whole Carrots & Snow Peas Farm Fresh Mixtures (Birds Eye) | ⅔ cup | 38 | 0 |
| Chinese Style International Recipe (Birds Eye) | ½ cup | 68 | tr |

| FOOD | PORTION | CALORIES | CHOLESTEROL |
|---|---|---|---|
| Chinese Style Stir Fry Vegetable (Birds Eye) | ½ cup | 36 | 0 |
| Chow Mein Style International Recipe (Birds Eye) | ½ cup | 89 | tr |
| Corn, Green Beans & Pasta Curls in Light Cream Sauce (Birds Eye) | ½ cup | 107 | 1 |
| Garden Medley (Hanover) | ½ cup | 20 | 0 |
| Green Peas & Pearl Onions (Birds Eye) | ½ cup | 71 | 0 |
| Italian Style International Recipe (Birds Eye) | ½ cup | 101 | 0 |
| Japanese Style International Recipe (Birds Eye) | ½ cup | 88 | tr |
| Japanese Style Stir Fry Vegetable (Birds Eye) | ½ cup | 29 | 0 |
| Mandarin Style International Recipe (Birds Eye) | ½ cup | 86 | tr |
| Medley Vegetable Crisp (Ore Ida) | 3 oz | 160 | 5 |
| Mixed Vegetables (Birds Eye) | ½ cup | 58 | tr |
| Mixed Vegetables (Hanover) | ½ cup | 50 | 0 |

| FOOD | PORTION | CALORIES | CHOLESTEROL |
|------|---------|----------|-------------|
| Mixed Vegetables w/ Onion Sauce (Birds Eye) | ⅓ cup | 97 | tr |
| New England Style International Recipe (Birds Eye) | ½ cup | 124 | tr |
| Oriental Blend (Hanover) | ½ cup | 25 | 0 |
| Pasta Primavera Style International Recipe (Birds Eye) | ½ cup | 121 | 3 |
| Peas & Cauliflower in Cream Sauce (Budget Gourmet) | 5.75 oz | 170 | 20 |
| Peas & Pearl Onions w/ Cream Sauce (Birds Eye) | ½ cup | 137 | 4 |
| Peas & Potatoes w/ Cream Sauce (Birds Eye) | ½ cup | 126 | 1 |
| Peas & Water Chestnuts Oriental (Budget Gourmet) | 5 oz | 120 | 5 |
| Peppers & Onions (Southland) | 2 oz | 15 | 0 |
| Rutabaga & Yellow Turnips (Southland) | 4 oz | 50 | 0 |
| San Francisco Style International Recipe (Birds Eye) | ½ cup | 90 | tr |
| Soup Mix Vegetables (Southland) | 3.2 oz | 50 | 0 |

| FOOD | PORTION | CALORIES | CHOLESTEROL |
|------|---------|----------|-------------|
| Spring Vegetables in Cheese Sauce (Budget Gourmet) | 5 oz | 90 | 20 |
| Stew Vegetables (Ore Ida) | 3 oz | 60 | 0 |
| Stew Vegetables (Southland) | 4 oz | 60 | 0 |
| Succotash (Hanover) | ½ cup | 80 | 0 |
| Summer Vegetables (Hanover) | ½ cup | 35 | 0 |
| Vegetables for Soup (Hanover) | ½ cup | 60 | 0 |
| Vegetables New England Recipe (Budget Gourmet) | 5.5 oz | 210 | 20 |
| mixed; cooked | ½ cup | 54 | 0 |
| mixed; not prep | 10 oz pkg | 201 | 0 |
| peas & carrots; cooked | ½ cup | 38 | 0 |
| peas & carrots; not prep | ½ cup | 37 | 0 |
| peas & onions; not prep | ½ cup | 48 | 0 |
| peas and onions; cooked | ½ cup | 40 | 0 |
| succotash | 10 oz pkg | 265 | 0 |
| succotash; cooked | ½ cup | 79 | 0 |
| **HOME RECIPE** | | | |
| caponata | ¼ cup | 28 | 0 |
| succotash | ½ cup | 111 | 0 |
| **JUICE** | | | |
| Beefamato (Mott's) | 6 oz | 80 | 0 |

| FOOD | PORTION | CALORIES | CHOLESTEROL |
|---|---|---|---|
| Clamato (Mott's) | 6 oz | 96 | 0 |
| vegetable cocktail | 6 fl oz | 34 | 0 |

## VINEGAR

| FOOD | PORTION | CALORIES | CHOLESTEROL |
|---|---|---|---|
| Apple Cider (White House) | 2 Tbsp | 4 | 0 |
| White Distilled (White House) | 2 Tbsp | 4 | 0 |

## WAFFLES

| FOOD | PORTION | CALORIES | CHOLESTEROL |
|---|---|---|---|
| FROZEN READY-TO-USE | | | |
| Raisins, Bran & Whole Grain, Nutri-Grain (Eggo) | 1 | 130 | 0 |
| HOME RECIPE | | | |
| waffle | 7" diam | 282 | 70 |
| waffle | 9" sq | 602 | 150 |
| MIX | | | |
| mix; as prep w/ egg & milk | 1 waffle (2.6 oz) | 210 | 0 |

## WALNUTS

| FOOD | PORTION | CALORIES | CHOLESTEROL |
|---|---|---|---|
| Black Walnuts (Planters) | 1 oz | 190 | 0 |
| English Walnuts, Whole, Halves or Pieces (Planters) | 1 oz | 190 | 0 |

| FOOD | PORTION | CALORIES | CHOLESTEROL |
|------|---------|----------|-------------|
| Walnut Topping (Kraft) | 1 Tbsp | 90 | 0 |
| black, dried | 1 oz | 172 | 0 |
| black, dried; chopped | 1 cup | 759 | 0 |
| English, dried | 1 oz | 182 | 0 |
| English, dried; chopped | 1 cup | 770 | 0 |

## WATERCHESTNUTS

CANNED
| Chinese; sliced | ½ cup | 35 | 0 |

## WATERCRESS
(*see also* CRESS)

FRESH
| raw; chopped | ½ cup | 2 | 0 |

## WATERMELON

| seeds, dried | 1 oz | 158 | 0 |
| watermelon; diced | 1 cup | 50 | 0 |

## WAX BEANS

CANNED
| Cut Wax Beans (Owatonna) | ½ cup | 20 | 0 |
| Golden Cut Premium (S&W) | ½ cup | 20 | 0 |
| Wax Beans (Libby) | ½ cup | 20 | 0 |
| Wax Beans (Seneca) | ½ cup | 20 | 0 |

| FOOD | PORTION | CALORIES | CHOLESTEROL |
|------|---------|----------|-------------|

# WHALE

**FRESH**
| | | | |
|------|---------|----------|-------------|
| raw | 3.5 oz | 156 | 15 |

# WHELK (SNAIL)

**FRESH**
| | | | |
|------|---------|----------|-------------|
| cooked | 3 oz | 233 | 110 |
| raw | 3 oz | 117 | 55 |

# WHIPPED TOPPINGS
(*see also* CREAM)

| FOOD | PORTION | CALORIES | CHOLESTEROL |
|------|---------|----------|-------------|
| Cool Whip (Non-Dairy) | 1 Tbsp | 11 | tr |
| Cool Whip Extra Creamy Dairy | 1 Tbsp | 16 | tr |
| D-Zerta w/ NutraSweet; as prep | 1 Tbsp | 7 | tr |
| D-Zerta; as prep | ¼ cup | 47 | tr |
| Dream Whip; as prep | 1 Tbsp | 9 | tr |
| Real Cream Topping (Kraft) | ¼ cup | 25 | 10 |
| Whipped Topping (Kraft) | ¼ cup | 35 | 0 |
| Whipped Topping; as prep (Estee) | 1 Tbsp | 4 | 0 |
| cream, pressurized | 1 Tbsp | 8 | 2 |
| cream, pressurized | 1 cup | 154 | 46 |
| frzn, non-dairy | ¼ cup | 60 | 0 |

| FOOD | PORTION | CALORIES | CHOLESTEROL |
|------|---------|----------|-------------|
| frzn, non-dairy | 1 Tbsp | 13 | 0 |
| non-dairy, powdered | 1 Tbsp | 8 | tr |
| non-dairy, pressurized | 1 Tbsp | 11 | 0 |
| pressurized, non-dairy | ¼ cup | 46 | 0 |

## WHITE BEANS

| FOOD | PORTION | CALORIES | CHOLESTEROL |
|------|---------|----------|-------------|
| **CANNED** | | | |
| white | 1 cup | 306 | 0 |
| **DRIED** | | | |
| cooked | 1 cup | 249 | 0 |
| raw | 1 cup | 674 | 0 |
| small white, raw | 1 cup | 723 | 0 |
| small white; cooked | 1 cup | 253 | 0 |

## WHITEFISH

| FOOD | PORTION | CALORIES | CHOLESTEROL |
|------|---------|----------|-------------|
| **FRESH** | | | |
| raw | 3 oz | 114 | 51 |
| raw | 1 fillet (6.9 oz) | 266 | 119 |
| **SMOKED** | | | |
| whitefish | 1 oz | 39 | 9 |
| whitefish | 3 oz | 92 | 28 |

## WHITING

| FOOD | PORTION | CALORIES | CHOLESTEROL |
|------|---------|----------|-------------|
| **FRESH** | | | |
| cooked | 1 fillet (2.5 oz) | 83 | 60 |

| FOOD | PORTION | CALORIES | CHOLESTEROL |
|---|---|---|---|
| cooked | 3 oz | 98 | 71 |
| raw | 3 oz | 77 | 57 |
| raw | 1 fillet (3.2 oz) | 83 | 61 |

## WINE
(*see also* WINE COOLERS)

| | | | |
|---|---|---|---|
| dessert | 2 oz | 90 | 0 |
| red | 3.5 oz | 74 | 0 |
| rose | 3.5 oz | 73 | 0 |
| sherry | 2 oz | 84 | 0 |
| vermouth, dry | 3.5 oz | 105 | 0 |
| vermouth, sweet | 3.5 oz | 167 | 0 |
| white | 3.5 oz | 70 | 0 |

## WINE COOLERS

| | | | |
|---|---|---|---|
| Bartles & Jaymes | 12 oz | 192 | 0 |

## WINGED BEANS

DRIED
| | | | |
|---|---|---|---|
| cooked | 1 cup | 252 | 0 |
| raw | 1 cup | 745 | 0 |

## WOLFFISH

FRESH
| | | | |
|---|---|---|---|
| Atlantic, raw | 3 oz | 82 | 39 |
| Atlantic, raw | ½ fillet (5.4 oz) | 147 | 70 |

| FOOD | PORTION | CALORIES | CHOLESTEROL |
|------|---------|----------|-------------|

# YAM
   (*see also* SWEET POTATO)

CANNED
| | | | |
|------|---------|----------|-------------|
| Candied<br>(S&W) | ½ cup | 180 | 0 |
| Yams Golden Cut in Syrup<br>(Sugary Sam) | ½ cup | 110 | 0 |
| Yams Golden Whole in Heavy<br>Syrup<br>(Trappey's) | ½ cup | 130 | 0 |
| Yams Southern Whole in<br>Extra Heavy Syrup<br>(S&W) | ½ cup | 139 | 0 |

FRESH
| | | | |
|------|---------|----------|-------------|
| mountain yam, Hawaii, raw;<br>cubed | ½ cup | 46 | 0 |
| mountain yam, Hawaii;<br>cooked | ½ cup | 59 | 0 |
| yam; cubed, cooked | ½ cup | 79 | 0 |

# YARDLONG BEANS

DRIED
| | | | |
|------|---------|----------|-------------|
| cooked | 1 cup | 202 | 0 |
| raw | 1 cup | 580 | 0 |

# YEAST

| | | | |
|------|---------|----------|-------------|
| baker's dry active | 1 pkg<br>(7 g) | 20 | 0 |
| brewer's dry | 1 Tbsp | 25 | 0 |

| FOOD | PORTION | CALORIES | CHOLESTEROL |
|------|---------|----------|-------------|

## YELLOW BEANS

DRIED
| | | | |
|------|---------|----------|-------------|
| cooked | 1 cup | 254 | 0 |
| raw | 1 cup | 676 | 0 |

## YOGURT
(*see also* YOGURT DRINKS; YOGURT, FROZEN)

Yoplait yogurt made in and/or distributed from California will have a slightly different fat content to comply with California law.

| FOOD | PORTION | CALORIES | CHOLESTEROL |
|------|---------|----------|-------------|
| All Flavors (TCBY) | 5 oz | 160 | 11–15 |
| Amaretto Almond Yo Creme (Yoplait) | 5 oz | 240 | 30 |
| Apple Cinnamon Breakfast Yogurt (Yoplait) | 6 oz | 220 | 10 |
| Apple Original (Yoplait) | 4 oz | 120 | 5 |
| Apple Original (Yoplait) | 6 oz | 190 | 10 |
| Banana Strawberry Non-Fat Lite (Colombo) | 8 oz | 190 | 5 |
| Banana Custard Style (Yoplait) | 6 oz | 190 | 20 |
| Banana Fruit-on-the-Bottom (Dannon) | 8 oz | 240 | 10 |
| Bavarian Chocolate Yo Creme (Yoplait) | 5 oz | 270 | 30 |

| FOOD | PORTION | CALORIES | CHOLESTEROL |
|------|---------|----------|-------------|
| Berries Breakfast Yogurt (Yoplait) | 6 oz | 230 | 10 |
| Black Cherry (Breyers) | 8 oz | 270 | 15 |
| Black Cherry Lowfat (Light N'Lively) | 6 oz | 180 | 5 |
| Blueberry (Breyers) | 8 oz | 260 | 15 |
| Blueberry (Dannon) | 8 oz | 200 | 10 |
| Blueberry (Yoplait 150) | 6 oz | 150 | 5 |
| Blueberry Custard Style (Yoplait) | 6 oz | 190 | 20 |
| Blueberry Fruit-on-the-Bottom (Dannon) | 8 oz | 240 | 10 |
| Blueberry Fruit-on-the-Bottom (Dannon) | 4.4 oz | 130 | 5 |
| Blueberry Lowfat (Light N'Lively) | 6 oz | 180 | 5 |
| Blueberry Non-Fat Lite (Colombo) | 8 oz | 160 | 5 |
| Blueberry Original (Yoplait) | 4 oz | 120 | 5 |
| Blueberry Original (Yoplait) | 6 oz | 190 | 10 |
| Boysenberry Fruit-on-the-Bottom (Dannon) | 8 oz | 240 | 10 |
| Boysenberry Original (Yoplait) | 4 oz | 120 | 5 |

| FOOD | PORTION | CALORIES | CHOLESTEROL |
|---|---|---|---|
| Cherries Jubilee (Yoplait) | 5 oz | 220 | 30 |
| Cherry (Yoplait 150) | 6 oz | 150 | 5 |
| Cherry Custard Style (Yoplait) | 6 oz | 180 | 20 |
| Cherry Fruit-on-the-Bottom (Dannon) | 8 oz | 240 | 10 |
| Cherry Fruit-on-the-Bottom (Dannon) | 4.4 oz | 130 | 5 |
| Cherry Original (Yoplait) | 4 oz | 120 | 5 |
| Cherry w/ Almonds Breakfast Yogurt (Yoplait) | 6 oz | 210 | 10 |
| Coffee (Dannon) | 8 oz | 200 | 10 |
| Coffee/Lowfat (Friendship) | 8 oz | 210 | 14 |
| Dutch Apple Fruit-on-the-Bottom (Dannon) | 8 oz | 240 | 10 |
| Exotic Fruit Fruit-on-the-Bottom (Dannon) | 8 oz | 240 | 10 |
| Fruit Cocktail Non-Fat Lite (Colombo) | 8 oz | 160 | 5 |
| Lemon (Dannon) | 8 oz | 200 | 10 |
| Lemon Custard Style (Yoplait) | 6 oz | 190 | 20 |

| FOOD | PORTION | CALORIES | CHOLESTEROL |
|---|---|---|---|
| Lemon Original (Yoplait) | 4 oz | 120 | 5 |
| Mixed Berries Extra Smooth (Dannon) | 4.4 oz | 130 | 10 |
| Mixed Berries Fruit-on-the-Bottom (Dannon) | 8 oz | 240 | 10 |
| Mixed Berries Fruit-on-the-Bottom (Dannon) | 4.4 oz | 130 | 5 |
| Mixed Berries Hearty Nuts & Raisins (Dannon) | 8 oz | 260 | 10 |
| Mixed Berry (Breyers) | 8 oz | 270 | 15 |
| Mixed Berry Custard Style (Yoplait) | 6 oz | 180 | 20 |
| Mixed Berry Original (Yoplait) | 4 oz | 120 | 5 |
| Orange Original (Yoplait) | 4 oz | 120 | 5 |
| Orchard Fruit Hearty Nuts & Raisins (Dannon) | 8 oz | 260 | 10 |
| Peach (Breyers) | 8 oz | 270 | 15 |
| Peach (Yoplait 150) | 6 oz | 150 | 5 |
| Peach Lowfat (Light N'Lively) | 6 oz | 180 | 5 |
| Peach Non-Fat Lite (Colombo) | 8 oz | 190 | 5 |

| FOOD | PORTION | CALORIES | CHOLESTEROL |
|------|---------|----------|-------------|
| Peach Original (Yoplait) | 4 oz | 120 | 5 |
| Peach Fruit-on-the-Bottom (Dannon) | 8 oz | 240 | 10 |
| Pina Colada Fruit-on-the-Bottom (Dannon) | 8 oz | 240 | 10 |
| Pina Colada Original (Yoplait) | 4 oz | 120 | 5 |
| Pina Colada Original (Yoplait) | 4 oz | 120 | 5 |
| Pineapple (Breyers) | 8 oz | 270 | 15 |
| Pineapple Lowfat (Light N'Lively) | 6 oz | 180 | 5 |
| Pineapple Original (Yoplait) | 4 oz | 120 | 5 |
| Plain (Breyers) | 8 oz | 190 | 20 |
| Plain (Friendship) | 8 oz | 170 | 30 |
| Plain (Yoplait) | 4 oz | 80 | 10 |
| Plain (Yoplait) | 6 oz | 120 | 15 |
| Plain Lowfat (Dannon) | 8 oz | 140 | 15 |
| Plain Non-Fat (Dannon) | 8 oz | 110 | <5 |
| Raspberries & Cream (Yoplait) | 5 oz | 230 | 30 |

| FOOD | PORTION | CALORIES | CHOLESTEROL |
|---|---|---|---|
| Raspberry (Dannon) | 8 oz | 200 | 10 |
| Raspberry (Yoplait 150) | 6 oz | 150 | 5 |
| Raspberry Custard Style (Yoplait) | 6 oz | 190 | 20 |
| Raspberry Original (Yoplait) | 4 oz | 120 | 5 |
| Raspberry Original (Yoplait) | 4 oz | 120 | 5 |
| Raspberry Extra Smooth (Dannon) | 4.4 oz | 130 | 10 |
| Raspberry Fruit-on-the-Bottom (Dannon) | 8 oz | 240 | 10 |
| Raspberry Fruit-on-the-Bottom (Dannon) | 4.4 oz | 130 | 5 |
| Red Raspberry (Breyers) | 8 oz | 260 | 15 |
| Red Raspberry Lowfat (Light N'Lively) | 6 oz | 170 | 5 |
| Strawberries Romanoff (Yoplait) | 5 oz | 220 | 30 |
| Strawberry (Breyers) | 8 oz | 270 | 15 |
| Strawberry (Dannon) | 8 oz | 200 | 10 |
| Strawberry (Yoplait 150) | 6 oz | 150 | 5 |
| Strawberry Banana (Breyers) | 8 oz | 280 | 15 |

| FOOD | PORTION | CALORIES | CHOLESTEROL |
|------|---------|----------|-------------|
| Strawberry Banana (Dannon) | 8 oz | 200 | 10 |
| Strawberry Banana Breakfast Yogurt (Yoplait) | 6 oz | 240 | 10 |
| Strawberry Banana Fruit-on-the-Bottom (Dannon) | 4.4 oz | 130 | 5 |
| Strawberry Banana Lowfat (Light N'Lively) | 6 oz | 200 | 5 |
| Strawberry Custard Style (Yoplait) | 6 oz | 190 | 20 |
| Strawberry Extra Smooth (Dannon) | 4.4 oz | 130 | 10 |
| Strawberry Fruit-on-the-Bottom (Dannon) | 8 oz | 240 | 10 |
| Strawberry Fruit-on-the-Bottom (Dannon) | 4.4 oz | 130 | 5 |
| Strawberry Lowfat (Light N'Lively) | 6 oz | 180 | 5 |
| Strawberry Non-Fat Lite (Colombo) | 8 oz | 190 | 5 |
| Strawberry Original (Yoplait) | 4 oz | 120 | 5 |
| Strawberry w/ Almonds Breakfast Yogurt (Yoplait) | 6 oz | 210 | 10 |
| Strawberry-Banana (Yoplait 150) | 6 oz | 150 | 5 |

| FOOD | PORTION | CALORIES | CHOLESTEROL |
| --- | --- | --- | --- |
| Strawberry-Banana Original (Yoplait) | 4 oz | 120 | 5 |
| Strawberry-Rhubarb Original (Yoplait) | 4 oz | 120 | 5 |
| Sunrise Peach Breakfast Yogurt (Yoplait) | 6 oz | 230 | 10 |
| Tropical Fruits Breakfast Yogurt (Yoplait) | 6 oz | 230 | 10 |
| Vanilla (Dannon) | 8 oz | 200 | 10 |
| Vanilla (Dannon) | 4.4 oz | 110 | 5 |
| Vanilla Bean (Breyers) | 8 oz | 230 | 7 |
| Vanilla Custard Style (Yoplait) | 6 oz | 180 | 20 |
| Vanilla Hearty Nuts & Raisins (Dannon) | 8 oz | 270 | 10 |
| Vanilla Lowfat (Friendship) | 8 oz | 210 | 14 |
| With Fruit Lowfat (Friendship) | 8 oz | 230 | 14 |
| coffee, lowfat | 1 cup | 193 | 11 |
| coffee, lowfat | 4 oz | 97 | 6 |
| coffee, lowfat | 8 oz | 194 | 11 |
| fruit, all flavors, lowfat | 1 cup | 232 | 9 |
| fruit, lowfat | 4 oz | 113 | 5 |
| fruit, lowfat | 8 oz | 225 | 10 |
| plain | 4 oz | 70 | 14 |

| FOOD | PORTION | CALORIES | CHOLESTEROL |
|---|---|---|---|
| plain | 8 oz | 139 | 29 |
| plain lowfat | 1 cup | 143 | 14 |
| plain lowfat | 4 oz | 72 | 7 |
| plain lowfat | 8 oz | 144 | 14 |
| plain skim milk | 1 cup | 127 | 5 |
| plain skim milk | 4 oz | 63 | 2 |
| plain skim milk | 8 oz | 127 | 4 |
| plain whole milk | 1 cup | 138 | 30 |
| vanilla lowfat | 8 oz | 194 | 11 |
| vanilla lowfat | 4 oz | 97 | 6 |
| vanilla lowfat | 1 cup | 193 | 11 |

## YOGURT DRINKS

| FOOD | PORTION | CALORIES | CHOLESTEROL |
|---|---|---|---|
| Exotic Fruit Dan'up (Dannon) | 8 oz | 190 | 10 |
| Mixed Berry Dan'up (Dannon) | 8 oz | 190 | 10 |
| Raspberry Dan'up (Dannon) | 8 oz | 190 | 10 |
| Strawberry Banana Dan'up (Dannon) | 8 oz | 190 | 10 |
| Strawberry Dan'up (Dannon) | 8 oz | 190 | 10 |

## YOGURT, FROZEN

| FOOD | PORTION | CALORIES | CHOLESTEROL |
|---|---|---|---|
| Black Cherry (Sealtest) | ½ cup | 100 | 5 |
| Peach (Sealtest) | ½ cup | 100 | 5 |

| FOOD | PORTION | CALORIES | CHOLESTEROL |
|------|---------|----------|-------------|
| Red Raspberry (Sealtest) | ½ cup | 100 | 5 |
| Strawberry (Sealtest) | ½ cup | 100 | 5 |
| Vanilla (Colombo) | 4 oz | 99 | 7 |

## YORKSHIRE PUDDING

| | | | |
|------|---------|----------|-------------|
| Yorkshire pudding (home recipe) | 3" sq | 171 | 86 |

## ZABAGLIONE
(*see* CUSTARD)

## ZABAIONE
(*see* CUSTARD)

## ZUCCHINI

| | | | |
|------|---------|----------|-------------|
| CANNED<br>Italian Style (S&W) | ½ cup | 45 | 0 |
| Italian style | ½ cup | 33 | 0 |
| FRESH<br>cooked; sliced | ½ cup | 14 | 0 |
| raw, sliced | ½ cup | 9 | 0 |
| FROZEN<br>Zucchini Vegetable Crisp (Ore Ida) | 3 oz | 150 | 5 |

| FOOD | PORTION | CALORIES | CHOLESTEROL |
|---|---|---|---|
| Zucchini Sliced (Southland) | 3.2 oz | 15 | 0 |
| cooked | ½ cup | 19 | 0 |
| HOME RECIPE | | | |
| croquettes | ½ cup | 118 | 75 |
| sticks | ½ cup | 81 | 18 |

# PART II

---

# Restaurant, Take-Out and Fast-Food Chains

| FOOD | PORTION | CALORIES | CHOLESTEROL |
|---|---|---|---|
| **ARBY'S** | | | |
| Bac'n Cheddar Deluxe | 1 | 561 | 78 |
| Beef'n Cheddar | 1 | 490 | 51 |
| Chicken Breast Sandwich | 1 | 595 | 57 |
| Chicken Club Sandwich | 1 | 621 | 108 |
| Chicken Roasted Breast | 1 | 254 | 200 |
| Chicken Roasted Leg | 1 | 319 | 214 |
| Chicken Salad Sandwich | 1 | 386 | 30 |
| Chicken Salad & Croissant | 1 | 472 | 12 |
| Chicken Salad w/ Tomato & Lettuce | 1 | 515 | 12 |
| French Fries | 1 reg | 211 | 6 |
| Hot Ham 'n Cheese | 1 reg | 353 | 50 |
| Potato Superstuffed Broccoli & Cheese | 1 | 541 | 24 |
| Potato Superstuffed Deluxe | 1 | 648 | 72 |
| Potato Superstuffed Mushroom & Cheese | 1 | 506 | 21 |
| Potato Superstuffed Taco | 1 | 619 | 145 |
| Potato Baked Plain | 1 | 290 | 0 |
| Potato Cakes | 1 | 201 | 1 |
| Roast Beef | 1 | 350 | 39 |
| Roast Beef Deluxe | 1 | 486 | 59 |
| Roast Beef Jr | 1 | 218 | 20 |
| Roast Beef King | 1 | 467 | 49 |
| Roast Beef Super | 1 | 501 | 40 |
| Shake, Chocolate | 1 | 384 | 32 |

| FOOD | PORTION | CALORIES | CHOLESTEROL |
|---|---|---|---|
| Shake, Jamocha | 1 | 424 | 31 |
| Shake, Vanilla | 1 | 295 | 30 |
| Tossed Salad, Plain | 1 | 44 | 0 |
| Tossed Salad w/ 20 Calorie Italian Dressing | 1 | 57 | 0 |
| Turkey Deluxe | 1 | 375 | 39 |

## BASKIN-ROBBINS

| | | | |
|---|---|---|---|
| Chocolate Ice Cream | 1 scoop | 270 | 37 |
| Jamoca Almond Fudge Ice Cream | 1 scoop | 270 | 32 |
| Low, Lite 'N Luscious Chunky Banana | 4 oz | 100 | 3 |
| Low, Lite 'N Luscious Jamoca Chip | 4 oz | 110 | 3 |
| Low, Lite 'N Luscious Pineapple Coconut | 4 oz | 110 | 3 |
| Pralines 'N Cream Ice Cream | 1 scoop | 280 | 36 |
| Vanilla Frozen Yogurt | 4 oz | 124 | 8 |
| Vanilla Ice Cream | 1 scoop | 240 | 52 |

## BRAZIER
(*see* DAIRY QUEEN)

## BURGER KING

| | | | |
|---|---|---|---|
| 7-UP | 1 reg | 144 | 0 |
| Apple Pie | 1 | 305 | 4 |
| Bacon Double Cheeseburger | 1 | 510 | 104 |
| Breakfast Croissan'wich w/ Bacon | 1 | 355 | 249 |

| FOOD | PORTION | CALORIES | CHOLESTEROL |
|------|---------|----------|-------------|
| Breakfast Croissan'wich w/ Ham | 1 | 335 | 262 |
| Breakfast Croissan'wich w/ Sausage | 1 | 538 | 293 |
| Cheeseburger | 1 | 317 | 48 |
| Chicken Specialty Sandwich | 1 | 688 | 82 |
| Chicken Tenders | 6 pieces | 204 | 47 |
| Coffee, black | 6 oz | 2 | 0 |
| Diet Pepsi | 1 reg | 1 | 0 |
| French Fries | 1 reg | 227 | 14 |
| French Toast Sticks | 1 serving | 499 | 74 |
| Great Danish | 1 | 500 | 6 |
| Ham & Cheese Specialty Sandwich | 1 | 471 | 70 |
| Hamburger | 1 | 275 | 37 |
| Milk, 2% | 8 oz | 121 | 18 |
| Milk, Whole | 8 oz | 157 | 35 |
| Onion Rings | 1 reg | 274 | 0 |
| Orange Juice | 6 oz | 80 | 0 |
| Pepsi-Cola | 1 reg | 159 | 0 |
| Salad Dressing, 1000 Island | 3 Tbsp | 117 | 17 |
| Salad Dressing, Bleu Cheese | 3 Tbsp | 156 | 22 |
| Salad Dressing, House | 3 Tbsp | 130 | 11 |
| Salad Dressing, Italian, Reduced Calorie | 3 Tbsp | 14 | 0 |
| Salad w/o Dressing | 1 reg | 28 | 0 |
| Scrambled Egg Platter | 1 | 468 | 370 |

| FOOD | PORTION | CALORIES | CHOLESTEROL |
|---|---|---|---|
| Scrambled Egg Platter w/ Bacon | 1 | 536 | 378 |
| Scrambled Egg Platter w/ Sausage | 1 | 702 | 420 |
| Whaler Fish Sandwich | 1 | 488 | 77 |
| Whopper Double Beef | 1 | 863 | 168 |
| Whopper Double Beef w/ Cheese | 1 | 946 | 191 |
| Whopper Jr. Sandwich | 1 | 322 | 41 |
| Whopper Jr. Sandwich w/ Cheese | 1 | 364 | 52 |
| Whopper Sandwich | 1 | 628 | 90 |
| Whopper Sandwich w/ Cheese | 1 | 711 | 113 |

## CARL'S JR.

| FOOD | PORTION | CALORIES | CHOLESTEROL |
|---|---|---|---|
| BAKERY SELECTIONS | | | |
| Chocolate Cake | 1 piece | 380 | 70 |
| Chocolate Chip Cookies | 2.5 oz | 353 | 15 |
| Danish | 1 | 300 | 0 |
| Muffin, Blueberry | 1 | 256 | 34 |
| Muffin, Bran | 1 | 220 | 50 |
| BEVERAGES | | | |
| Iced Tea | 1 reg | 2 | 0 |
| Milk, 2% | 10 oz | 175 | 0 |
| Orange Juice | 1 sm | 94 | 0 |
| Shake | 1 reg | 353 | 17 |
| Soda | 1 reg | 243 | 0 |
| Soda, Diet | 1 reg | 2 | 0 |

| FOOD | PORTION | CALORIES | CHOLESTEROL |
|------|---------|----------|-------------|
| **BREAKFAST ITEMS** | | | |
| Bacon | 2 strips | 50 | 8 |
| English Muffin w/ Margarine | 1 | 180 | 0 |
| French Toast Dips w/o syrup | 1 serving | 480 | 54 |
| Hash Brown Nuggets | 1 serving | 170 | 10 |
| Hot Cakes w/ Margarine w/o Syrup | 1 serving | 360 | 15 |
| Sausage | 1 patty | 190 | 25 |
| Scrambled Eggs | 1 serving | 120 | 245 |
| Sunrise Sandwich w/ Bacon | 1 | 370 | 120 |
| Sunrise Sandwich w/ Sausage | 1 | 500 | 165 |
| **REGULAR MENU SELECTIONS** | | | |
| American Cheese | ½ oz | 63 | 16 |
| California Roast Beef 'n Swiss | 1 | 360 | 130 |
| Cheeseburger Double Western Bacon | 1 | 890 | 145 |
| Cheeseburger Western Bacon | 1 | 630 | 105 |
| Chicken Club Sandwich Charbroiler | 1 | 510 | 85 |
| Chicken Sandwich Charbroiler BBQ | 1 | 320 | 50 |
| Country Fried Steak Sandwich | 1 | 610 | 45 |
| Filet of Fish Sandwich | 1 | 550 | 90 |
| French Fries | 1 reg | 360 | 15 |
| Hamburger, Famous Star | 1 | 590 | 45 |
| Hamburger, Happy Star | 1 | 220 | 45 |
| Hamburger, Old Time Star | 1 | 400 | 80 |
| Hamburger, Super Star | 1 | 770 | 125 |

| FOOD | PORTION | CALORIES | CHOLESTEROL |
|---|---|---|---|
| Onion Rings | 1 serving | 310 | 10 |
| Potato w/ Bacon & Cheese | 1 | 650 | 45 |
| Potato w/ Broccoli & Cheese | 1 | 470 | 10 |
| Potato Fiesta | 1 | 550 | 40 |
| Potato Lite | 1 | 250 | 0 |
| Potato w/ Sour Cream & Chives | 1 | 350 | 10 |
| Potato w/ Cheese | 1 | 550 | 40 |
| Swiss Cheese | ½ oz | 57 | 16 |
| Zucchini | 1 serving | 300 | 10 |

### SALADS AND DRESSINGS

| FOOD | PORTION | CALORIES | CHOLESTEROL |
|---|---|---|---|
| Dressing, Blue Cheese | 1 oz | 151 | 18 |
| Dressing, French, Reduced Calorie | 1 oz | 38 | 0 |
| Dressing, House | 1 oz | 110 | 10 |
| Dressing, Italian | 1 oz | 120 | 0 |
| Dressing, 1000 Island | 1 oz | 110 | 5 |
| Salad-to-Go, Chef | 1 | 180 | 63 |
| Salad-to-Go, Chicken | 1 | 206 | 83 |
| Salad-to-Go, Garden | 1 | 46 | 7 |
| Salad-to-Go, Taco | 1 | 356 | 99 |

### SOUPS

| FOOD | PORTION | CALORIES | CHOLESTEROL |
|---|---|---|---|
| Boston Clam Chowder | 7 oz | 140 | 22 |
| Cream of Broccoli | 7 oz | 140 | 22 |
| Lumber Jack Mix Vegetable | 7 oz | 70 | 3 |
| Old Fashioned Chicken Noodle | 7 oz | 80 | 14 |

| FOOD | PORTION | CALORIES | CHOLESTEROL |
|------|---------|----------|-------------|
| **CHICK-FIL-A** | | | |
| Carrot-Raisin Salad | 2.7 oz | 116 | 6 |
| Carrot-Raisin Salad | 13 oz | 570 | 30 |
| Chick-fil-A Nuggets | 8 pack | 287 | 62 |
| Chick-fil-A Nuggets | 12 pack | 430 | 92 |
| Chick-fil-A Sandwich | 1 | 426 | 66 |
| Chick-fil-A, no bun | 3.6 oz | 219 | 42 |
| Chicken Salad Cup | 3.4 oz | 309 | 21 |
| Chicken Salad Plate | 1 | 475 | 97 |
| Chicken Salad Sandwich (Wheat) | 1 | 449 | 50 |
| Coleslaw | 4 oz | 175 | 13 |
| Coleslaw | 15 oz | 718 | 52 |
| Fudge Brownie w/ Nuts | 1 | 369 | 0 |
| Hearty Breast of Chicken Soup | 8.5 oz | 152 | 46 |
| Ice Cream | 4.5 oz | 134 | 24 |
| Iced Tea, Unsweetened | 9 oz | 3 | 0 |
| Lemon Pie | 1 slice | 329 | 7 |
| Lemonade | 10 oz | 124 | tr |
| Orange Juice | 6 oz | 82 | 0 |
| Potato Salad | 4 oz | 198 | 6 |
| Potato Salad | 16 oz | 850 | 23 |
| Waffle Potato Fries | 1 reg | 270 | 8 |
| **DAIRY QUEEN/BRAZIER** | | | |
| FOOD SELECTION All White Chicken Nuggets | 1 serving | 276 | 39 |

| FOOD | PORTION | CALORIES | CHOLESTEROL |
|---|---|---|---|
| Chicken Breast Fillet | 1 | 608 | 78 |
| Chicken Breast Fillet w/ Cheese | 1 | 661 | 87 |
| DQ Hounder | 1 | 480 | 80 |
| DQ Hounder w/ Cheese | 1 | 533 | 89 |
| DQ Hounder w/ Chili | 1 | 575 | 89 |
| Double Hamburger | 1 | 530 | 85 |
| Double Hamburger w/ Cheese | 1 | 650 | 95 |
| Fish Fillet | 1 | 430 | 40 |
| Fish Fillet w/ Cheese | 1 | 483 | 49 |
| French Fries | 1 reg | 200 | 10 |
| French Fries | 1 lg | 320 | 15 |
| Hot Dog | 1 | 280 | 45 |
| Hot Dog w/ Cheese | 1 | 330 | 55 |
| Hot Dog w/ Chili | 1 | 320 | 55 |
| Onion Rings | 1 reg | 280 | 15 |
| Single Hamburger | 1 | 360 | 45 |
| Single Hamburger w/ Cheese | 1 | 410 | 50 |
| Super Hot Dog | 1 | 520 | 80 |
| Super Hot Dog w/ Cheese | 1 | 580 | 100 |
| Super Hot Dog w/ Chili | 1 | 570 | 100 |
| Triple Hamburger | 1 | 710 | 135 |
| Triple Hamburger w/ Cheese | 1 | 820 | 145 |
| | | | |
| **ICE CREAM** | | | |
| Banana Split | 1 | 540 | 30 |
| Buster Bar | 1 | 460 | 10 |

| FOOD | PORTION | CALORIES | CHOLESTEROL |
|------|---------|----------|-------------|
| Chipper Sandwich | 1 | 318 | 13 |
| Cone | 1 sm | 140 | 10 |
| Cone | 1 reg | 240 | 15 |
| Cone | 1 lg | 340 | 25 |
| DQ Sandwich | 1 | 140 | 5 |
| Dilly Bar | 1 | 210 | 10 |
| Dipped Cone | 1 sm | 190 | 10 |
| Dipped Cone | 1 reg | 340 | 20 |
| Dipped Cone | 1 lg | 510 | 30 |
| Double Delight | 1 | 490 | 25 |
| Float | 1 | 410 | 20 |
| Freeze | 1 | 500 | 30 |
| Fudge Nut Bar | 1 | 406 | 10 |
| Heath Blizzard | 1 | 800 | 65 |
| Hot Fudge Brownie Delight | 1 | 600 | 20 |
| Malt | 1 sm | 406 | 10 |
| Malt | 1 reg | 520 | 35 |
| Malt | 1 lg | 760 | 50 |
| Mr. Misty | 1 sm | 190 | 0 |
| Mr. Misty | 1 reg | 250 | 0 |
| Mr. Misty | 1 lg | 340 | 0 |
| Mr. Misty Float | 1 | 390 | 20 |
| Mr. Misty Freeze | 1 | 500 | 30 |
| Mr. Misty Kiss | 1 | 70 | 0 |
| Parfait | 1 | 430 | 30 |
| Peanut Buster Parfait | 1 | 740 | 30 |

| FOOD | PORTION | CALORIES | CHOLESTEROL |
|------|---------|----------|-------------|
| Shake | 1 sm (10 oz) | 490 | 35 |
| Shake | 1 reg (15 oz) | 710 | 50 |
| Shake | 1 lg (17 oz) | 831 | 60 |
| Shake | 1 xlg (21 oz) | 990 | 70 |
| Strawberry Shortcake | 1 | 540 | 30 |
| Sundae | 1 sm | 190 | 10 |
| Sundae | 1 reg | 310 | 20 |

## DOMINO'S PIZZA
(see also PIZZA, SHAKEY'S)

| FOOD | PORTION | CALORIES | CHOLESTEROL |
|------|---------|----------|-------------|
| 10" PIZZA | | | |
| Double Cheese | 2 slices | 284 | 24 |
| Double Cheese, Pepperoni | 2 slices | 331 | 35 |
| Ground Beef | 2 slices | 250 | 21 |
| Ground Beef, Pepperoni | 2 slices | 297 | 32 |
| Mushroom, Sausage | 2 slices | 248 | 18 |
| Pepperoni | 2 slices | 265 | 23 |
| Pepperoni, Mushroom | 2 slices | 267 | 23 |
| Pepperoni, Sausage | 2 slices | 293 | 29 |
| Plain Cheese | 2 slices | 218 | 12 |
| Sausage | 2 slices | 246 | 18 |
| 14" PIZZA | | | |
| Double Cheese | 2 slices | 365 | 31 |
| Double Cheese, Pepperoni | 2 slices | 427 | 45 |

| FOOD | PORTION | CALORIES | CHOLESTEROL |
|---|---|---|---|
| Ground Beef | 2 slices | 321 | 26 |
| Ground Beef, Pepperoni | 2 slices | 382 | 40 |
| Mushroom, Sausage | 2 slices | 322 | 24 |
| Pepperoni | 2 slices | 343 | 29 |
| Pepperoni, Mushroom | 2 slices | 346 | 29 |
| Pepperoni, Sausage | 2 slices | 380 | 38 |
| Plain Cheese | 2 slices | 281 | 15 |
| Sausage | 2 slices | 318 | 24 |
| **LARGE PIZZA** | | | |
| Double Cheese | 2 slices | 700 | 42 |
| Double Cheese, Pepperoni | 2 slices | 778 | 60 |
| Ground Beef | 2 slices | 527 | 34 |
| Ground Beef, Pepperoni | 2 slices | 605 | 52 |
| Mushroom, Sausage | 2 slices | 532 | 33 |
| Pepperoni | 2 slices | 556 | 39 |
| Pepperoni, Mushroom | 2 slices | 550 | 39 |
| Pepperoni, Sausage | 2 slices | 606 | 51 |
| Plain Cheese | 2 slices | 478 | 21 |
| Sausage | 2 slices | 528 | 33 |
| **SMALL PIZZA** | | | |
| Double Cheese | 2 slices | 480 | 35 |
| Double Cheese, Pepperoni | 2 slices | 453 | 46 |
| Ground Beef | 2 slices | 361 | 30 |
| Ground Beef, Pepperoni | 2 slices | 431 | 46 |
| Mushroom, Sausage | 2 slices | 365 | 28 |
| Pepperoni | 2 slices | 384 | 34 |
| Pepperoni, Mushroom | 2 slices | 388 | 34 |

| FOOD | PORTION | CALORIES | CHOLESTEROL |
|------|---------|----------|-------------|
| Pepperoni, Sausage | 2 slices | 431 | 44 |
| Plain Cheese | 2 slices | 314 | 17 |
| Sausage | 2 slices | 360 | 35 |

## *DRUTHER'S INTERNATIONAL*

| FOOD | PORTION | CALORIES | CHOLESTEROL |
|------|---------|----------|-------------|
| Bacon and Egg Biscuit | 1 | 258 | 253 |
| Bacon and Egg Plate; fried | 1 | 721 | 500 |
| Bacon and Egg Plate; scrambled | 1 | 742 | 501 |
| Biscuits and Gravy | 1 serving | 331 | 3 |
| Cheeseburger | 1 | 380 | 69 |
| Chicken Snack, Thigh, Drumstick | 1 snack | 925 | 77 |
| Chicken Snack, Wing, Breast | 1 snack | 970 | 159 |
| Deluxe Quarter Hamburger | 1 | 660 | 127 |
| Double Cheeseburger | 1 | 500 | 105 |
| Eight Piece Chicken Dinner | 1 | 3664 | 601 |
| Fish and Chips | 1 dinner | 729 | 112 |
| Fish Dinner | 1 | 770 | 117 |
| Fish Sandwich | 1 | 349 | 56 |
| Ham and Egg Biscuit | 1 | 217 | 256 |
| Ham and Egg Plate | 1 | 681 | 511 |
| Ham and Egg Plate; scrambled | 1 | 703 | 511 |
| Hamburger | 1 | 327 | 55 |
| Sausage and Egg Biscuit | 1 | 246 | 257 |
| Sausage and Egg Plate; fried | 1 | 741 | 515 |
| Sausage and Egg Plate; scrambled | 1 | 762 | 515 |

| FOOD | PORTION | CALORIES | CHOLESTEROL |
|---|---|---|---|
| Three Piece Chicken Dinner, Thigh, Breast, Wing | 1 | 1309 | 271 |
| Three Piece Chicken Dinner, Thigh, Breat, Drumstick | 1 | 1281 | 273 |
| Twelve Piece Chicken Dinner | 1 | 5496 | 982 |
| Two Piece Chicken Dinner | 1 | 925 | 157 |
| Two Piece Chicken Dinner, Breast, Wing | 1 | 970 | 159 |
| Two Sausages/Two Biscuits | 1 meal | 358 | 34 |

## DUNKIN' DONUTS
(see also DOUGHNUT)

| FOOD | PORTION | CALORIES | CHOLESTEROL |
|---|---|---|---|
| CROISSANT | | | |
| Almond | 1 | 435 | 2 |
| Chocolate | 1 | 502 | 2 |
| Plain | 1 | 291 | 2 |
| DOUGHNUT | | | |
| Apple Filled w/ Cinnamon Sugar | 1 | 219 | 1 |
| Bavarian Creme Filled | 1 | 226 | 2 |
| Bavarian Filled w/ Chocolate Frosting | 1 | 231 | 1 |
| Blueberry Filled | 1 | 196 | 1 |
| Chocolate Frosted Yeast Ring | 1 | 246 | 1 |
| Chocolate Cake Ring w/ Glaze | 1 | 324 | 2 |
| Coconut Coated Cake Ring | 1 | 417 | 2 |
| French Cruller w/ Glaze | 1 | 201 | 16 |
| Honey Dipped Coffee Roll | 1 | 348 | 1 |
| Honey Dipped Cruller | 1 | 370 | 2 |

| FOOD | PORTION | CALORIES | CHOLESTEROL |
|---|---|---|---|
| Honey Dipped Yeast Ring | 1 | 208 | 2 |
| Jelly Filled | 1 | 274 | 2 |
| Lemon Filled | 1 | 221 | 1 |
| Munchkin Cake w/ Powdered Sugar | 1 | 69 | tr |
| Munchkin Chocolate w/ Glaze | 1 | 88 | 1 |
| Munchkin Yeast w/ Glaze | 1 | 43 | tr |
| Plain Cake Ring | 1 | 319 | 2 |
| Sugared Jelly Stick | 1 | 332 | 2 |
| MISCELLANEOUS Biscuit | 1 | 332 | tr |
| Brownie | 1 | 280 | 20 |
| Chocolate Chip Cookie | 1 | 129 | 6 |
| Macaroon | 1 | 351 | 3 |
| MUFFIN Apple Spice | 1 | 327 | 26 |
| Banana Nut | 1 | 327 | 23 |
| Blueberry | 1 | 263 | 21 |
| Bran | 1 | 353 | 12 |
| Cherry | 1 | 317 | 31 |
| Corn | 1 | 347 | 25 |

## *HARDEE'S*

| | | | |
|---|---|---|---|
| American Cheese | ½ oz | 47 | 12 |
| Apple Turnover | 1 | 282 | tr |
| Bacon Cheeseburger | 1 | 556 | 60 |
| Big Cookie | 1 | 278 | 9 |

| FOOD | PORTION | CALORIES | CHOLESTEROL |
|---|---|---|---|
| Big Country Breakfast Ham Platter | 1 | 665 | 369 |
| Big Country Breakfast Platter | 1 | 716 | 350 |
| Big Country Breakfast Sausage Platter | 1 | 940 | 442 |
| Big Deluxe | 1 | 503 | 50 |
| Biscuit | 1 | 257 | 0 |
| Biscuit Gravy | 4 oz | 144 | 21 |
| Biscuit w/ Bacon & Egg | 1 | 405 | 369 |
| Biscuit w/ Cheese | 1 | 304 | 12 |
| Biscuit w/ Cinnamon 'N' Raisin | 1 | 276 | tr |
| Biscuit w/ Country Ham | 1 | 328 | 12 |
| Biscuit w/ Egg | 1 | 334 | 160 |
| Biscuit w/ Sausage | 1 | 426 | 17 |
| Biscuit w/ Sausage & Egg | 1 | 503 | 177 |
| Biscuit w/ Steak | 1 | 491 | 16 |
| Biscuit w/ Sugar Cured Ham | 1 | 299 | 17 |
| Canadian Sunrise | 1 | 489 | 253 |
| Cheeseburger | 1 | 309 | 28 |
| Cheeseburger, ¼ lb | 1 | 511 | 77 |
| Chicken Fillet | 1 | 510 | 57 |
| Egg | 1 oz | 77 | 160 |
| Fisherman's Fillet | 1 | 469 | 80 |
| French Fries | 1 reg | 239 | tr |
| French Fries | 1 lg | 406 | tr |
| Hamburger | 1 | 276 | 22 |
| Hash Rounds | 1 | 200 | 10 |

| FOOD | PORTION | CALORIES | CHOLESTEROL |
|------|---------|----------|-------------|
| Hot Ham 'N' Cheese | 1 | 376 | 59 |
| Jelly | 1 Tbsp | 49 | 0 |
| Milkshake | 11 oz | 391 | tr |
| Mushroom 'N' Swiss | 1 | 512 | 86 |
| Roast Beef Sandwich | 1 | 312 | 68 |
| Roast Beef Sandwich, Big | 1 | 440 | 86 |
| Salad Chef | 1 | 277 | 179 |
| Salad Side | 1 | 21 | tr |
| Turkey Club | 1 | 426 | 45 |

## *JACK-IN-THE-BOX*

| FOOD | PORTION | CALORIES | CHOLESTEROL |
|------|---------|----------|-------------|
| Bacon Cheeseburger | 1 | 705 | 85 |
| Breakfast Jack | 1 | 307 | 203 |
| Cheeseburger | 1 | 325 | 41 |
| Cheesecake | 1 | 309 | 63 |
| Chicken Strips | 4 pieces | 349 | 68 |
| Chicken Strips | 6 pieces | 523 | 103 |
| Chicken Supreme | 1 | 524 | 82 |
| Club Pita (no sauce) | 1 | 277 | 43 |
| Coca-Cola Classic | 12 oz | 144 | 0 |
| Coffee, black | 8 oz | 2 | 0 |
| Crescent, Canadian | 1 | 452 | 226 |
| Crescent, Sausage | 1 | 584 | 187 |
| Crescent, Supreme | 1 | 547 | 178 |
| Diet Coke | 12 oz | 8 | 0 |
| Dinner, Chicken Strip (no sauce) | 1 | 689 | 100 |

| FOOD | PORTION | CALORIES | CHOLESTEROL |
|------|---------|----------|-------------|
| Dinner, Shrimp (no sauce) | 1 | 731 | 157 |
| Dinner, Sirloin Steak (no sauce) | 1 | 699 | 75 |
| Dr Pepper | 12 oz | 144 | 0 |
| Dressing, Buttermilk House | 1 pkg | 181 | 10 |
| Dressing, Reduced Calorie French | 1 pkg | 80 | 0 |
| Dressing, Thousand Island | 1 pkg | 156 | 11 |
| Dressing, Bleu Cheese | 1 pkg | 131 | 9 |
| Egg Rolls | 3 pieces | 405 | 30 |
| Egg Rolls | 5 pieces | 675 | 50 |
| Fajita Pita | 1 | 278 | 30 |
| Fish Supreme | 1 | 554 | 66 |
| French Fries | 1 reg | 221 | 8 |
| French Fries | 1 lg | 353 | 13 |
| French Fries | 1 jumbo | 442 | 16 |
| Grape Jelly | 1 pkg | 38 | 0 |
| Guacamole | 1 oz | 55 | 0 |
| Ham & Swiss Burger | 1 | 754 | 106 |
| Hamburger | 1 | 288 | 26 |
| Hash Brown | 1 | 116 | 3 |
| Hot Apple Turnover | 1 | 410 | 15 |
| Hot Club Supreme | 1 | 524 | 82 |
| Iced Tea | 12 oz | 3 | 0 |
| Jumbo Jack | 1 | 584 | 73 |
| Jumbo Jack w/ Cheese | 1 | 677 | 102 |
| Lowfat Milk | 8 oz | 122 | 18 |

| FOOD | PORTION | CALORIES | CHOLESTEROL |
|---|---|---|---|
| Milk Shake, Chocolate | 1 reg | 330 | 25 |
| Milk Shake, Vanilla | 1 reg | 320 | 25 |
| Moby Jack | 1 | 444 | 47 |
| Monterey Burger | 1 | 865 | 152 |
| Mushroom Burger | 1 | 470 | 64 |
| Nachos, Cheese | 1 serving | 571 | 37 |
| Nachos, Supreme | 1 serving | 787 | 59 |
| Onion Rings | 1 serving | 383 | 27 |
| Orange Juice | 6 oz | 80 | 0 |
| Pancake Platter | 1 | 612 | 99 |
| Pancake Syrup | 1 pkg | 121 | 0 |
| Pizza Pocket | 1 | 497 | 32 |
| Ramblin' Root Beer | 12 oz | 176 | 0 |
| Salad, Chef | 1 | 295 | 107 |
| Salad, Pasta & Seafood | 1 | 394 | 48 |
| Salad, Side | 1 | 51 | tr |
| Salad, Taco | 1 | 377 | 102 |
| Salsa | 1 oz | 8 | 0 |
| Sauce, A-1 Steak | 1 pkg | 35 | 0 |
| Sauce, BBQ | 1 pkg | 39 | tr |
| Sauce, Mayo-Mustard | 1 pkg | 124 | 10 |
| Sauce, Mayo-Onion | 1 pkg | 143 | 20 |
| Sauce, Seafood Cocktail | 1 pkg | 57 | 0 |
| Sauce, Sweet & Sour | 1 pkg | 39 | 0 |
| Scrambled Egg Platter | 1 | 662 | 354 |
| Shrimp | 10 pieces | 270 | 84 |

| FOOD | PORTION | CALORIES | CHOLESTEROL |
|------|---------|----------|-------------|
| Shrimp | 15 pieces | 404 | 126 |
| Sprite | 12 oz | 144 | 0 |
| Swiss & Bacon Burger | 1 | 678 | 127 |
| Taco | 1 | 191 | 21 |
| Taco, Super | 1 | 288 | 37 |
| Ultimate Cheeseburger | 1 | 942 | 127 |

## KENTUCKY FRIED CHICKEN

| CHICKEN DISHES | | | |
|------|---------|----------|-------------|
| Extra Crispy Center Breast | 1 | 353 | 93 |
| Extra Crispy Drumstick | 1 | 173 | 65 |
| Extra Crispy Side Breast | 1 | 354 | 66 |
| Extra Crispy Thigh | 1 | 371 | 121 |
| Extra Crispy Wing | 1 | 218 | 63 |
| Kentucky Nugget Sauce, Barbecue | 1 oz | 35 | 1 |
| Kentucky Nugget Sauce, Honey | 1 oz | 49 | 1 |
| Kentucky Nugget Sauce, Mustard | 1 oz | 36 | 1 |
| Kentucky Nugget Sauce, Sweet & Sour | 1 oz | 58 | 1 |
| Kentucky Nuggets | 1 nugget | 46 | 12 |
| Original Center Breast | 1 | 257 | 93 |
| Original Drumstick | 1 | 147 | 81 |
| Original Side Breast | 1 | 276 | 96 |
| Original Thigh | 1 | 278 | 122 |
| Original Wing | 1 | 181 | 67 |

| FOOD | PORTION | CALORIES | CHOLESTEROL |
|---|---|---|---|
| **SIDE DISHES** | | | |
| Baked Beans | 1 portion | 105 | 1 |
| Buttermilk Biscuit | 1 | 269 | 1 |
| Chicken Gravy | 1 serving | 59 | 2 |
| Coleslaw | 1 serving | 103 | 4 |
| Corn on the Cob | 1 ear | 176 | 1 |
| Kentucky Fries | 1 reg | 268 | 2 |
| Mashed Potatoes | 1 serving | 59 | 1 |
| Mashed Potatoes w/ Gravy | 1 serving | 62 | 1 |
| Potato Salad | 1 serving | 141 | 11 |

## *LONG JOHN SILVER'S*

| FOOD | PORTION | CALORIES | CHOLESTEROL |
|---|---|---|---|
| 2 Piece Fish & Fryes | 1 | 651 | 75 |
| 2 Piece Kitchen Breaded Fish Dinner | 1 | 818 | 76 |
| 3 Piece Fish Dinner | 1 | 1180 | 119 |
| 3 Piece Fish & Fryes | 1 | 853 | 106 |
| 3 Piece Kitchen Breaded Fish Dinner | 1 | 940 | 101 |
| 3 Piece Chicken Planks Dinner | 1 | 885 | 25 |
| 4 Piece Chicken Planks Dinner | 1 | 1037 | 25 |
| 6 Piece Chicken Nuggets Dinner | 1 | 699 | 25 |
| Batter Fried Fish | 1 | 202 | 31 |
| Batter Fried Shrimp | 1 | 47 | 17 |
| Batter Fried Shrimp Dinner | 1 | 711 | 127 |
| Clam Chowder | 1 | 128 | 17 |

| FOOD | PORTION | CALORIES | CHOLESTEROL |
|------|---------|----------|-------------|
| Clam Dinner | 1 | 955 | 27 |
| Coleslaw | 1 | 182 | 12 |
| Fish & Chicken | 1 | 935 | 56 |
| Fish & More | 1 | 978 | 88 |
| Fish Sandwich Platter | 1 | 835 | 75 |
| Fryes | 1 reg | 247 | 13 |
| Hush Puppies | 1 | 145 | 1 |
| Kitchen Breaded Fish | 1 | 122 | 25 |
| Ocean Chef Salad | 1 | 229 | 64 |
| Oyster Dinner | 1 | 789 | 55 |
| Scallop Dinner | 1 | 747 | 37 |
| Seafood Platter | 1 | 976 | 95 |
| Seafood Salad | 1 | 426 | 113 |

## McDONALD'S

BEVERAGES

| Coca-Cola Classic | 16 oz | 190 | 0 |
|------|---------|----------|-------------|
| Diet Coke | 16 oz | 1 | 0 |
| Grapefruit Juice | 6 oz | 80 | 0 |
| Milk, 2% | 8 oz | 121 | 18 |
| Milk Shake, Chocolate | 10 oz | 388 | 41 |
| Milk Shake, Strawberry | 10 oz | 384 | 41 |
| Milk Shake, Vanilla | 10 oz | 354 | 41 |
| Orange Drink | 16 oz | 177 | 0 |
| Orange Juice | 6 oz | 80 | 0 |
| Sprite | 16 oz | 190 | 0 |

| FOOD | PORTION | CALORIES | CHOLESTEROL |
|---|---|---|---|
| **BREAKFAST ITEMS** | | | |
| Biscuit w/ Bacon, Egg & Cheese | 1 | 449 | 336 |
| Biscuit w/ Biscuit Spread | 1 | 260 | 1 |
| Biscuit w/ Sausage | 1 | 440 | 49 |
| Biscuit w/ Sausage & Egg | 1 | 529 | 358 |
| Egg McMuffin | 1 | 293 | 299 |
| English Muffin w/ Butter | 1 | 169 | 9 |
| Hashbrown Potatoes | 1 | 131 | 9 |
| Hotcakes w/ Butter & Syrup | 1 portion | 413 | 21 |
| Pork Sausage | 1.7 oz | 180 | 48 |
| Sausage McMuffin | 1 | 372 | 64 |
| Sausage McMuffin w/ Egg | 1 | 451 | 336 |
| Scrambled Eggs | 1 portion | 157 | 545 |
| | | | |
| **DESSERTS** | | | |
| Apple Pie | 1 | 262 | 6 |
| Cone, Soft Serve | 1 | 144 | 16 |
| Cookies, Chocolate Chip | 1 pkg | 325 | 4 |
| Cookies, McDonaldland | 1 pkg | 288 | 0 |
| Danish, Apple | 1 | 389 | 25 |
| Danish, Cinnamon Raisin | 1 | 445 | 34 |
| Danish, Iced Cheese | 1 | 395 | 47 |
| Danish, Raspberry | 1 | 414 | 26 |
| Sundae, Hot Caramel | 1 | 343 | 35 |
| Sundae, Hot Fudge | 1 | 313 | 28 |
| Sundae, Strawberry | 1 | 283 | 27 |

| FOOD | PORTION | CALORIES | CHOLESTEROL |
|---|---|---|---|
| **MAIN MENU SELECTIONS** | | | |
| Big Mac | 1 | 562 | 103 |
| Cheeseburger | 1 | 308 | 53 |
| Chicken McNuggets | 1 portion | 288 | 65 |
| Filet-O-Fish | 1 | 442 | 50 |
| French Fries | 1 reg | 220 | 9 |
| French Fries | 1 lg | 312 | 12 |
| Hamburger | 1 | 257 | 37 |
| McD.L.T. | 1 | 674 | 112 |
| McNuggets Sauce, Barbeque | 1 oz | 53 | 0 |
| McNuggets Sauce, Honey | 1 oz | 46 | 0 |
| McNuggets Sauce, Hot Mustard | 1 oz | 66 | 5 |
| McNuggets Sauce, Sweet & Sour | 1 oz | 57 | 0 |
| Quarter Pounder | 1 | 517 | 118 |
| **SALADS AND DRESSINGS** | | | |
| 1000 Island Dressing | ½ oz | 78 | 8 |
| Bacon Bits | .1 oz | 16 | 0 |
| Bleu Cheese Dressing | ½ oz | 69 | 6 |
| Chef Salad | 1 | 231 | 152 |
| Chicken Salad Oriental | 1 | 141 | 78 |
| Chow Mein Noodles | .3 oz | 45 | 2 |
| Croutons | .4 oz | 52 | 0 |
| French Dressing | ½ oz | 58 | 0 |
| Lite Vinaigrette Dressing | ½ oz | 15 | 0 |
| Oriental Dressing | ½ oz | 24 | 0 |
| Ranch Dressing | ½ oz | 83 | 5 |

| FOOD | PORTION | CALORIES | CHOLESTEROL |
|------|---------|----------|-------------|
| Shrimp Salad | 1 | 104 | 193 |
| Side Salad | 1 | 57 | 53 |

## RAX

MEXICAN BAR
| Banana Pepper Rings | 1 Tbsp | 2 | tr |
| Cheese Sauce, Nacho | 3.5 oz | 470 | 11 |
| Cheese Sauce, Regular | 3.5 oz | 420 | 11 |
| Green Onions | ¼ cup | 10 | 0 |
| Japapeno Peppers | 1 oz | 6 | 0 |
| Olives | 3.5 oz | 110 | 0 |
| Refried Beans | 3 oz | 120 | 2 |
| Sour Topping | 3.5 oz | 130 | tr |
| Spanish Rice | 3.5 oz | 90 | tr |
| Spicy Meat Sauce | 3.5 oz | 80 | 12 |
| Taco Sauce | 3.5 oz | 30 | tr |
| Taco Shell | 1 | 40 | tr |
| Tomatoes | 1 oz | 6 | 0 |
| Tortilla Chips | 1 oz | 140 | tr |
| Tortillas | 1 | 110 | tr |

MISCELLANEOUS
| Cherry Coke | 10 oz | 120 | 0 |
| Chocolate Chip Cookie | 1 | 130 | tr |
| Coca-Cola | 10 oz | 120 | 0 |
| Coffee, decafe, black | 6 oz | 2 | 0 |
| Coffee, regular, black | 6 oz | 2 | 0 |
| Creamer, Non-Dairy | ⅜ oz | 14 | 0 |

| FOOD | PORTION | CALORIES | CHOLESTEROL |
|---|---|---|---|
| Diet Coke | 10 oz | tr | 0 |
| Drive-Thru Salad, Chef Salad w/o dressing | 1 | 230 | 322 |
| Drive-Thru Salad, Garden w/o dressing | 1 | 160 | 273 |
| Fanta Root Beer | 10 oz | 120 | 0 |
| Hot Cocoa Mix | 10 oz | 110 | tr |
| Hot Tea | 6 oz | tr | 0 |
| Iced Tea | 6 oz | tr | 0 |
| Milk, 2% | 8 oz | 110 | 20 |
| Milk, Whole | 8 oz | 150 | 30 |
| Milk Shake, Chocolate | 1 | 560 | 63 |
| Milk Shake, Strawberry | 1 | 560 | 62 |
| Milk Shake, Vanilla | 1 | 500 | 58 |
| Sprite | 10 oz | 110 | 0 |
| Whipped Topping | 1 dip | 50 | 2 |
| PASTA BAR | | | |
| Alfredo Sauce | 3.5 oz | 80 | 10 |
| Chicken Noodle Soup | 3.5 oz | 40 | 10 |
| Creme of Broccoli Soup | 3.5 oz | 50 | tr |
| Parmesan Cheese Substitute | 1 oz | 80 | tr |
| Pasta Shells | 3.5 oz | 170 | 0 |
| Pasta/Vegetable Blend | 3.5 oz | 100 | 0 |
| Rainbow Rotine | 3.5 oz | 180 | 2 |
| Spaghetti | 3.5 oz | 140 | 0 |
| Spaghetti Sauce | 3.5 oz | 80 | tr |
| Spaghetti Sauce w/ Meat | 3.5 oz | 150 | tr |

| FOOD | PORTION | CALORIES | CHOLESTEROL |
|---|---|---|---|
| **POTATOES** | | | |
| BBQ Potato | 1 | 730 | 18 |
| Cheese & Bacon Potato | 1 | 780 | 23 |
| Cheese & Broccoli Potato | 1 | 760 | 11 |
| Chili & Cheese Potato | 1 | 700 | 25 |
| French Fries, salted or unsalted | 1 reg | 260 | 4 |
| French Fries, salted or unsalted | 1 lg | 390 | 6 |
| Plain | 1 | 270 | 0 |
| Plain w/ margarine | 1 | 370 | 0 |
| Sour Topping Potato | 1 | 400 | tr |
| **SALAD BAR** | | | |
| Alfalfa Sprouts | 1 oz | 8 | 0 |
| Applesauce | 1 cup | 100 | 0 |
| Bacon Bits | .5 oz | 40 | 12 |
| Banana Chips | 1 oz | 100 | 0 |
| Beets | 1 cup | 60 | 0 |
| Blue Cheese Dressing | 1 Tbsp | 50 | 8 |
| Broccoli | ½ cup | 16 | 0 |
| Cabbage | 1 cup | 16 | 0 |
| Cantaloupe | 2 pieces | 16 | 0 |
| Carrots | ¼ cup | 8 | 0 |
| Cauliflower | ½ cup | 16 | 0 |
| Celery | 1 Tbsp | 14 | 0 |
| Cheddar Cheese Tidbits | 1 oz | 160 | tr |
| Cherry Peppers | 1 Tbsp | 6 | 0 |
| Chow Mein Noddles | 1 oz | 140 | tr |

| FOOD | PORTION | CALORIES | CHOLESTEROL |
|---|---|---|---|
| Coconut | 1 oz | 160 | 0 |
| Coleslaw | 3.5 oz | 70 | tr |
| Cottage Cheese | 1 cup | 250 | 47 |
| Crackers (Saltines) | 2 | 16 | tr |
| Croutons | .5 oz | 50 | tr |
| Cucumbers | 4 slices | 2 | 0 |
| Eggs | 1.5 oz | 70 | 267 |
| French Dressing | 1 Tbsp | 60 | tr |
| Garbanzo Beans | ½ cup | 360 | 0 |
| Gelatin, Lime | ½ cup | 90 | 0 |
| Gelatin, Strawberry | ½ cup | 90 | 0 |
| Grapefruit Sections | 1 cup | 80 | 0 |
| Grapes | 1 cup | 100 | 0 |
| Green Peppers | ¼ cup | 8 | 0 |
| Honeydew Melons | 2 pieces | 25 | 0 |
| Italian Dressing | 1 Tbsp | 50 | tr |
| Kale | 1 oz | 16 | 0 |
| Kidney Beans | 1 cup | 220 | 0 |
| Lettuce | 1 leaf | 2 | 0 |
| Lite Blue Cheese Dressing | 1 Tbsp | 35 | 3 |
| Lite French Dressing | 1 Tbsp | 40 | tr |
| Lite Italian Dressing | 1 Tbsp | 30 | 5 |
| Lite Thousand Island Dressing | 1 Tbsp | 40 | 5 |
| Macaroni Salad | 3.5 oz | 160 | tr |
| Mushrooms | ¼ cup | 4 | 0 |
| Oil | 1 Tbsp | 130 | 0 |

| FOOD | PORTION | CALORIES | CHOLESTEROL |
| --- | --- | --- | --- |
| Onions | ¼ cup | 12 | 0 |
| Pasta Salad | 3.5 oz | 80 | tr |
| Peaches | 2 slices | 16 | 0 |
| Peas | 1 oz | 25 | 0 |
| Pickle Spear | 1 | 8 | 0 |
| Pineapple, canned | 3.5 oz | 100 | 0 |
| Pineapple, fresh | 1 slice | 45 | 0 |
| Poppy Seed Dressing | 1 Tbsp | 60 | 6 |
| Potato Salad | 1 cup | 260 | 7 |
| Pudding, Butterscotch | 3.5 oz | 140 | 2 |
| Pudding, Chocolate | 3.5 oz | 140 | 2 |
| Pudding, Vanilla | 3.5 oz | 140 | 2 |
| Radishes | .5 oz | 2 | 0 |
| Ranch Dressing | 1 Tbsp | 45 | 5 |
| Red Cabbage | ¼ cup | 4 | 0 |
| Sesame Sticks | 1 oz | 150 | 0 |
| Shredded Imitation Cheddar Cheese | 1 oz | 90 | 6 |
| Soynuts | 1 oz | 120 | 0 |
| Strawberries | 2 oz | 18 | 0 |
| Sunflower Seeds w/ Raisins | 1 oz | 130 | 0 |
| Thousand Island Dressing | 1 Tbsp | 70 | 8 |
| Three Bean Salad | ½ cup | 100 | 0 |
| Tomatoes | 1 oz | 6 | 0 |
| Turkey Bits | 2 oz | 70 | 49 |
| Vinegar | 1 Tbsp | 2 | 0 |
| Watermelon | 2 pieces | 18 | 0 |

| FOOD | PORTION | CALORIES | CHOLESTEROL |
|---|---|---|---|
| **SANDWICHES AND INGREDIENTS** | | | |
| American Slices | 1 slice | 60 | 15 |
| BBC | 1 | 720 | 137 |
| BBC Sauce | .75 oz | 140 | 41 |
| BBQ Meat Topping | 3.25 oz | 140 | 24 |
| BBQ Sandwich | 1 | 420 | 24 |
| Bacon | 1 slice | 80 | 30 |
| Banana Pepper Rings | 1 Tbsp | 2 | tr |
| Bun | 1 sm | 180 | tr |
| Double Works Burger | 1 | 440 | 50 |
| Fish | 3.5 oz | 230 | tr |
| Fish Sandwich | 1 | 460 | tr |
| Ham | 2.5 oz | 70 | 24 |
| Ham & Swiss Sandwich | 1 | 430 | 37 |
| Hamburger | 1 | 130 | 25 |
| Hamburger Seasoning Salt | 1 sprinkle | tr | tr |
| Horseradish Sauce | .75 oz | 10 | tr |
| Kaiser Bun | 4" | 180 | tr |
| Kaiser Bun | 6" | 280 | tr |
| Ketchup | 1 Tbsp | 6 | tr |
| Mayonnaise | .75 oz | 150 | tr |
| Mustard | 1 Tbsp | 4 | tr |
| Onions | 3 rings | 4 | 0 |
| Onions, Diced | ¼ cup | 18 | 0 |
| Philly Vegetables | 2 oz | 30 | tr |
| Philly Beef & Cheese Sandwich | 1 | 470 | 49 |

| FOOD | PORTION | CALORIES | CHOLESTEROL |
|---|---|---|---|
| Pickle Slices | 4 slices | 2 | 0 |
| Pickle Spears | 1 | 8 | 0 |
| Regular BBQ Sauce | 1 oz | 40 | tr |
| Roast Beef | 2.8 oz | 140 | 36 |
| Roast Beef Sandwich | 1 lg | 570 | 36 |
| Roast Beef Sandwich | 1 reg | 320 | 36 |
| Roast Beef Sandwich (Uncle Al) | 1 sm | 260 | 19 |
| Shredded Lettuce | ¼ cup | 2 | 0 |
| Smokey BBQ Sauce | 1 oz | 40 | tr |
| Sweet Pickle Relish | 1 Tbsp | 20 | tr |
| Swiss | 1 slice | 30 | 13 |
| Tartar Sauce | .5 oz | 50 | tr |
| Tomato | 1 slice | 2 | 0 |
| Turkey | 2.5 oz | 80 | 27 |
| Turkey & Bacon Club | 1 | 470 | 87 |
| Works Burger | 1 | 310 | 25 |

## *RED LOBSTER*

All of the following are for a cooked portion unless otherwise noted.

| | | | |
|---|---|---|---|
| Atlantic Cod | 1 lunch serving | 100 | 70 |
| Atlantic Ocean Perch | 1 lunch serving | 130 | 75 |
| Blacktip Shark | 1 lunch serving | 150 | 60 |
| Calamari; breaded & fried | 1 lunch serving | 360 | 140 |

| FOOD | PORTION | CALORIES | CHOLESTEROL |
|---|---|---|---|
| Calico Scallops | 1 lunch serving | 180 | 115 |
| Catfish | 1 lunch serving | 170 | 85 |
| Cherrystone Clams | 1 lunch serving | 130 | 80 |
| Chicken Breast | 4 oz before cooking | 120 | 65 |
| Deep Sea Scallops | 1 lunch serving | 130 | 50 |
| Flounder | 1 lunch serving | 100 | 70 |
| Grouper | 1 lunch serving | 110 | 65 |
| Haddock | 1 lunch serving | 110 | 85 |
| Halibut | 1 lunch serving | 110 | 60 |
| Hamburger | 5 oz before cooking | 320 | 105 |
| King Crab Legs | 1 lb | 170 | 100 |
| Langostino | 1 lunch serving | 120 | 210 |
| Lemon Sole | 1 lunch serving | 120 | 65 |
| Mackerel | 1 lunch serving | 190 | 100 |
| Maine Lobster | 1¼ lb | 240 | 310 |
| Mako Shark | 1 lunch serving | 140 | 100 |

| FOOD | PORTION | CALORIES | CHOLESTEROL |
|---|---|---|---|
| Monkfish | 1 lunch serving | 110 | 80 |
| Mussels | 3 oz | 70 | 50 |
| Norwegian Salmon | 1 lunch serving | 230 | 80 |
| Oysters, raw | 6 | 110 | 60 |
| Pollack | 1 lunch serving | 120 | 90 |
| Porterhouse Steak | 18 oz before cooking | 1420 | 290 |
| Rainbow Trout | 1 lunch serving | 170 | 90 |
| Red Rockfish | 1 lunch serving | 90 | 85 |
| Red Snapper | 1 lunch serving | 110 | 70 |
| Rock Lobster | 1 tail | 230 | 200 |
| Shrimp | 8–12 pieces | 120 | 230 |
| Sirloin Steak | 7 oz before cooking | 570 | 140 |
| Snow Crab Legs | 1 lb | 150 | 130 |
| Sockeye Salmon | 1 lunch serving | 160 | 50 |
| Strip Steak | 7 oz before cooking | 690 | 140 |
| Swordfish | 1 lunch serving | 100 | 100 |

| FOOD | PORTION | CALORIES | CHOLESTEROL |
|------|---------|----------|-------------|
| Tilefish | 1 lunch serving | 100 | 80 |
| Yellowfin Tuna | 1 lunch serving | 180 | 70 |

## *ROY ROGERS*

| FOOD | PORTION | CALORIES | CHOLESTEROL |
|------|---------|----------|-------------|
| Bacon Cheeseburger | 1 | 581 | 103 |
| Biscuit | 1 | 231 | 5 |
| Breakfast Crescent Sandwich | 1 | 401 | 148 |
| Breakfast Crescent Sandwich w/ Bacon | 1 | 431 | 156 |
| Breakfast Crescent Sandwich w/ Ham | 1 | 442 | 305 |
| Breakfast Crescent Sandwich w/ Sausage | 1 reg | 449 | 168 |
| Breakfast Crescent Sandwich w/ Sausage | 1 lg | 608 | 94 |
| Brownie | 1 | 264 | 10 |
| Cheeseburger | 1 | 563 | 95 |
| Chicken Breast | 4.8 oz | 412 | 118 |
| Chicken Breast & Wing | 6.5 oz | 604 | 165 |
| Chicken Leg | 1.8 oz | 140 | 40 |
| Chicken Nuggets | 6 nuggets | 267 | 51 |
| Chicken Thigh | 3.2 oz | 296 | 85 |
| Chicken Thigh & Leg | 5 oz | 436 | 125 |
| Chicken Wing | 1.7 oz | 192 | 47 |
| Coffee, black | 1 reg | 0 | 0 |

| FOOD | PORTION | CALORIES | CHOLESTEROL |
|---|---|---|---|
| Coke | 12 oz | 145 | 0 |
| Coleslaw | 1 reg | 110 | 5 |
| Danish, Apple | 1 | 249 | 15 |
| Danish, Cheese | 1 | 254 | 11 |
| Danish, Cherry | 1 | 271 | 11 |
| Diet Coke | 12 oz | 1 | 0 |
| French Fries | 1 reg | 268 | 42 |
| French Fries | 1 lg | 357 | 56 |
| Hamburger | 1 | 456 | 73 |
| Hot Chocolate | 6 oz | 123 | 35 |
| Hot Topped Potato w/ Bacon 'n Cheese | 1 | 397 | 34 |
| Hot Topped Potato w/ Broccoli 'n Cheese | 1 | 376 | 19 |
| Hot Topped Potato w/ Oleo | 1 | 274 | 0 |
| Hot Topped Potato w/ Sour Cream 'n Chives | 1 | 408 | 31 |
| Hot Topped Potato w/ Taco Beef 'n Cheese | 1 | 463 | 37 |
| Hot Topped Potato, Plain | 1 | 211 | 0 |
| Ice Tea | 1 reg | 0 | 0 |
| Large Roast Beef Sandwich | 1 | 360 | 73 |
| Large Roast Beef Sandwich w/ Cheese | 1 | 467 | 95 |
| Macaroni Salad | 1 reg | 186 | 5 |
| Milk, Whole | 8 oz | 150 | 33 |
| Orange Juice | 7 oz | 99 | 0 |
| Orange Juice | 10 oz | 136 | 0 |

| FOOD | PORTION | CALORIES | CHOLESTEROL |
|------|---------|----------|-------------|
| Pancake Platter w/ Syrup, Butter | 1 | 452 | 53 |
| Pancake Platter w/ Syrup, Butter, Bacon | 1 | 493 | 63 |
| Pancake Platter w/ Syrup, Butter, Ham | 1 | 506 | 73 |
| Pancake Platter w/ Syrup, Butter, Sausage | 1 | 608 | 94 |
| Potato Salad | 1 reg | 107 | 5 |
| RR Bar Burger | 1 | 611 | 115 |
| Roast Beef Sandwich | 1 | 317 | 55 |
| Roast Beef Sandwich w/ Cheese | 1 | 424 | 77 |
| Shake, Chocolate | 1 | 358 | 37 |
| Shake, Strawberry | 1 | 315 | 37 |
| Shake, Vanilla | 1 | 306 | 40 |
| Strawberry Shortcake | 1 | 447 | 28 |
| Sundae, Caramel | 1 | 293 | 23 |
| Sundae, Hot Fudge | 1 | 337 | 23 |
| Sundae, Strawberry | 1 | 216 | 23 |
| SALAD BAR | | | |
| Beets, Sliced | ¼ cup | 16 | 0 |
| Broccoli | ½ cup | 20 | 0 |
| Carrots, Shredded | ¼ cup | 42 | 0 |
| Croutons | 2 Tbsp | 70 | 0 |
| Cucumbers | 5–6 slices | 4 | 0 |
| Green Peas | ¼ cup | 7 | 0 |

| FOOD | PORTION | CALORIES | CHOLESTEROL |
|------|---------|----------|-------------|
| Green Peppers | 2 Tbsp | 4 | 0 |
| Lettuce | 1 cup | 10 | 0 |
| Mushrooms | ¼ cup | 5 | 0 |
| Sunflower Seeds | 2 Tbsp | 157 | 0 |
| Tomatoes | 3 slices | 20 | 0 |

## SHAKEY'S

(*see also* PIZZA, DOMINO'S PIZZA)

All servings are based on 1 slice from a 12″ pie cut into 10 slices.

PIZZA

| FOOD | PORTION | CALORIES | CHOLESTEROL |
|------|---------|----------|-------------|
| Homestyle Shakey's Special | 1 slice | 384 | 29 |
| Homestyle Cheese | 1 slice | 303 | 21 |
| Homestyle w/ Onion, Green Peppers, Olives, Mushrooms | 1 slice | 320 | 21 |
| Homestyle w/ Pepperoni | 1 slice | 343 | 27 |
| Homestyle w/ Sausage, Mushrooms | 1 slice | 343 | 24 |
| Homestyle w/ Sausage, Pepperoni | 1 slice | 374 | 24 |
| Thick Crust, Cheese Only | 1 slice | 170 | 13 |
| Thick Crust, Shakey's Special | 1 slice | 208 | 18 |
| Thick Crust w/ Pepperoni | 1 slice | 185 | 17 |
| Thick Crust w/ Sausage, Mushrooms | 1 slice | 179 | 15 |
| Thick Crust w/ Sausage, Pepperoni | 1 slice | 177 | 19 |
| Thick Crust w/ Green Pepper, Black Olives, Mushrooms | 1 slice | 162 | 13 |
| Thin Crust, Cheese Only | 1 slice | 133 | 14 |

| FOOD | PORTION | CALORIES | CHOLESTEROL |
| --- | --- | --- | --- |
| Thin Crust, Shakey's Special | 1 slice | 171 | 16 |
| Thin Crust w/ Pepperoni | 1 slice | 148 | 14 |
| Thin Crust w/ Sausage, Mushroom | 1 slice | 141 | 13 |
| Thin Crust w/ Sausage, Pepperoni | 1 slice | 166 | 17 |
| Thin Crust w/ Onion, Green Pepper, Black Olives, Mushroom | 1 slice | 125 | 11 |

## *TACO BELL*

| | | | |
| --- | --- | --- | --- |
| Bellbeefer | 1 | 312 | 39 |
| Bellbeefer, Green | 1 | 306 | 39 |
| Burrito, Double Beef Supreme, Green | 1 | 459 | 59 |
| Burrito Supreme Platter | 1 | 774 | 79 |
| Burrito Supreme Platter, Green | 1 | 762 | 79 |
| Burrito, Bean | 1 | 360 | 14 |
| Burrito, Bean, Green | 1 | 354 | 14 |
| Burrito, Beef | 1 | 402 | 59 |
| Burrito, Beef, Green | 1 | 396 | 59 |
| Burrito, Combo | 1 | 381 | 36 |
| Burrito, Combo, Green | 1 | 375 | 36 |
| Burrito, Double Beef Supreme | 1 | 464 | 59 |
| Burrito Supreme | 1 | 422 | 35 |
| Burrito Supreme, Green | 1 | 416 | 35 |
| Cinnamon Crispas | 1 | 266 | 2 |

| FOOD | PORTION | CALORIES | CHOLESTEROL |
|---|---|---|---|
| Enchirito | 1 | 382 | 56 |
| Enchirito, Green | 1 | 370 | 56 |
| Fabulous Steak Fajita | 1 | 235 | 14 |
| Fabulous Steak Fajita w/ Guacamole | 1 | 269 | 14 |
| Fabulous Steak Fajita w/ Sour Cream | 1 | 281 | 14 |
| Mexican Pizza | 1 | 714 | 81 |
| Nachos | 1 | 356 | 9 |
| Nachos Bellgrande | 1 | 719 | 43 |
| Pico De Gallo | 1 | 8 | tr |
| Pintos & Cheese | 1 | 194 | 19 |
| Pintos & Cheese, Green | 1 | 189 | 19 |
| Ranch Dressing | 2½ oz | 236 | 35 |
| Salsa | 3 oz. | 18 | 0 |
| Seafood Salad w/o Dressing | 1 | 648 | 82 |
| Seafood Salad w/o Dressing & Shell | 1 | 216 | 81 |
| Seafood Salad w/ Ranch Dressing | 1 | 884 | 117 |
| Taco | 1 | 184 | 32 |
| Taco Bellgrande | 1 | 351 | 55 |
| Taco Bellgrande Platter | 1 | 1002 | 80 |
| Taco Bellgrande Platter, Green | 1 | 990 | 80 |
| Taco Light | 1 | 411 | 57 |
| Taco Light Platter | 1 | 1062 | 82 |
| Taco Light Platter, Green | 1 | 1051 | 82 |
| Taco Salad w/ Ranch Dressing | 1 | 1167 | 121 |

| FOOD | PORTION | CALORIES | CHOLESTEROL |
|---|---|---|---|
| Taco Salad w/ Salsa | 1 | 949 | 85 |
| Taco Salad w/o Beans | 1 | 822 | 80 |
| Taco Salad w/o Salsa | 1 | 931 | 85 |
| Taco Salad w/o Shell | 1 | 524 | 82 |
| Taco Sauce | 1 pkg | 2 | 0 |
| Taco Sauce, Hot | 1 pkg | 3 | 0 |
| Taco, Soft | 1 | 228 | 32 |
| Tostada | 1 | 243 | 18 |
| Tostada, Beefy | 1 | 322 | 40 |
| Tostada, Beefy, Green | 1 | 316 | 40 |
| Tostada, Green | 1 | 238 | 18 |

## WENDY'S

### SANDWICH TOPPINGS

All Wendy's sandwiches are custom-made. The following list of sandwich toppings allows you to calculate the cholesterol and calories in any sandwich you order.

| FOOD | PORTION | CALORIES | CHOLESTEROL |
|---|---|---|---|
| Single Hamburger Patty, no bun | 1 (4 oz) | 210 | 75 |
| Bacon | 1 strip | 30 | 5 |
| Big Classic | 1 | 470 | 80 |
| Biscuit, Buttermilk | 1 | 320 | tr |
| Breakfast Potatoes | 1 | 360 | 20 |
| Breakfast Sandwich | 1 | 370 | 200 |
| Bun, Kaiser | 1 | 180 | 5 |
| Bun, Multi-Grain | 1 | 140 | tr |
| Bun, White | 1 | 140 | tr |
| Chicken Breast Fillet | 1 | 200 | 60 |

| FOOD | PORTION | CALORIES | CHOLESTEROL |
|---|---|---|---|
| Chicken Fried Steak | 1 | 580 | 95 |
| Chili | 1 reg | 240 | 25 |
| Chocolate Chip Cookie | 1 | 320 | 5 |
| Coca-Cola | 8 oz | 100 | 0 |
| Coffee, Decaffeinated, black | 6 oz | 2 | 0 |
| Coffee, black | 6 oz | 2 | 0 |
| Creamer, Non- Dairy | ⅜ oz | 14 | 0 |
| Crispy Chicken Nuggets; cooked in animal/ vegetable oil | 6 pieces | 290 | 55 |
| Crispy Chicken Nuggets; cooked in vegetable oil | 6 pieces | 310 | 50 |
| Diet Coke | 8 oz | 0 | 0 |
| Diet Pepsi | 8 oz | 0 | 0 |
| Dr Pepper | 8 oz | 100 | 0 |
| Egg, Fried | 1 egg | 90 | 230 |
| Eggs, Scrambled | 2 eggs | 190 | 450 |
| Fish Fillet | 1 | 210 | 45 |
| French Fries; cooked in vegetable oil | 1 reg | 300 | 5 |
| French Fries; cooked in animal /vegetable oil | 1 reg | 310 | 15 |
| French Toast | 2 slices | 400 | 115 |
| French Toast, Apple Topping | 1 pkg | 130 | 0 |
| French Toast, Blueberry Topping | 1 pkg | 60 | 0 |
| French Toast, Syrup | 1 pkg | 140 | 0 |
| Frosty Dairy Dessert | 1 sm | 400 | 50 |
| Grape Jelly | 1 pkg | 40 | 0 |

| FOOD | PORTION | CALORIES | CHOLESTEROL |
|---|---|---|---|
| Half & Half | ⅜ oz | 14 | 5 |
| Hot Chocolate | 6 oz | 110 | tr |
| Kid's Meal Hamburger | 1 | 200 | 35 |
| Lemonade | 12 oz | 160 | 0 |
| Milk, 2% | 8 oz | 110 | 20 |
| Milk, Chocolate | 8 oz | 190 | 25 |
| Milk, Whole | 8 oz | 140 | 30 |
| Mountain Dew | 8 oz | 110 | 0 |
| Nuggets Sauce, Barbecue | 1 pkg | 50 | 0 |
| Nuggets Sauce, Honey | 1 pkg | 45 | 0 |
| Nuggets Sauce, Sweet & Sour | 1 pkg | 45 | 0 |
| Nuggets Sauce, Sweet Mustard | 1 pkg | 50 | 0 |
| Omelet #1 | 1 | 290 | 355 |
| Omelet #2 | 1 | 250 | 450 |
| Omelet #3 | 1 | 280 | 525 |
| Omelet #4 | 1 | 210 | 460 |
| Orange Juice | 6 oz | 80 | 0 |
| Pepsi-Cola | 8 oz | 110 | 0 |
| Sausage Gravy | 6 oz | 440 | 85 |
| Sausage Patty | 1 | 200 | 45 |
| Slice, Lemon-Lime | 8 oz | 100 | 0 |
| Slice, Mandarin Orange | 8 oz | 110 | 0 |
| Taco Salad | 1 | 430 | 45 |
| Taco Sauce | 1 pkg | 10 | 0 |
| Tea, Hot or Iced | 6 oz hot 12 oz iced | 0 | 0 |

| FOOD | PORTION | CALORIES | CHOLESTEROL |
|---|---|---|---|
| Toast, Wheat w/ Margarine | 2 slices | 190 | 5 |
| Toast, White | 2 slices | 250 | 20 |
| **GARDEN SPOT SALAD BAR** | | | |
| Alfalfa Sprouts | 1 oz | 8 | 0 |
| American Cheese | 1 oz | 90 | 5 |
| Bacon Bits | 1 tsp | 10 | tr |
| Blueberries | 1 Tbsp | 6 | 0 |
| Breadsticks | 2 | 35 | tr |
| Broccoli | ½ cup | 12 | 0 |
| Cabbage, Red | ¼ cup | 4 | 0 |
| Cantaloupe | 2 pieces (2 oz) | 18 | 0 |
| Carrots | ¼ cup | 10 | 0 |
| Cauliflower | ½ cup | 12 | 0 |
| Celery | 1 Tbsp | tr | 0 |
| Cheddar Cheese (imitation) | 1 oz | 80 | tr |
| Cherry Tomatoes, Pickled | 1 Tbsp | 14 | 0 |
| Coleslaw | ¼ cup | 80 | 40 |
| Cottage Cheese | ½ cup | 110 | 20 |
| Cucumbers | 4 slices | 2 | 0 |
| Eggs; hard cooked, chopped | 1 Tbsp | 30 | 90 |
| Grapefruit | 2 oz | 10 | 0 |
| Grapes | ¼ cup | 30 | 0 |
| Green Peas | 1 oz | 25 | 0 |
| Green Peppers | ¼ cup | 8 | 0 |
| Honeydew Melon | 2 pieces (2 oz) | 20 | 0 |
| Jalapeno Peppers | 1 Tbsp | 9 | 0 |

| FOOD | PORTION | CALORIES | CHOLESTEROL |
|------|---------|----------|-------------|
| Lettuce | 1 cup | 8 | 0 |
| Mozzarella Cheese (imitation) | 1 oz | 90 | tr |
| Mushrooms | ¼ cup | 4 | 0 |
| Oranges | 2 oz | 25 | 0 |
| Parmesan, Grated | 1 oz | 130 | 20 |
| Pasta Salad | ¼ cup | 130 | 5 |
| Peaches | 2 pieces | 17 | 0 |
| Pepper Rings, Pickled | 1 Tbsp | 2 | 0 |
| Pineapple Chunks | ½ cup | 70 | 0 |
| Provolone Cheese | 1 oz | 90 | tr |
| Radishes | ½ oz | 2 | 0 |
| Red Onions | 3 rings | 2 | 0 |
| Salad Dressing, Blue Cheese | 1 Tbsp | 60 | 10 |
| Salad Dressing, Celery Seed | 1 Tbsp | 70 | 5 |
| Salad Dressing, French Style | 1 Tbsp | 70 | 0 |
| Salad Dressing, Golden Italian | 1 Tbsp | 50 | 0 |
| Salad Dressing, Oil | 1 Tbsp | 120 | 0 |
| Salad Dressing, Ranch | 1 Tbsp | 50 | 5 |
| Salad Dressing, Reduced Calorie Bacon/Tomato | 1 Tbsp | 45 | tr |
| Salad Dressing, Reduced Calorie Creamy Cucumber | 1 Tbsp | 50 | tr |
| Salad Dressing, Reduced Calorie Italian | 1 Tbsp | 25 | 0 |
| Salad Dressing, Reduced Calorie Thousand Island | 1 Tbsp | 54 | 5 |
| Salad Dressing, Thousand Island | 1 Tbsp | 70 | 10 |

| FOOD | PORTION | CALORIES | CHOLESTEROL |
| --- | --- | --- | --- |
| Salad Dressing, Wine Vinegar | 1 Tbsp | 2 | 0 |
| Strawberries | 2 oz | 18 | 0 |
| Sunflower Seeds & Raisins | 1 oz | 140 | 0 |
| Swiss Cheese (imitation) | 1 oz | 90 | 5 |
| Tomatoes | 1 oz | 6 | 0 |
| Watermelon | 2 pieces (2 oz) | 18 | 0 |

HOT STUFFED BAKED POTATOES

| FOOD | PORTION | CALORIES | CHOLESTEROL |
| --- | --- | --- | --- |
| Bacon & Cheese | 1 | 570 | 22 |
| Broccoli & Cheese | 1 | 500 | 23 |
| Cheese | 1 | 590 | 22 |
| Chili & Cheese | 1 | 510 | 22 |
| Plain | 1 | 250 | 0 |
| Sour Cream & Chives | 1 | 460 | 15 |

SANDWICH TOPPINGS

| FOOD | PORTION | CALORIES | CHOLESTEROL |
| --- | --- | --- | --- |
| American Cheese | 1 sice | 60 | 15 |
| Bacon | 1 strip | 30 | 5 |
| Ketchup | 1 tsp | 6 | 0 |
| Lettuce | 1 leaf | 2 | 0 |
| Mayonnaise | 1 Tbsp | 90 | 10 |
| Mustard | 1 tsp | 4 | 0 |
| Onion | 3 rings | 2 | 0 |
| Pickles, Dill | 4 slices | 2 | 0 |
| Tomatoes | 1 slice | 2 | 0 |

## ZANTIGO

| FOOD | PORTION | CALORIES | CHOLESTEROL |
| --- | --- | --- | --- |
| Beef Enchilada | 1 | 315 | 49 |

| FOOD | PORTION | CALORIES | CHOLESTEROL |
|------|---------|----------|-------------|
| Cheese Enchilada | 1 | 390 | 63 |
| Hot Chilito | 1 | 329 | 32 |
| Mild Chilito | 1 | 330 | 26 |
| Taco | 1 | 198 | 31 |
| Taco Burrito | 1 | 415 | 44 |

# APPENDIX

# Baby Foods

# BABY FOODS

Strained foods packed for infant feeding are often used to feed adults when they cannot chew regular foods. It is for this reason that we include the following products. It is neither necessary nor desirable to limit cholesterol intake in infant and toddler diets.

| FOOD | PORTION | CALORIES | CHOLESTEROL |
|---|---|---|---|
| **CEREAL** | | | |
| Baby Cereal (Health Valley) | 1 oz | 60 | 0 |
| Baby Cereal Brown Rice (Health Valley) | 1 oz | 60 | 0 |
| **BAKED GOODS** | | | |
| Animal Shaped Cookies (Gerber) | 2 | 60 | tr |
| Arrowroot Cookies (Gerber) | 2 | 50 | tr |
| Pretzels (Gerber) | 2 | 50 | 0 |
| Toddler Biter Biscuits (Gerber) | 1 | 50 | tr |
| Zwieback Toast (Gerber) | 2 | 60 | tr |
| **CHUNKY FOODS** | | | |
| Homestyle Noodles & Beef (Gerber) | 6 oz | 150 | 14 |
| Macaroni Alphabets w/ Beef & Tomato Sauce (Gerber) | 6.25 oz | 130 | 13 |

| FOOD | PORTION | CALORIES | CHOLESTEROL |
|---|---|---|---|
| Noodles & Chicken w/ Carrots & Peas (Gerber) | 6 oz | 100 | 20 |
| Rice w/ Beef & Tomato Sauce (Gerber) | 6.25 oz | 150 | 12 |
| Saucy Rice w/ Chicken (Gerber) | 6 oz | 150 | 18 |
| Spaghetti Tomato Sauce & Beef (Gerber) | 6.25 oz | 160 | 10 |
| Vegetables & Beef (Gerber) | 6.25 oz | 140 | 10 |
| Vegetables & Chicken (Gerber) | 6.25 oz | 140 | 16 |
| Vegetables & Ham (Gerber) | 6.25 oz | 120 | 10 |
| Vegetables & Turkey (Gerber) | 6.25 oz | 110 | 20 |
| **JUNIOR AND TODDLER MEATS** | | | |
| Beef (Gerber) | 3.5 oz | 110 | 27 |
| Chicken (Gerber) | 3.5 oz | 140 | 58 |
| Chicken Sticks (Gerber) | 2.5 oz | 120 | 65 |
| Ham (Gerber) | 3.5 oz | 120 | 29 |
| Meat Sticks (Gerber) | 2.5 oz | 110 | 33 |
| Turkey (Gerber) | 3.5 oz | 130 | 53 |

| FOOD | PORTION | CALORIES | CHOLESTEROL |
|---|---|---|---|
| Turkey Sticks (Gerber) | 2.5 oz | 120 | 61 |
| Veal (Gerber) | 3.5 oz | 100 | 27 |
| JUNIOR DESSERTS | | | |
| Dutch Apple (Gerber) | 6 oz | 128 | 7 |
| Fruit Dessert (Gerber) | 6 oz | 128 | 0 |
| Hawaiian Delight (Gerber) | 6 oz | 105 | 3 |
| Peach Cobbler (Gerber) | 6 oz | 128 | 0 |
| Vanilla Custard Pudding (Gerber) | 6 oz | 128 | 23 |
| JUNIOR DINNERS | | | |
| Beef Egg Noodle Dinner (Gerber) | 7.5 oz | 140 | 12 |
| Beef w/ Vegetables (Gerber) | 4.5 oz | 130 | 13 |
| Chicken Noodle Dinner (Gerber) | 7.5 oz | 120 | 18 |
| Chicken w/ Vegetables (Gerber) | 4.5 oz | 130 | 21 |
| Ham w/ Vegetables (Gerber) | 4.5 oz | 110 | 13 |
| Macaroni Tomato Beef Dinner (Gerber) | 7.5 oz | 130 | 8 |
| Spaghetti Tomato Sauce Beef Dinner (Gerber) | 7.5 oz | 140 | 9 |

| FOOD | PORTION | CALORIES | CHOLESTEROL |
|---|---|---|---|
| Split Peas w/ Ham Dinner (Gerber) | 7.5 oz | 150 | 5 |
| Turkey Rice Dinner (Gerber) | 7.5 oz | 120 | 24 |
| Turkey w/ Vegetables (Gerber) | 4.5 oz | 140 | 15 |
| Vegetable Bacon Dinner (Gerber) | 7.5 oz | 180 | 7 |
| Vegetable Beef Dinner (Gerber) | 7.5 oz | 140 | 9 |
| Vegetable Chicken Dinner (Gerber) | 7.5 oz | 120 | 17 |
| Vegetable Ham Dinner (Gerber) | 7.5 oz | 140 | 9 |
| Vegetable Lamb Dinner (Gerber) | 7.5 oz | 140 | 6 |
| Vegetable Turkey Dinner (Gerber) | 7.5 oz | 120 | 24 |

STRAINED DESSERTS

| FOOD | PORTION | CALORIES | CHOLESTEROL |
|---|---|---|---|
| Banana Apple (Gerber) | 4.5 oz | 90 | 0 |
| Cherry Vanilla Pudding (Gerber) | 4.5 oz | 90 | 3 |
| Chocolate Custard Pudding (Gerber) | 4.5 oz | 110 | 14 |
| Dutch Apple (Gerber) | 4.5 oz | 100 | 4 |
| Fruit Dessert (Gerber) | 4.5 oz | 100 | 0 |
| Hawaiian Dessert (Gerber) | 4.5 oz | 120 | 2 |

| FOOD | PORTION | CALORIES | CHOLESTEROL |
|---|---|---|---|
| Orange Pudding (Gerber) | 4.5 oz | 110 | 11 |
| Peach Cobbler (Gerber) | 4.5 oz | 100 | 0 |
| Vanilla Custard Pudding (Gerber) | 4.5 oz | 100 | 15 |
| STRAINED DINNERS Beef Egg Noodle Dinner (Gerber) | 4.5 oz | 90 | 6 |
| Beef w/ Vegetables (Gerber) | 4.5 oz | 120 | 11 |
| Chicken Noodle Dinner (Gerber) | 4.5 oz | 80 | 10 |
| Chicken w/ Vegetables (Gerber) | 4.5 oz | 140 | 18 |
| Ham w/ Vegetables (Gerber) | 4.5 oz | 100 | 12 |
| Macaroni Cheese Dinner (Gerber) | 4.5 oz | 90 | 3 |
| Macaroni Tomato Beef Dinner (Gerber) | 4.5 oz | 90 | 3 |
| Turkey Rice Dinner (Gerber) | 4.5 oz | 80 | 15 |
| Turkey w/ Vegetables (Gerber) | 4.5 oz | 130 | 17 |
| Vegetable Bacon Dinner (Gerber) | 4.5 oz | 100 | 4 |
| Vegetable Beef Dinner (Gerber) | 4.5 oz | 80 | 5 |
| Vegetable Chicken Dinner (Gerber) | 4.5 oz | 80 | 7 |

| FOOD | PORTION | CALORIES | CHOLESTEROL |
|---|---|---|---|
| Vegetable Ham Dinner (Gerber) | 4.5 oz | 80 | 4 |
| Vegetable Lamb Dinner (Gerber) | 4.5 oz | 90 | 3 |
| Vegetable Liver Dinner (Gerber) | 4.5 oz | 60 | 29 |
| Vegetable Turkey Dinner (Gerber) | 4.5 oz | 70 | 12 |

## STRAINED MEATS AND EGG YOLKS

| FOOD | PORTION | CALORIES | CHOLESTEROL |
|---|---|---|---|
| Beef (Gerber) | 3.5 oz | 100 | 29 |
| Chicken (Gerber) | 3.5 oz | 100 | 61 |
| Egg Yolks (Gerber) | 2.25 oz | 128 | 398 |
| Ham (Gerber) | 3.5 oz | 110 | 24 |
| Lamb (Gerber) | 3.5 oz | 100 | 38 |
| Pork (Gerber) | 3.5 oz | 110 | 35 |
| Turkey (Gerber) | 3.5 oz | 130 | 58 |
| Veal (Gerber) | 3.5 oz | 100 | 25 |